Laparoscopic Surgery in Urology

Yushi Zhang • Xin Zhao
Editors

Laparoscopic Surgery in Urology

Cases and Analysis

Springer

中国协和医科大学出版社
Peking Union Medical College Press

Editors
Yushi Zhang
Department of Urology
Peking Union Medical College Hospital
Beijing, China

Xin Zhao
Department of Urology
Peking Union Medical College Hospital
Beijing, China

ISBN 978-981-96-8597-4 ISBN 978-981-96-8598-1 (eBook)
https://doi.org/10.1007/978-981-96-8598-1

The original submitted manuscript has been translated into English. The translation was done using artificial intelligence. A subsequent revision was performed by the author(s) to further refine the work and to ensure that the translation is appropriate concerning content and scientific correctness. It may, however, read stylistically different from a conventional translation.

Translation from the Chinese language edition: "协和泌尿外科腹腔镜手术例释" by Yushi Zhang and Xin Zhao, © Peking Union Medical College Press 2023. Published by Peking Union Medical College Press. All Rights Reserved.

Jointly published with Peking Union Medical College Press
The print edition is not for sale in China (Mainland). Customers from China (Mainland) please order the print book from: Peking Union Medical College Press.

This Springer imprint is published by the registered company Springer Nature Singapore Pte Ltd.
The registered company address is: 152 Beach Road, #21-01/04 Gateway East, Singapore 189721, Singapore

Foreword I

As the former director of the Urology Department of Peking Union Medical College Hospital and the pioneer who introduced laparoscopic technology to the department, I have watched the younger generation of doctors grow and the progress and maturity of urological laparoscopic technology. I am honored to write the preface for "Laparoscopic Surgery in Urology: Cases and Analysis." This book aims to integrate clinical practice with theory, providing a useful reference for the new forces in the medical field.

"Without accumulating steps, there is no way to reach a thousand miles; without accumulating small streams, there is no way to become a river or sea." This sentence profoundly explains that the foundation of any success comes from accumulation and continuous effort. Urological laparoscopic surgery, as a combination of technology and clinical science, is constantly developing and growing in the daily practice of countless excellent doctors. We advocate starting from clinical reality, focusing on the inheritance and innovation of technology, and inspiring more young doctors to continuously improve in this field.

In "Laparoscopic Surgery in Urology: Cases and Analysis," we hope to not only impart medical techniques but also pass on the spirit of medicine. The skill of surgery lies not only in the use of instruments but also in the doctor's thorough understanding of the physiological structure of the human body, comprehensive understanding of the patient, and continuous reflection, summarization, and improvement in practice.

The authors of this book have carefully selected a series of clinical cases, using the real world as a teaching background, conveying a spirit of facing challenges and climbing the peak of science. We hope to inspire a new generation of doctors to think independently, continue to explore, pioneer, and innovate, and make their mark in this field.

I would like to take this opportunity to express my heartfelt thanks to all the authors who have worked hard on this "Laparoscopic Surgery in Urology: Cases and Analysis." Finally, I would like to offer some advice to young doctors.

1. Climb the peak and never stop: In the field of medicine, due to the rapid development of laparoscopic technology in urology, we need to maintain keen insight, be brave to accept new knowledge and technology, and continuously improve our technical level.

2. Seek truth from facts and pursue reality: In the process of exploration and learning, we must base ourselves on real cases, learn from experience and lessons, form our unique insights, and thus enhance our practical operation ability.
3. Focus on patients and put people first: The ultimate purpose of medicine is to benefit patients. We should always focus on the needs and interests of patients, put the safety and health of patients first, and achieve mutual progress between doctors and patients.
4. Be humble and learn, and continue to progress: Medicine is a science that requires lifelong learning and research. We need to have a humble and eager to learn attitude, constantly learn, reflect and summarize, and strive to achieve higher achievements in the field of medicine.
5. Explore and innovate, carry forward the spirit of medicine: Bravely exert your imagination and creativity, constantly explore new fields and methods of medicine, and make greater contributions to the development of medical career.

I wish every reader could gain useful knowledge when reading this book, feel the inheritance of the spirit of medicine, and contribute to the progress of the field of urology.

Peking Union Medical College Hospital Hanzhong Li
Beijing, China

Foreword II

I am honored to introduce this distinctive monograph to respected readers. This book brings together the knowledge and experience of many frontline urologists. Unlike traditional surgical monographs, it focuses on real cases in the hope of being closer to clinical reality and providing a practical surgical atlas based on cases.

The aim of this book is to allow readers to fully understand the principles and techniques of various laparoscopic urological surgeries through specific surgical cases, and to demonstrate the surgical thinking and techniques used in different cases through detailed descriptions and high-quality illustrations.

A distinctive feature of this book is its practicality, providing readers with a real and rich learning experience. It carefully selects a variety of cases, some surgeries may not be perfect, but they provide a real picture of laparoscopic surgery; emphasizing the importance of learning from real cases, it aims to help readers master the knowledge and skills needed to deal with specific problems in clinical practice, as well as the ability to adjust surgical thinking and methods according to actual conditions during the operation.

To further optimize the learning experience, this book includes a rich video library that complements the text, allowing readers the opportunity to witness the surgical process firsthand and provide a more immersive learning experience. It hopes to bridge the gap between theoretical knowledge and practical application, fostering a deeper understanding of laparoscopic techniques and principles among young doctors.

In addition to a large number of surgical images and videos, this book also includes expert commentary on potential complications and postoperative management related to urological laparoscopic surgery. This information can help readers identify potential surgical risks, formulate appropriate strategies to ensure the best therapeutic effect for patients, and fully understand the postoperative recovery process.

This book focuses on presenting real case handling processes, a method that sets it apart from traditional scientific monographs. Readers can see shortcomings from specific surgical processes and review the entire surgical process through postoperative expert commentary. We believe this approach will be welcomed by both novices and experienced practitioners, enabling them to quickly improve their skills, overcome challenges, and ultimately improve patient prognosis.

I would like to express my deep gratitude to all those who have contributed their professional knowledge, insights, and focus on urological laparoscopic surgery to this book. They are committed to advancing the field and sharing knowledge and experience with the future generation of urologists, which is truly commendable. At the same time, I would like to thank our readers for choosing this book. I believe this book will be a valuable resource in your pursuit of excellence in the field of urological laparoscopic surgery.

As you begin to read this book, I encourage you to embrace the successes and imperfections of these surgical cases. Through reflection, continuous improvement, and the combination of theoretical knowledge and practical experience, you will undoubtedly make real progress in the field of urological laparoscopic surgery.

Peking Union Medical College Hospital
Beijing, China

Zhigang Ji

Preface

As the main editors of this book, we are very honored to introduce this practical work to you. We have compiled real cases from clinical practice to provide a valuable surgical guide for urologists. The writing of this book aims to provide doctors engaged in urology with practical experience, skill transfer, and expert advice, helping them improve their surgical skills and ultimately provide better medical services to patients.

This book is divided into two parts, covering a comprehensive explanation from the establishment of laparoscopic surgery position and channel to specific surgical cases. In the writing process, we particularly focus on practicality and richness of cases, striving to make this book a powerful assistant and useful reference material for urologists.

The first part is about the positioning and channel establishment in laparoscopic surgery, including the first and second chapters. In this section, we elaborate on the choice of position and the techniques of channel establishment in laparoscopic surgery. In addition, we also discuss the important role of patient positioning and Trocar placement in achieving the best surgical view and surgical results. Through a comprehensive analysis of these key steps, we hope to lay a solid foundation for readers to better understand and master the techniques and essentials of positioning and channel establishment in laparoscopic surgery.

The second part is about specific surgical cases. This section focuses on urological laparoscopic cases, aiming to reflect real surgical cases. Each case is divided into sections including case summary, imaging data, preoperative assessment, surgical process, and postoperative expert commentary, providing rich practical experience and useful tips. We have carefully selected surgical cases involving various organs such as the adrenal gland, kidney, bladder, and prostate, demonstrating the wide application scenarios of urological laparoscopic surgery. Through analyzing and reflecting on these cases, we hope that readers can fully understand the techniques, challenges, and details of urological laparoscopic surgery, thereby improving their surgical skills.

In terms of the writing style of this book, we have used detailed text descriptions, exquisite pictures, and detailed expert commentary, striving to present each surgical process clearly and vividly. At the same time, the book also includes actual surgical videos. Readers can scan the QR code to watch the surgical process, better understand and master the essentials of the surgery.

We hope that "Laparoscopic Surgery in Urology: Cases and Analysis" can become a powerful assistant for urologists, helping them to genuinely improve their surgical techniques and provide patients with higher quality medical services. Here, we would like to thank all the editors and participants of this book. It is their hard work and professionalism that have made this work possible.

Beijing, China Yushi Zhang
Beijing, China Xin Zhao

Contents

Contributors

Main Reviewers

Hanzhong Li Beijing Union Medical College Hospital, Beijing, China

Zhigang Ji Beijing Union Medical College Hospital, Beijing, China

Chief Editors

Yushi Zhang Beijing Union Medical College Hospital, Beijing, China

Xin Zhao Beijing Union Medical College Hospital, Beijing, China

Associate Editors

Wenda Wang Beijing Union Medical College Hospital, Beijing, China

Jiaquan Zhou Hainan Affiliated Hospital of Hainan Medical University, Hainan, China

Editorial Board

Wenda Wang Beijing Union Medical College Hospital, Beijing, China

Dong Wang Beijing Union Medical College Hospital, Beijing, China

Jianhua Deng Beijing Union Medical College Hospital, Beijing, China

Jie Dong Beijing Union Medical College Hospital, Beijing, China

Xuebing Zhang Beijing Union Medical College Hospital, Beijing, China

Jiaquan Zhou Hainan Affiliated Hospital of Hainan Medical University, Hainan, China

Zixing Ye Beijing Union Medical College Hospital, Beijing, China

Xin Zhao Beijing Union Medical College Hospital, Beijing, China

Yang Zhao Beijing Union Medical College Hospital, Beijing, China

Yi Zhao Beijing Union Medical College Hospital, Beijing, China

Weifeng Xu Beijing Union Medical College Hospital, Beijing, China

Yihong Liu The 7th People's Hospital of Zhengzhou, Henan, China

Yushi Zhang Beijing Union Medical College Hospital, Beijing, China

Yanan Li Beijing Union Medical College Hospital, Beijing, China

Jingmin Zhou Beijing Union Medical College Hospital, Beijing, China

Dongxu Qiu Hunan Provincial People's Hospital the First Affiliated Hospital of Hunan Normal University, Changsha, China

Yi Qiao Beijing Union Medical College Hospital, Beijing, China

Guoyang Zheng Beijing Union Medical College Hospital, Beijing, China

Yi Xie Beijing Union Medical College Hospital, Beijing, China

Zhongming Huang Beijing Union Medical College Hospital, Beijing, China

Hua Fan Beijing Union Medical College Hospital, Beijing, China

Hao Yi People's Hospital of Tibet Autonomous Region, Tibet, China

Weigang Yan Beijing Union Medical College Hospital, Beijing, China

Jin Wen Beijing Union Medical College Hospital, Beijing, China

Secretary

Fei Peng Beijing Union Medical College Hospital, Beijing, China

Positioning in Laparoscopic Surgery

Xin Zhao

Regular Positioning in Laparoscopic Surgery

Positioning for Extraperitoneal (Retroperitoneal) Surgery

Positioning for Upper Urinary Tract Surgery via Retroperitoneal Approach

This position is mainly used for adrenal gland, kidney, and ureter surgeries. The common surgical position for open urological surgery in our country is the lateral position, with a retroperitoneal approach. Based on this, most laparoscopic upper urinary tract surgeries also adopt the lateral position with a retroperitoneal approach. Presently, this approach is suitable for most upper urinary tract surgeries, and its safety and ease of use have been confirmed.

The patient generally adopts a healthy side-lying position. A soft pad is placed under the waist, raising the lumbar bridge, to fully open the space between the rib edge and the iliac crest on the affected side, which is conducive to the establishment of the surgical space. An armrest is placed on the head side, and the healthy arm is placed on the armrest. Soft pads need to be placed under the head side and the healthy arm to prevent pressure on the face and brachial plexus nerves. The healthy side lower limb is bent at 90°, the affected side lower limb is fully extended, and the legs are in an "upper-extended and lower-flexed" position. A large soft pad needs to be placed at the knee joint between the two legs to prevent pressure from the protruding knee and ankle joints. A long cylindrical sandbag is placed on the back to prevent the patient from leaning back. A larger long cylindrical sandbag is placed on the chest to prevent the patient from leaning forward. Use restraint straps to fix the position at the pelvis and knee joints, and place cotton pads under the restraint straps to prevent local pressure (Figs. 1, 2, and 3).

The monitor is placed in front of the patient's head; the surgeon stands at the patient's buttocks, facing the monitor. The height of the monitor is

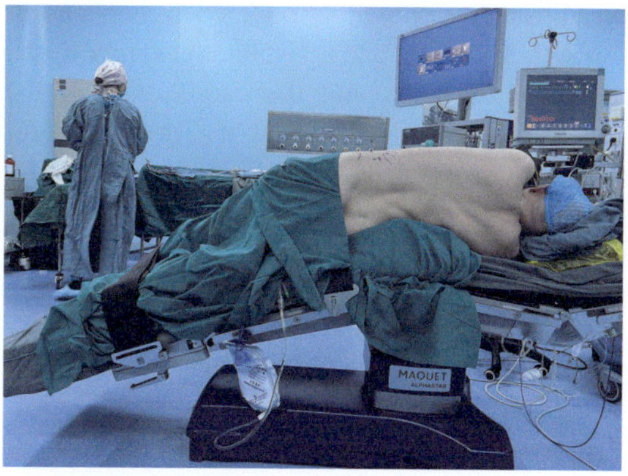

Fig. 1 Lateral position for upper urinary tract surgery (back view)

X. Zhao (✉)
Beijing Union Medical College Hospital,
Beijing, China

Y. Zhang, X. Zhao (eds.), *Laparoscopic Surgery in Urology*,
https://doi.org/10.1007/978-981-96-8598-1_1

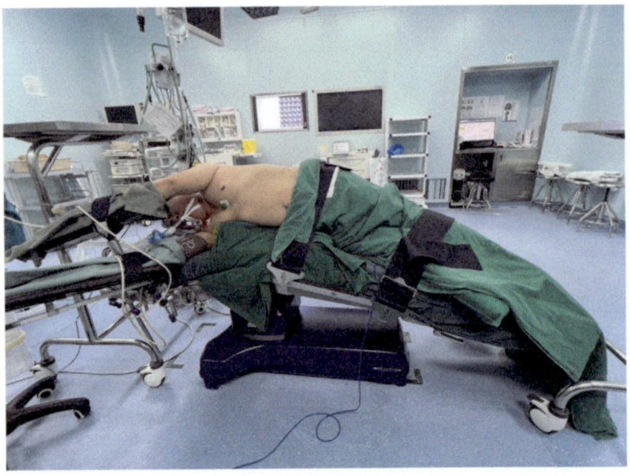

Fig. 2 Lateral position for upper urinary tract surgery (abdominal view)

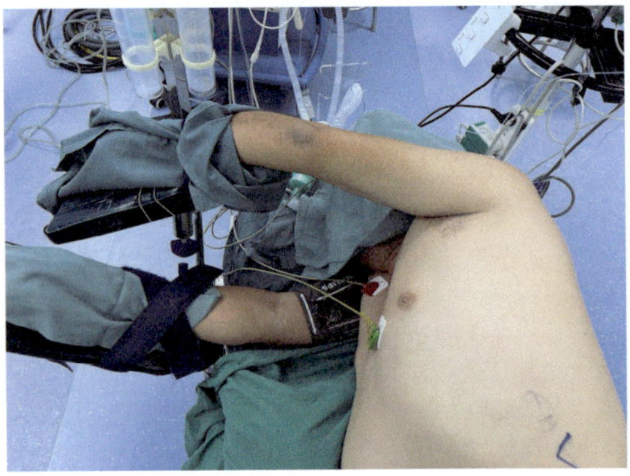

Fig. 3 Upper limb position in lateral position for upper urinary tract surgery

level with the surgeon's line of sight, and it can be adjusted appropriately for the surgeon's comfort. When there is one assistant, the surgeon is at the patient's back, and the assistant is at the patient's abdomen, acting as the mirror holder and assistant (Fig. 4). When there are two assistants, one assistant is at the patient's abdomen, and the mirror holder is at the surgeon's back (Figs. 5 and 6). At this time, the surgeon should wear a cape on the back to maintain good aseptic principles.

Extraperitoneal Lower Urinary Tract Surgery Position

This position is mainly used for radical prostatectomy. The patient is in a supine position, with shoulder blocks, head low, and feet high, and the head low angle is 15–20° (Fig. 7). A pad is placed

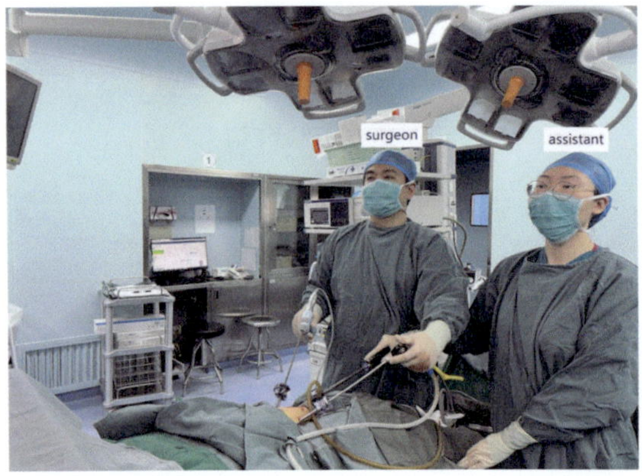

Fig. 4 Two-person operation position in lateral position for upper urinary tract surgery

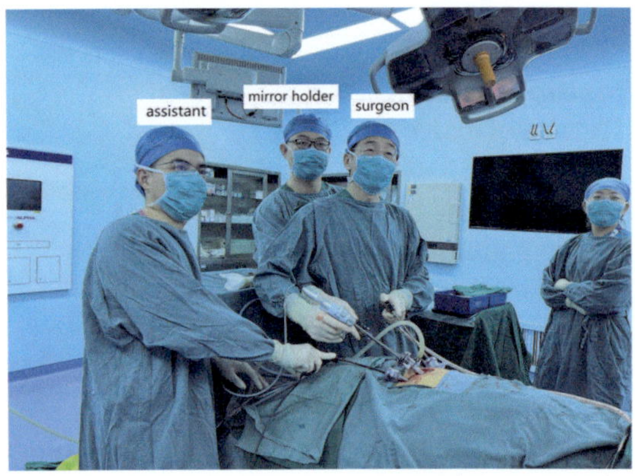

Fig. 5 Three-person operation position in lateral position for upper urinary tract surgery

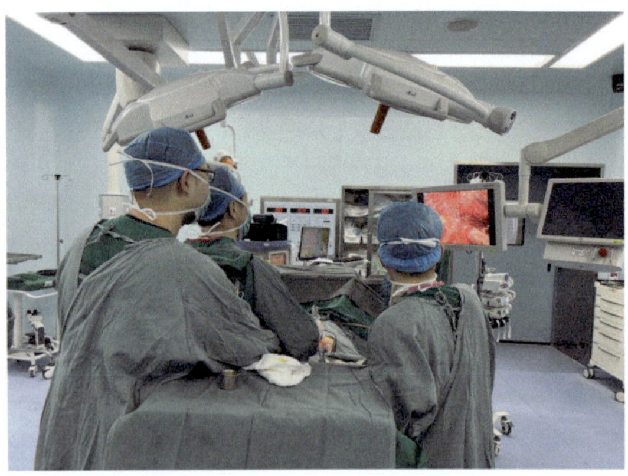

Fig. 6 Monitor position in lateral position for upper urinary tract surgery

under the buttocks, the knee joint is slightly bent, and a soft pad is placed under the popliteal fossa. The area above the knee joint and the chest are

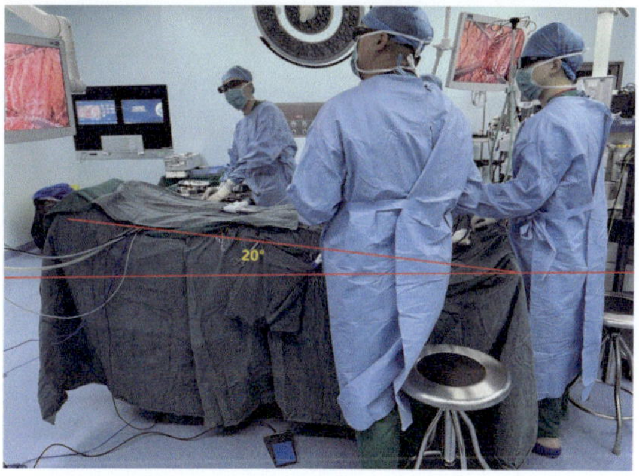

Fig. 7 Lateral position for lower urinary tract surgery

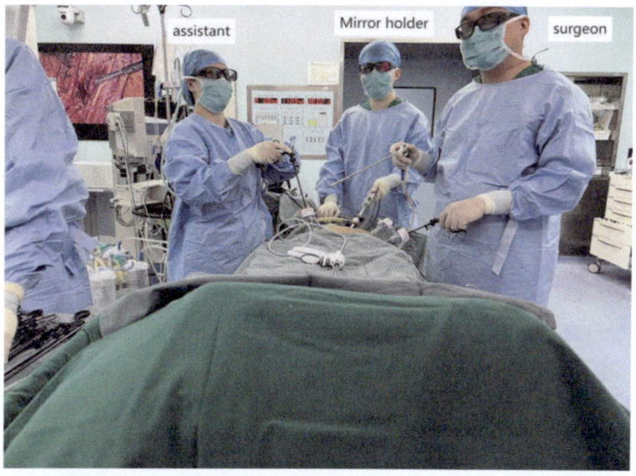

Fig. 8 Frontal position for lower urinary tract surgery

fixed with restraint straps, and the patient's hands are placed on the sides of the body. The monitor is placed at the patient's feet. The mirror holder stands at the patient's head, the surgeon stands on the patient's left side, and the assistant stands on the patient's right side (Fig. 8).

Abdominal Surgery Position

For the upper urinary tract surgery position through the abdominal cavity, the healthy side semi-lateral position is generally adopted (Fig. 9). The affected side is raised, forming a 45–60° angle with the bed surface. A cylindrical lumbar pad is placed on the back to prevent the patient from leaning back, which is conducive to the abdominal organs falling to the healthy side under the action of gravity, to better expose the surgical operation area. Slightly raise the lumbar bridge to moderately expand the operation area space, which is conducive to operation. Other requirements are the same as for the upper urinary tract surgery position through the retroperitoneal cavity (Figs. 10 and 11).

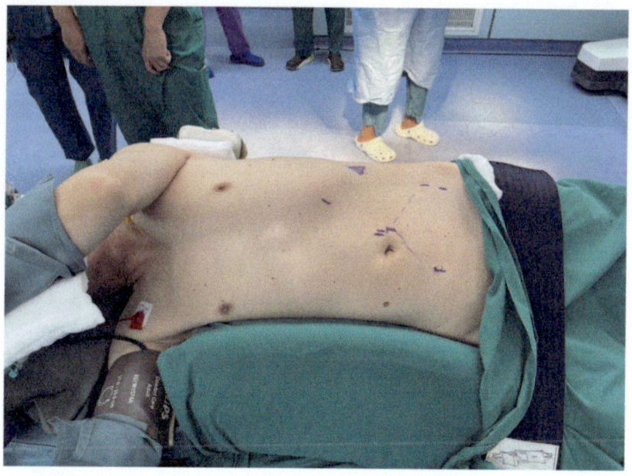

Fig. 9 Abdominal upper urinary tract position (overhead view)

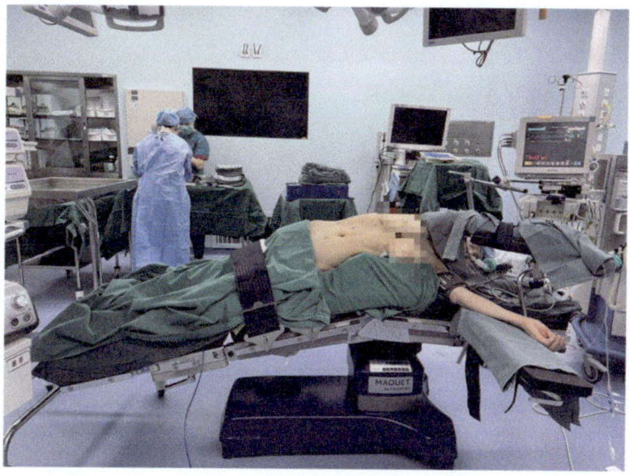

Fig. 10 Abdominal upper urinary tract position (lateral view)

The abdominal lower urinary tract surgical position is mainly used for bladder surgery. The method is the same as the lower urinary tract surgery through the extraperitoneal cavity, just establishing a channel through the abdominal cavity.

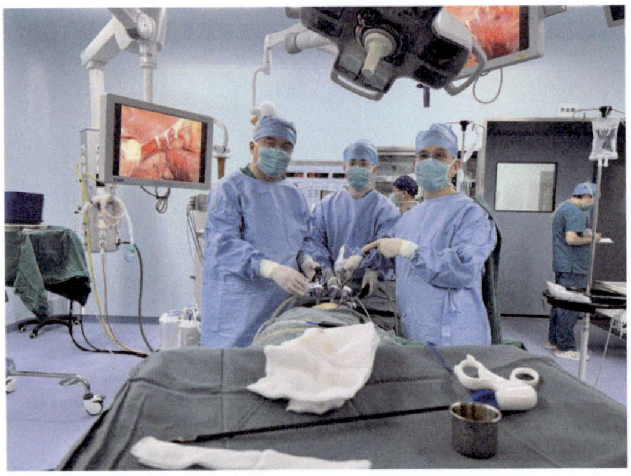

Fig. 11 Abdominal upper urinary tract position (surgeon's standing position)

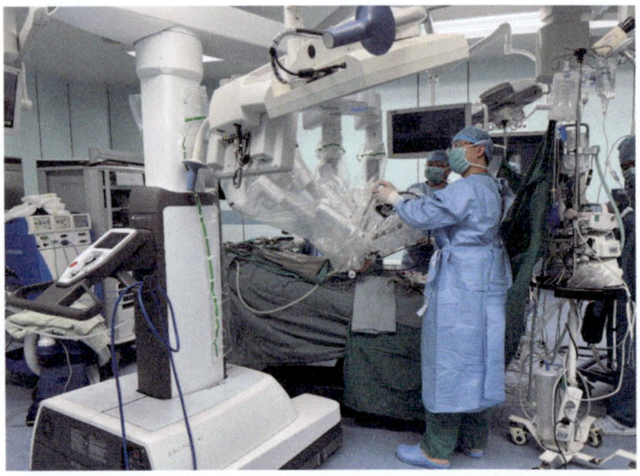

Fig. 12 Position for robot-assisted laparoscopic total bladder resection (lateral view)

Robotic-Assisted Laparoscopic Surgery Position

Extraperitoneal (Retroperitoneal) Surgical Operation Position

Retroperitoneal Upper Urinary Tract Robotic Surgery Position

Mainly used for kidney- and adrenal-related surgeries. This position is the same as the upper urinary tract surgery position in the retroperitoneal cavity, with the robot placed on the patient's head side.

Extraperitoneal Lower Urinary Tract Robotic Surgery Position

Mainly used for robot-assisted radical prostatectomy. This position is similar to the lower urinary tract surgery position in the extraperitoneal cavity, adopting a head-down and foot-up position, with a head-down angle of 10–15°.

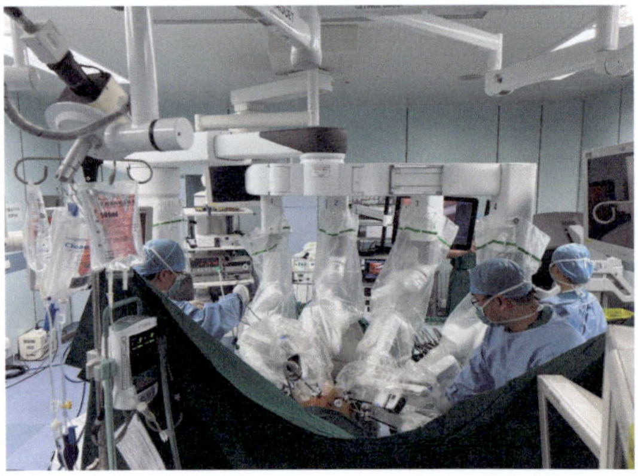

Fig. 13 Position for robot-assisted laparoscopic total bladder resection (head view)

Abdominal Surgical Operation Position

Abdominal Upper Urinary Tract Robotic Surgery Position

Mainly used for kidney- and adrenal-related surgeries. This position is the same as the abdominal upper urinary tract position.

Abdominal Lower Urinary Tract Robotic Surgery Position

Mainly used for bladder- and prostate-related surgeries. This position is the same as the abdominal lower urinary tract position (Figs. 12 and 13).

Establishment of Laparoscopic Surgical Operation Channel

Xin Zhao

Determination of Puncture Site

The puncture site is generally determined by using anatomical structures that are marked on the body surface. Commonly used body surface markers include the anterior axillary line, midaxillary line, posterior axillary line, iliac crest, anterior superior iliac spine, costal arch, umbilicus, xiphoid process, lateral edge of the rectus abdominis, and midclavicular line.

Establishment of Conventional Laparoscopic Surgical Operation Channel

Establishment of Retroperitoneal (Extraperitoneal) Surgical Operation Channel

The establishment of the retroperitoneal upper urinary tract surgical operation channel usually uses three or four holes. First, mark the iliac crest and ribs 11 and 12. The ① hole is located two transverse fingers above the iliac crest on the midaxillary line, parallel to the iliac crest, with a transverse incision of about 3 cm. The fingers assist in pushing the peritoneum and extraperitoneal fat as much as possible, placing a 10 mm trocar. Pay attention to apply force evenly, and push open in an arc shape to prevent tearing of the peritoneum (Fig. 1). For thin patients, special attention should be paid because their peritoneum is thin and often closer to the posterior axillary line, and an airbag can be used for expansion. Then, through the ① hole, the fingers assist in placing the ②, ③, and ④ trocar. The ② hole is located at the costovertebral angle, the tip of the 12th rib. It is located 1–2 cm below the tip of the 12th rib; depending on whether the lesion is closer to the ventral or dorsal side, it is placed one to two transverse fingers anterior to the psoas major muscle. Hole ③ is located 1 cm below the anterior axillary line. If it is necessary to place auxiliary hole ④, you can choose to align with hole ①; 5 cm outside hole ③, usually place a 5 mm trocar. Different trocar models are chosen according to different patient surgeries. The dominant hand chooses a 10 mm or 12 mm (partial nephrectomy,

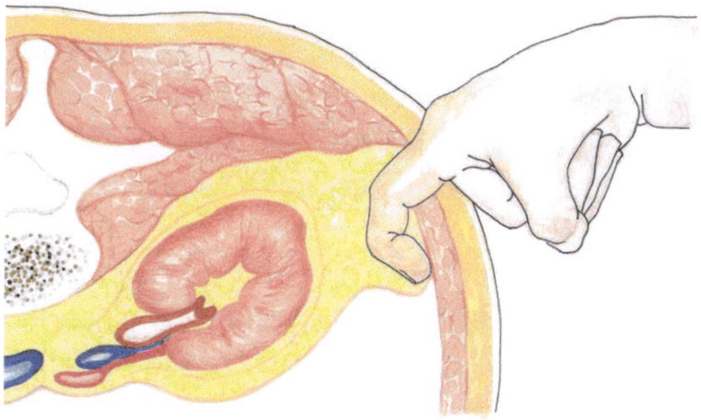

Fig. 1 Expanding the retroperitoneal space with fingers

X. Zhao (✉)
Beijing Union Medical College Hospital,
Beijing, China

Y. Zhang, X. Zhao (eds.), *Laparoscopic Surgery in Urology*,
https://doi.org/10.1007/978-981-96-8598-1_2

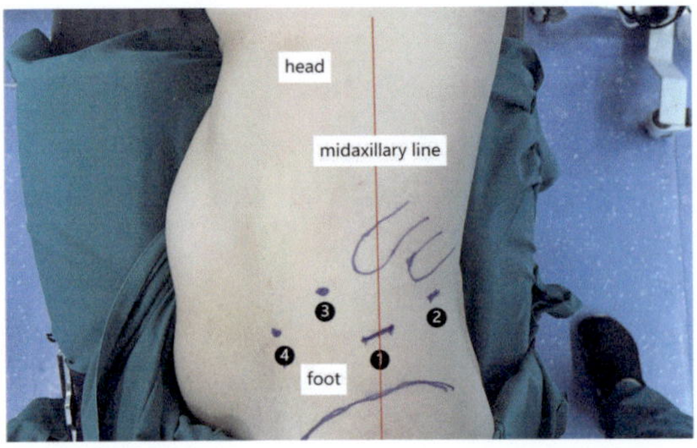

Fig. 2 Retroperitoneal upper urinary tract surgical operation channel location

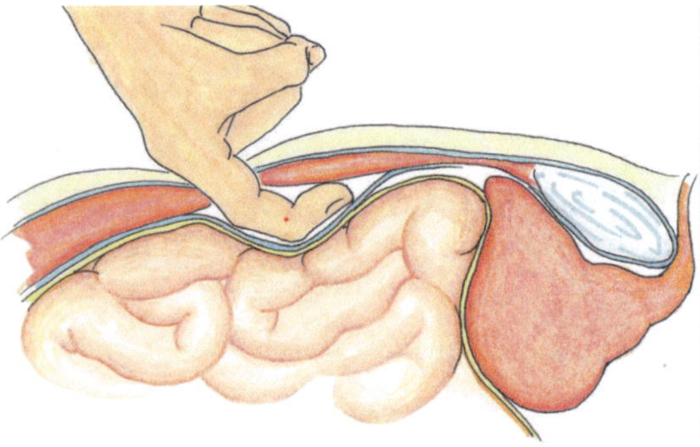

Fig. 3 Expanding the extraperitoneal space with fingers

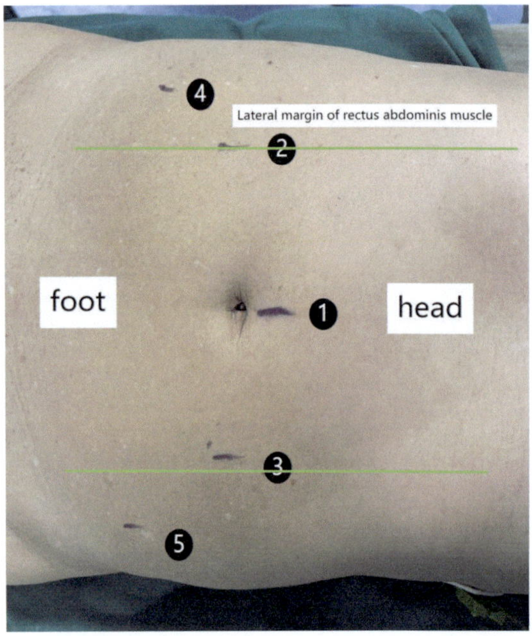

Fig. 4 Extraperitoneal approach lower urinary tract surgical operation channel location

because a bulldog vascular clamp needs to be placed) trocar. When placing trocars ②, ③, and ④ with the help of fingers, after cutting the skin, use a trocar with an inner core to penetrate the subcutaneous and muscle layers, with the tip pointing toward the surgical site, rotating downward with force, and applying force evenly and continuously. When the finger feels the tip of the trocar core, the finger slides to the side to insert the trocar. The trocars are arranged in a parallelogram, with the tip position pointing toward the surgical site (Fig. 2).

Establishing the Extraperitoneal Lower Urinary Tract Surgical Operation Channel

This channel is mainly used for radical prostatectomy. Typically, five trocars are placed in total for this surgery. The process begins with making a 3–4 cm midline longitudinal incision through the skin and subcutaneous tissue, located two transverse fingers below the navel. The tissues are then dissected layer by layer until the anterior sheath of the rectus abdominis is reached. Longitudinally cut the anterior sheath of the rectus abdominis, pull open the anterior sheath of the rectus abdominis, and the rectus abdominis can be seen. One centimeter beside the midline of the rectus abdominis, use your fingers to bluntly separate the rectus abdominis on both sides to reach the posterior sheath of the rectus abdominis, push down and back along the posterior sheath of the rectus abdominis to open the peritoneum or use an expander to expand the preperitoneal space, and establish the extraperitoneal space (Fig. 3). Place a 10 mm trocar ① as an observation hole, and suture the anterior sheath of the rectus abdominis, subcutaneous tissue, and skin sequentially to prevent air leakage. Maintain pneumoperitoneum pressure at about 15 mmHg, and insert a laparoscope. Under direct vision of the laparoscope, place a 12 mm trocar on the right side ② and a 5 mm trocar on the left side ③ two transverse fingers below the navel on the outer edge of the rectus abdominis. At the outer one-third of the line between the bilateral anterior superior iliac spine and the navel, place two 5 mm trocars (④ and ⑥). The trocars are arranged in an arc, with the tip pointing toward the surgical site (Fig. 4).

Establishing the Intraperitoneal Surgical Operation Channel

The establishment of the abdominal upper urinary tract surgical operation channel is mainly used for radical nephroureterectomy, as well as for the removal of larger tumors through the abdomen, such as large renal cell carcinoma, adrenal tumors, etc. The patient is positioned at a 45–60° oblique position, which can be adjusted through the operating table. First, determine the approximate body surface projection position of the surgical site. The rest of the trocar layout is roughly arc-shaped, with the operation site as the vertex. Due to different tumor positions trocar positions should be adjusted according to the tumor location, and the selectable trocar insertion points include ① two transverse fingers below the clavicle midline rib edge, ② one transverse finger below the sternum side line rib edge, ③ two transverse fingers above and below the outer edge of the rectus abdominis, ④ one-third of the outer line between the navel and the anterior superior iliac spine, ⑤ side of the navel or next to the navel, and ⑥ midpoint between the navel and the pubic symphysis; ⑦ sometimes a 5 mm trocar needs to be placed below the xiphoid process on the right side to block the liver. The position of the trocar can be selected according to the different conditions of the patient's lesions. The commonly used trocar positions in our hospital are ① 5 cm above the outer edge of the rectus abdominis (observation hole, 10 mm trocar), ② 2 cm below the clavicle midline rib edge (main operation hole, 10 mm trocar), ③ 3 cm below the anterior axillary line rib edge (auxiliary operation hole, 5 mm trocar), ④ 3–5 cm below the navel (auxiliary operation hole, dealing with the distal end of the ureter, 5 mm trocar), and ⑥ below the xiphoid process (auxiliary operation hole, blocking the liver, 5 mm trocar) (Fig. 5).

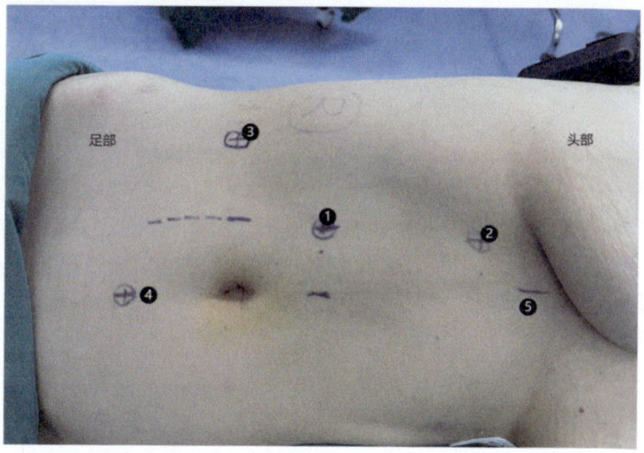

Fig. 5 Abdominal upper urinary tract surgical operation channel location

The establishment of the abdominal lower urinary tract surgical operation channel is mainly used for radical cystectomy. Usually, five trocars are placed. A 2 cm longitudinal incision is made 1 cm above the navel, and the layers are separated to the fascia. Two curved forceps are used to lift the fascia, and a scalpel is used to cut it open. The peritoneum can be seen by exploring downward. Find a place where the peritoneum is not adhered and cut it open. The finger is inserted into the abdominal cavity to explore and push away the adhered intestines. Under direct vision, the no. 1 trocar (10 mm) is inserted as the observation hole. The subcutaneous tissue and skin are sutured to prevent air leakage. Inflate to maintain an intra-abdominal pressure of about 15 mmHg, and insert a 30° laparoscope. Under laparoscopic direct vision, the main operation hole ②, 12 mm trocar (right side), and the auxiliary operation hole ③, 10 mm trocar (left side), are placed on the outer edge of the rectus abdominis at the level of the navel, respectively. Two 5 mm trocars ④ are placed at the outer one-third of the line between the bilateral anterior superior iliac spine and the navel, respectively. The trocars are arranged in an arc shape, with the tip pointing toward the surgical site (Fig. 6).

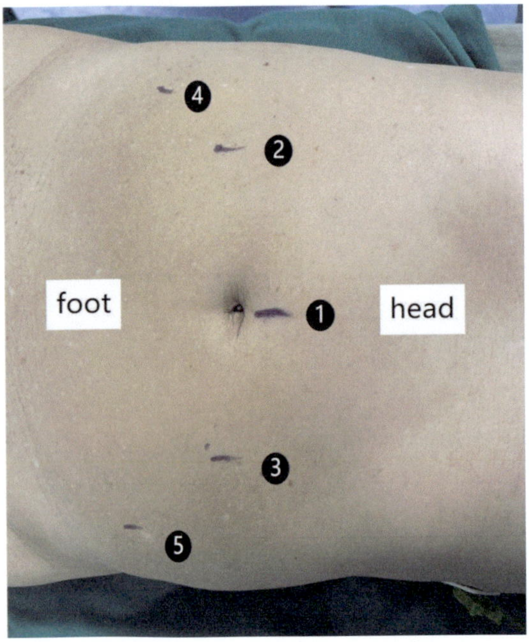

Fig. 6 Abdominal lower urinary tract surgical operation channel location

Establishment of Robotic-Assisted Laparoscopic Surgical Operation Channel

Establishment of Robotic-Assisted Extraperitoneal (Retroperitoneal) Surgical Operation Channel

Establishment of the Retroperitoneal Upper Urinary Tract Surgical Operation Channel

This type of surgery has the same indications as conventional retroperitoneal laparoscopic surgery. The patient is positioned on the healthy side, with the waist bridge raised. A 3 cm incision is made 2 cm above the axillary midline spinous process. After bluntly separating the muscles, enter the retroperitoneal space. After using a homemade balloon to push the peritoneum as far as possible to the abdominal side, an 8 mm lens hole trocar ② is placed 2 cm above the axillary midline spinous process, the robot lens is inserted, and pneumoperitoneum is established. Under direct vision of the lens, an 8 mm robot-specific trocar ①③ is placed at the level of the lens hole and 2 cm above the posterior axillary line spinous process, and then a 12 mm trocar ④ is placed 2 cm above the anterior axillary line spinous process as an auxiliary port. After all trocars are inserted, the robot is docked, and the robot-specific surgical instruments are inserted (Fig. 7).

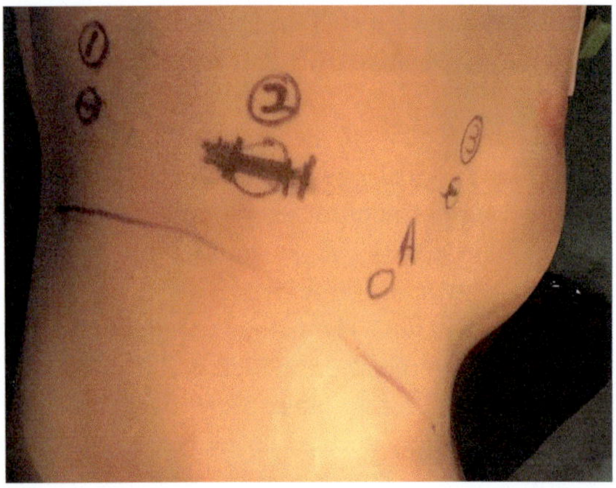

Fig. 7 Robotic retroperitoneal upper urinary tract surgical pathway site

The establishment of the robotic-assisted extraperitoneal lower urinary tract surgical pathway is mainly used for robotic-assisted radical prostatectomy. The establishment of this type of surgical pathway is similar to the establishment of the extraperitoneal lower urinary tract surgical pathway. It is less used in Peking Union Medical College Hospital (hereinafter referred to as "our hospital").

Establishment of the Robotic-Assisted Intraperitoneal Operation Channel

Establishment of the Robotic-Assisted Intraperitoneal Upper Urinary Tract Operation Channel

The establishment of this type of Operation Channel is the same as the conventional laparoscopic intraperitoneal surgery. The patient is placed in a 70° lateral decubitus position with the unaffected side up, and the waist bridge is raised. First, the approximate body surface projection position of the surgical site is determined. An 8 mm trocar is inserted 15–20 cm away from the surgical site, and 5 cm on the umbilical side, the robotic camera is inserted, and pneumoperitoneum is established. Under

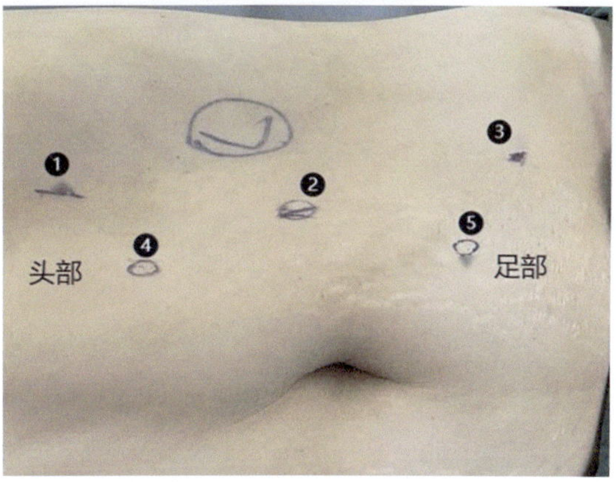

Fig. 8 Robotic-assisted intraperitoneal upper urinary tract surgical pathway site

direct vision of the camera, 8 mm trocars are inserted at 5 cm below the midclavicular line rib margin and 5 cm above the anterior superior iliac spine, and a 12 mm auxiliary trocar is inserted 5 cm on the head side of the camera port. If necessary, a 5 mm auxiliary trocar is inserted 5 cm on the foot side of the camera port (Fig. 8). When performing upper urinary tract surgery on the right side, if the liver obstructs the surgical site, a 5 mm trocar is placed below the xiphoid process to push the liver away. After all trocars are inserted, the robot is docked, and the robot-specific surgical instruments are inserted.

Establishment of the Robotic-Assisted Intraperitoneal Lower Urinary Tract Operation Channel

The establishment of this type of channel is the same as the conventional laparoscopic intraperitoneal lower urinary tract surgery. The patient is placed in a supine position with the head down. Pneumoperitoneum is established by puncturing two horizontal fingers above the umbilicus, and an 8 mm camera port trocar is inserted. The robotic camera is inserted. Under direct vision of the camera, 8 mm robotic-specific trocars are inserted at the lateral edge of the rectus abdominis on both sides at the umbilical level, and 2 cm above the anterior superior iliac spine on the right side, and a 12 mm trocar is inserted 2 cm above the anterior superior iliac spine on the left side as an auxiliary port (Fig. 9). After all trocars are inserted, the robot is docked, and the robot-specific surgical instruments are inserted.

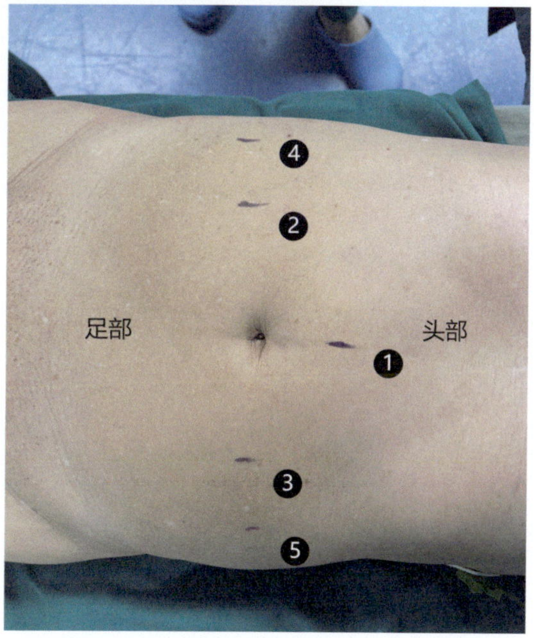

Fig. 9 Robotic-assisted intraperitoneal lower urinary tract surgical pathway site

Establishment of the Operation Channel for the Da Vinci Xi Robotic-Assisted Laparoscopic Surgery

The channel establishment of the da Vinci Xi robot is different from the previous Si model. To minimize the interference between the robotic arms, it is recommended to arrange the channels linearly. First, determine the target anatomical structure, and then establish the observation hole 10–20 cm away from the target anatomical structure (recommended about 20 cm). Draw a perpendicular line between the observation hole and the farthest point of the target anatomical structure. Mark the channel every 8 cm on the perpendicular line from the observation hole. Each trocar should be placed at least 2 cm away from any bony structure, and do not place the channel between other channels and the target anatomical structure. Place the auxiliary channel at least 7 cm away from the robotic arm channel, and do not place the auxiliary channel between the robotic arm channel and the target anatomical structure (Fig. 10).

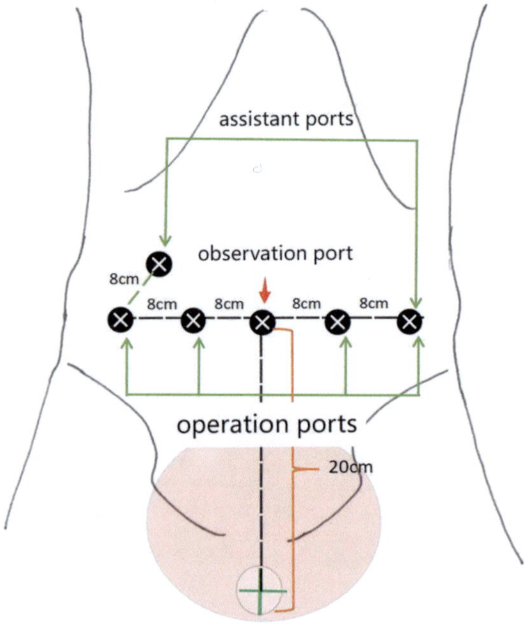

Fig. 10 Da Vinci Xi robotic surgical channel site

Adrenal Surgery: Case 1 Laparoscopic Transperitoneal Left Adrenalectomy

Zixing Ye

Chief Complaint

Hypertension for over 10 years, bilateral adrenal nodules found 6 months ago. History: male, 43 years old. The patient developed hypertension without obvious cause over 10 years ago, with the highest blood pressure 180/115 mmHg. After taking antihypertensive drugs, the blood pressure dropped to 150/90 mmHg, but no further treatment was sought. Six months ago, the patient's hypertension became poorly controlled. He sought treatment at another hospital, where an abdominal and pelvic CT scan revealed multiple nodules in both adrenal glands, suggesting adenomas. Nodules were visible in the medial limb and junction of the left adrenal gland, measuring approximately 15 mm × 14 mm and 5 mm × 4 mm, with clear boundaries. The plain CT values were about 2 HU and 3 HU, and the enhanced CT values were about 65 HU and 37 HU. A nodule was seen in the lateral limb of the right adrenal gland, measuring approximately 5 mm × 7 mm, with a clear boundary. The plain CT value was about 9 HU, and the enhanced CT value was about 30 HU (Fig. 1). Endocrine examination: aldosterone 485.3 pmol/L, renin activity 0.17 ng/(ml·h), ARR103; captopril test suggested that aldosterone levels could not be suppressed. The patient underwent adrenal venous sampling, which showed that the left side was the dominant side for aldosterone secretion. PET/CT suggested nodular thickening of the left adrenal gland with increased radioactive uptake, SUVm4.3; no increased radioactive uptake was seen in the right adrenal gland, suggesting that the left nodule was functional. The patient was then given spironolactone 20 mg bid, olmesartan medoxomil and

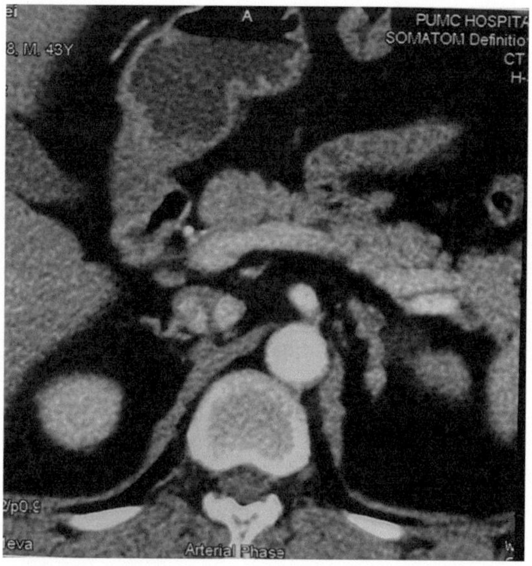

Fig. 1 Adrenal enhanced CT image

Supplementary Information The online version contains supplementary material available at https://doi.org/10.1007/978-981-96-8598-1_3.

Z. Ye (✉)
Beijing Union Medical College Hospital, Beijing, China
e-mail: yezixing@pumch.cn

Y. Zhang, X. Zhao (eds.), *Laparoscopic Surgery in Urology*, https://doi.org/10.1007/978-981-96-8598-1_3

amlodipine 20 mg qd, and bisoprolol 2.5 mg qd, and his blood pressure has been well controlled presently. During the course of the disease, the patient had no obvious symptoms such as headache, dizziness, limb weakness, numbness in the extremities, or palpitations.

Past History

None in particular.

Physical Examination

None in particular.

Imaging Data (Fig. 1)

Preoperative Assessment: The patient's imaging studies suggested multiple nodules in both adrenal glands. Adrenal venous sampling and PET/CT both suggested that the left side was dominant, suggesting that the multiple nodules in the left adrenal gland were likely endocrinologically functional. The indications for surgery were clear. After admission, routine preoperative examinations such as complete blood count, liver and renal function, coagulation function, and electrocardiogram were all normal. The surgical approach was laparoscopic transperitoneal left adrenalectomy.

Surgical Procedure

1. The patient was placed in the right lateral decubitus position with the waist bridge elevated. The surgical side was marked in the ward before surgery. Intubation general anesthesia was used. A urinary catheter was placed. Routine disinfection and draping were performed.
2. The retroperitoneal upper urinary tract surgical approach was used. In this case, a four-port approach was used (2 cm above the iliac crest on the midaxillary line, below the costal margin on the anterior axillary line, below the costal margin on the posterior axillary line, and between the trocars on the midaxillary line and anterior axillary line).
3. The pararenal fat was cleared, and the extraperitoneal fat was freed from top to bottom and flipped into the psoas fossa, clearly exposing the renal fascia (Fig. 2).
4. Open the renal fascia longitudinally along the peritoneal reflection, from the level below the diaphragm to the level above the iliac crest (Fig. 3).
5. Locate the kidney and free it upward along the surface of the kidney, completely separating the upper pole of the kidney from the adrenal gland.
6. Lift the adrenal gland upward and maintain a tension, free the central vein of the adrenal gland, and clamp it with a Hem-o-lok (Fig. 4).
7. Pull the left adrenal gland toward the dorsal side, and separate the adrenal gland within the avascular area between the peritoneum and the anterior layer of the renal fascia (Fig. 5).
8. Pull the left adrenal gland toward the ventral side, and separate the adrenal gland within the avascular area posterior to the posterior layer of the renal fascia.

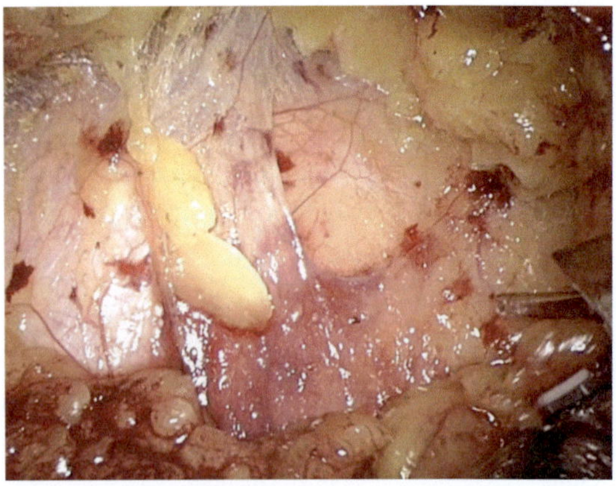

Fig. 2 Clearing of pararenal fat

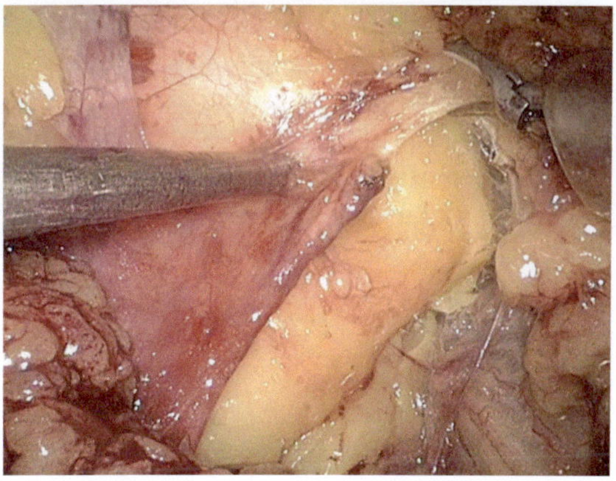

Fig. 3 Opening the renal fascia

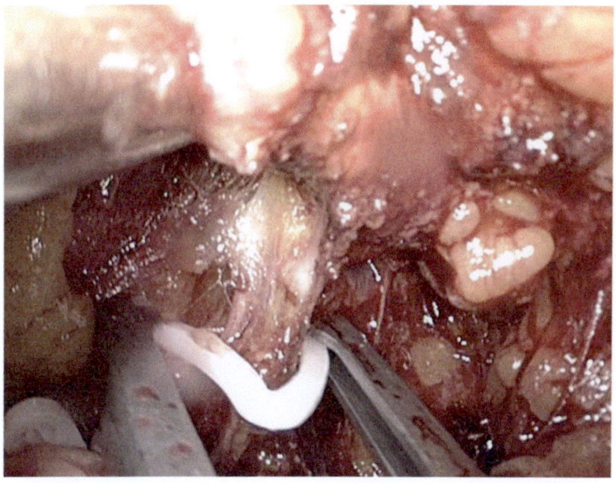

Fig. 4 Clamping and cutting the central vein of the left adrenal gland

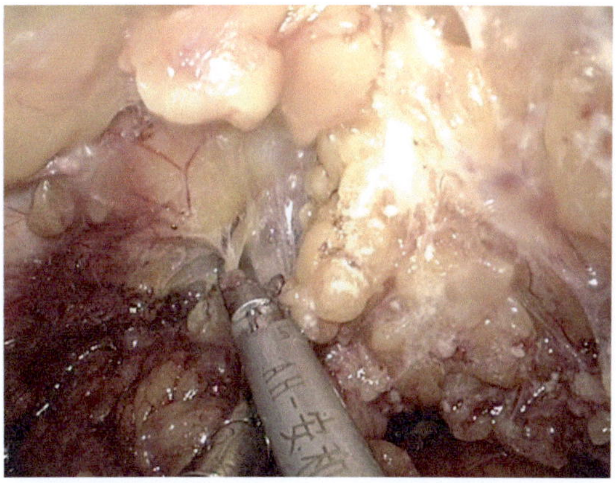

Fig. 5 Separating the ventral and dorsal sides of the adrenal gland

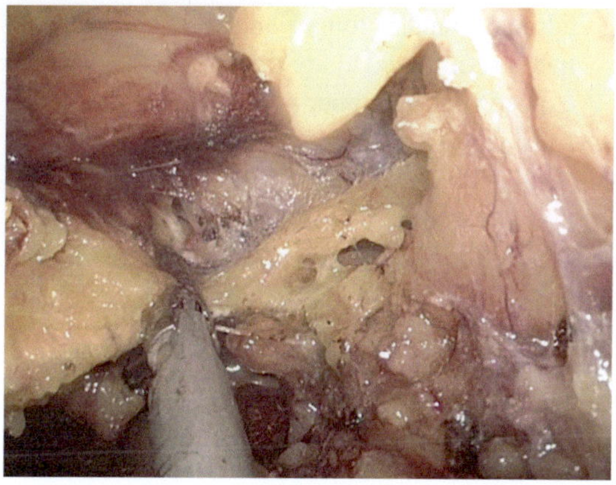

Fig. 6 Free the upper pole of the adrenal gland

9. Free the upper pole of the adrenal gland until the adrenal gland is completely removed (Fig. 6).
10. Carefully check the surgical field for active bleeding, place the specimen in a specimen bag, and remove it through the midaxillary line trocar.
11. Place one drainage tube in the adrenal fossa, count the gauze and instruments and close the incisions, and the operation is over.

Expert Comments

1. The key to anatomical resection of the adrenal gland is to find the adrenal gland and the avascular area around it and to find the loose connective tissue on the ventral and dorsal sides of the adrenal gland. Small vessels exist in the avascular area occationally, so it is important to use a combination of blunt and sharp dissection; In the area between the adrenal gland and the kidney, where the space is often narrow and arteries supplying the adrenal gland often pass through, sharp dissection should be the main method to avoid local bleeding affecting the surgical field.
2. Handling of the central vein of the left adrenal gland: Although the central vein of the left

adrenal gland is longer and relatively easy to handle compared to the right side, it is better to expose after the upper pole of the left kidney is fully freed. When freeing the central vein on the left side, special attention should be paid to avoid excessive traction to prevent damage to the central vein or even the renal vein.

3. The adrenal tissue is fragile and rich in blood supply, so direct clamping of the adrenal tissue should be avoided during surgery to prevent adrenal tissue rupture and bleeding, which can affect the surgical field. A certain amount of fat tissue can be retained around the adrenal gland for easier traction.

Adrenal Surgery: Case 2 Laparoscopic Retroperitoneal Right Adrenalectomy

Yanan Li

Chief Complaint

Bilateral adrenal tumors found during physical examination for over a year.

Medical History

Male, 65 years old. The patient had a CT scan at the end of 2020 during a physical examination, which showed tumors in the medial limbs of both adrenal glands, the larger one on the right side, about 42 mm, with no obvious discomfort. Subsequent annual physical examinations showed no significant changes in the tumors. In February 2022, the patient came to our hospital for treatment. Abdominopelvic enhanced CT suggested low-density lesions in both adrenal glands, with the largest cross section about 2.8 cm × 1.9 cm (left side) and 4.5 cm × 2.5 cm (right side), slightly enhanced after enhancement (Figs. 1 and 2). Endocrine examination: ACTH 9.9 pg/ml, 24 h urinary cortisol, renin, aldosterone, urinary catecholamines, and dehydroepiandrosterone sulfate (DS) were roughly normal, admitted to the hospital with the diagnosis of "adrenal tumor." Past history, family history, and physical examination were unremarkable.

Imaging Data (Figs. 1 and 2)

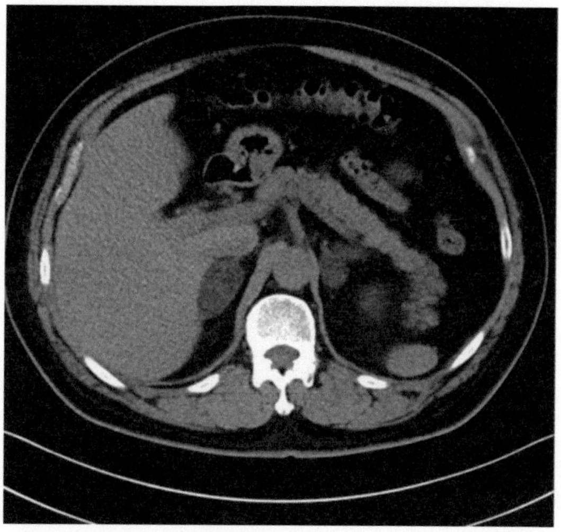

Fig. 1 Adrenal CT plain scan image

Supplementary Information The online version contains supplementary material available at https://doi.org/10.1007/978-981-96-8598-1_4.

Y. Li (✉)
Beijing Union Medical College Hospital, Beijing, China

Y. Zhang, X. Zhao (eds.), *Laparoscopic Surgery in Urology*, https://doi.org/10.1007/978-981-96-8598-1_4

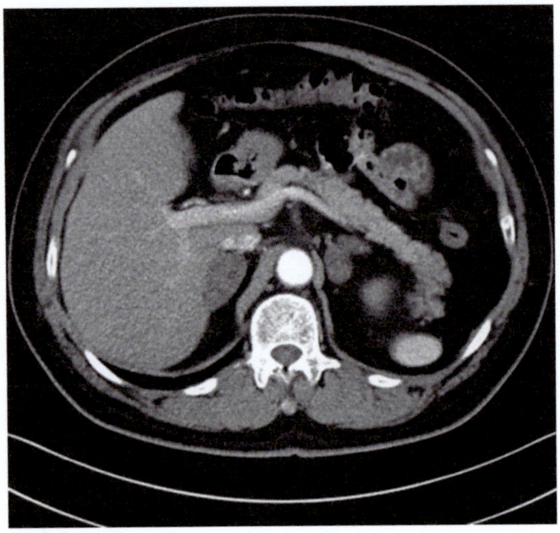

Fig. 2 Adrenal CT-enhanced image

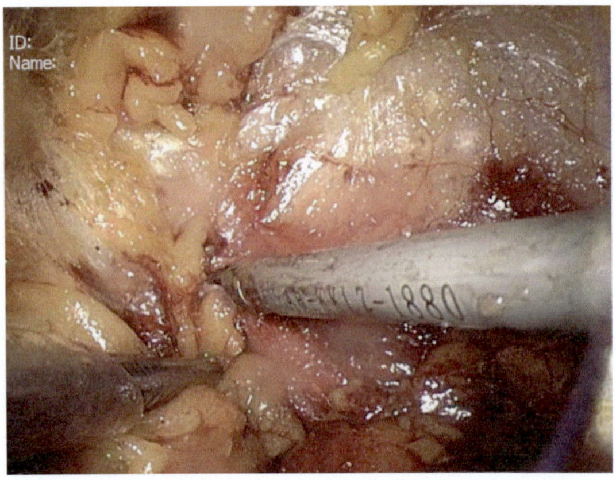

Fig. 3 Cleaning the extraperitoneal fat tissue

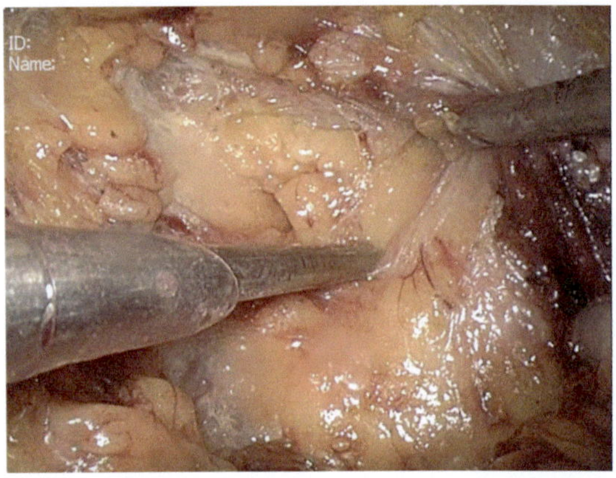

Fig. 4 Opening the renal fascia, exposing the perirenal tissue

Preoperative Assessment

The patient was found to have bilateral adrenal tumors during a physical examination. The imaging features were round low-density lesions, slightly enhanced after enhancement, with no discomfort complaints. The endocrine examination showed a decrease in ACTH. Considering the patient's history, laboratory tests, and imaging evaluation, the diagnosis of bilateral adrenal tumors (likely adenomas) and subclinical Cushing's syndrome was basically clear, and surgical treatment was recommended. The surgical method was laparoscopic right adrenalectomy.

Surgical Procedure

1. Adopt the retroperitoneal upper urinary tract surgical position. Mark the surgical side (right side) preoperatively. Intubation general anesthesia is used. A urinary catheter is placed. Routine disinfection and draping.
2. Establish a retroperitoneal upper urinary tract surgical access; this surgery uses four ports.
3. Clean the retroperitoneal fat. Gather the dorsal and ventral fat toward the midline, try to bluntly separate the whole fat, and flip the extraperitoneal fat down to the iliac fossa. When encountering nourishing blood vessels during separation, use an ultrasonic knife for electrocoagulation to prevent bleeding, and small fat particles can be sucked away with a suction device (Fig. 3).
4. Open the retroperitoneal space, expose the perirenal tissue, and see that the perirenal fat is abundant (Fig. 4).
5. Find the ventral surface of the kidney, and free the kidney along the ventral surface toward the head until the upper pole of the kidney (Fig. 5).
6. Differentiate the adrenal gland from the perirenal fat, separate the upper pole of the kidney from the adrenal kidney surface, press down the kidney, establish the operating

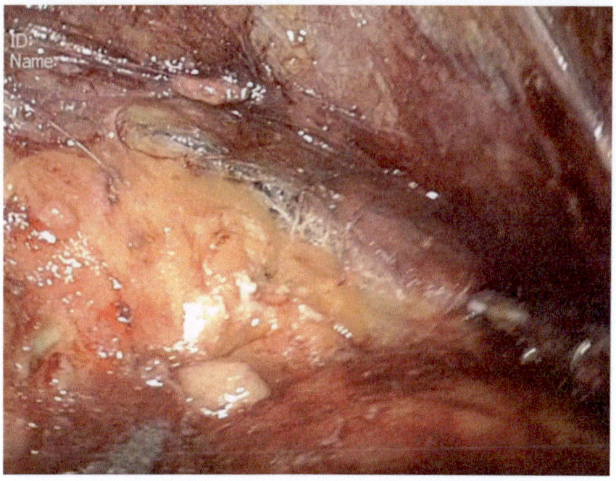

Fig. 5 Separating the ventral surface of the kidney

space, and simultaneously sever the small arteries below the adrenal gland (Fig. 6).

7. Separate the ventral surface of the adrenal gland from the liver surface (Fig. 7).
8. Locate the central vein of the right adrenal gland, and clamp and sever the central vein of the adrenal gland with Hem-o-lok (Fig. 8).
9. Continue to separate the dorsal surface of the adrenal gland, and completely peel off the adrenal gland (Fig. 9).
10. Check for bleeding points, place a drainage tube, close the wound, and the surgery is completed (Fig. 10). The postoperative specimen is shown in Fig. 11.

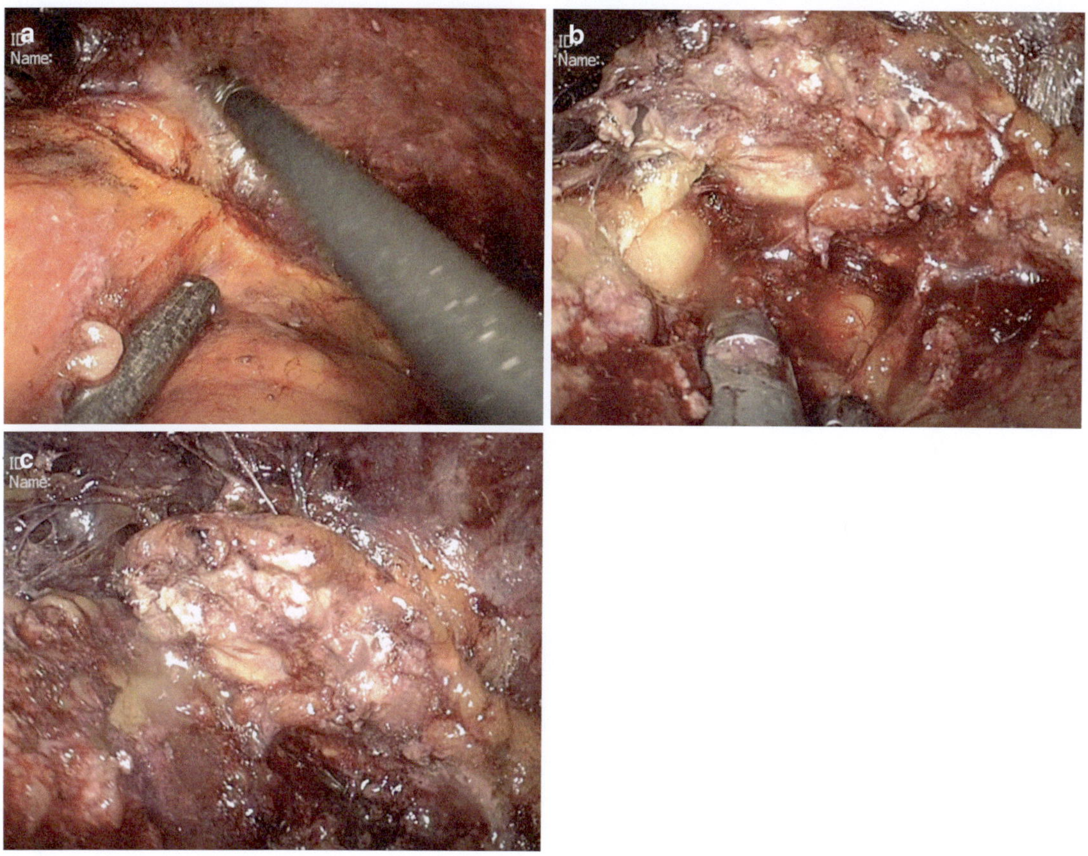

Fig. 6 (**a**–**c**) Separating the kidney and adrenal plane

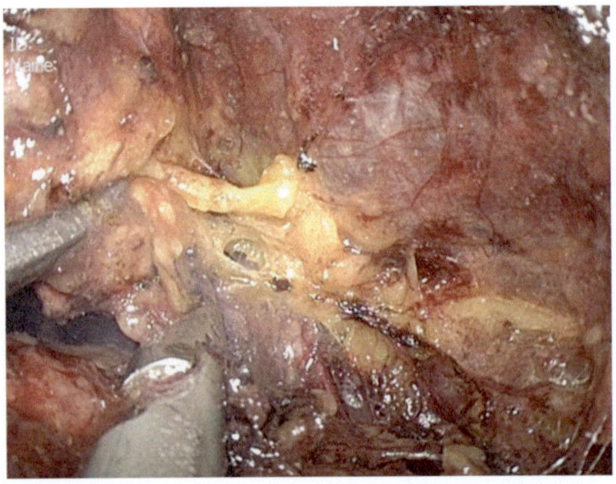

Fig. 7 Separating the adrenal and liver plane

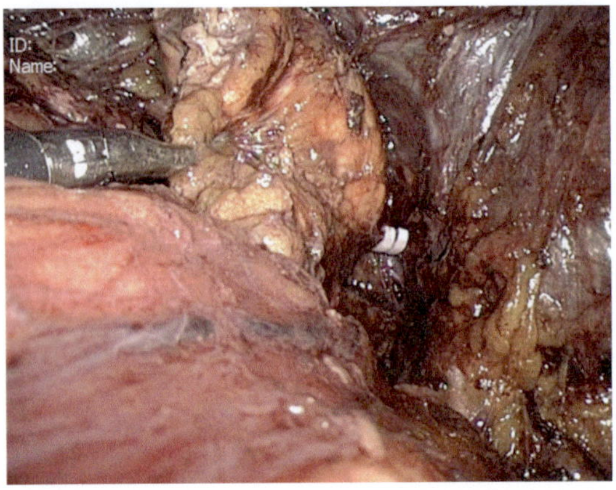

Fig. 8 Separating and severing the central vein of the adrenal gland

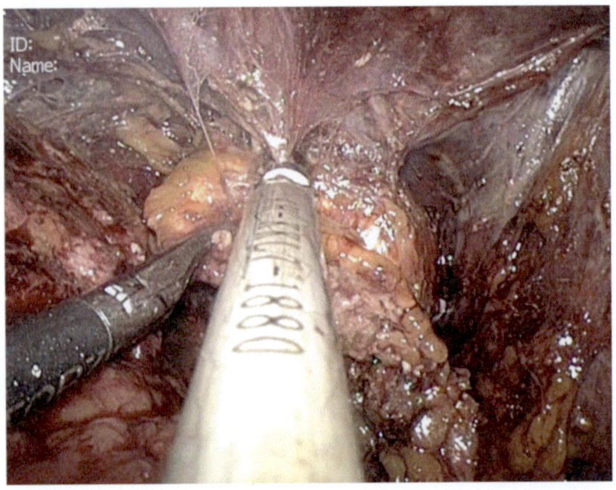

Fig. 9 Separating the dorsal surface of the adrenal gland

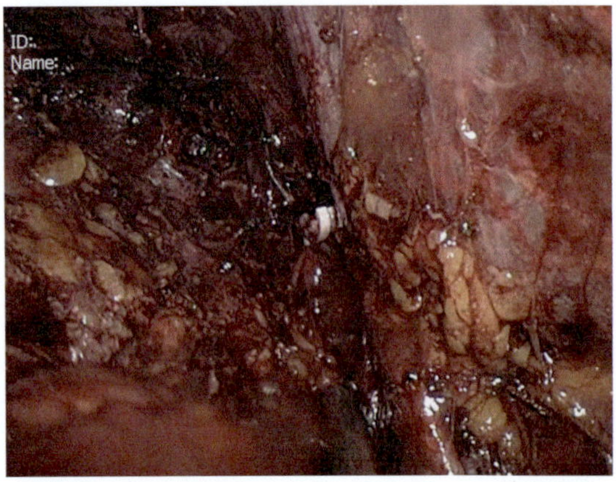

Fig. 10 Checking the wound

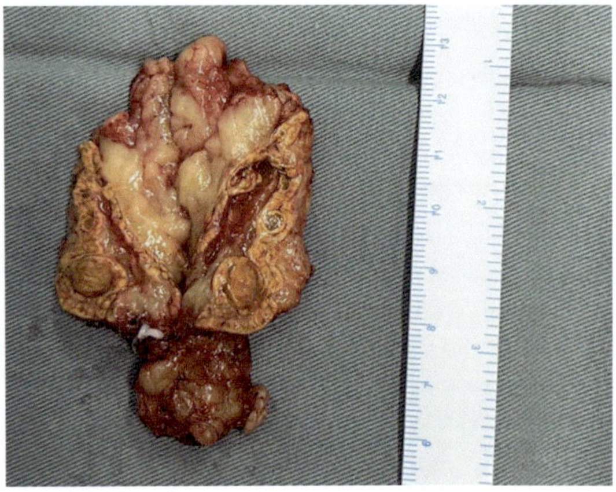

Fig. 11 Cross-sectional view of the right adrenal gland specimen

Expert Review

The goal of this case surgery is to completely remove the right adrenal gland. There are various surgical methods, and the key points of this case surgery method are as follows:

1. Establish the retroperitoneal space. When establishing the retroperitoneal space, pay attention to distinguish the position of the peritoneal fold to prevent damage to the peritoneum. If the peritoneal fold is unclear, you can open the renal fascia longitudinally as

close as possible to the psoas major muscle, you can open it 1–2 cm away from the psoas major muscle, and after confirming that the peritoneum is not damaged, you can open the renal fascia appropriately toward the abdominal side according to the need to provide a better operating space. After opening the renal fascia, you can bluntly tear the renal fascia in the direction of the peritoneal fold.

2. Locate the kidney. If the patient has too much fat, you can press the surface of the fat sac with a suction device to feel and locate the kidney.
3. Locate the adrenal gland. Use the kidney as an anatomical marker, separate along the kidney toward the head side, and locate the adrenal gland. If the perirenal fat is thick, you can temporarily not separate the perirenal fat sac and renal capsule, but separate them as a whole until the upper pole of the kidney, then separate the adrenal gland and perirenal fat, and separate the kidney surface of the adrenal gland. Press the kidney down to establish an operating space above the upper pole of the kidney.
4. Adrenal gland separation. First, separate the kidney surface, and then separate the liver surface. Be careful not to damage the liver capsule and cause bleeding, focus on handling the main blood vessel area of the adrenal gland, and separate it to a slightly deeper place to see the central vein of the right adrenal gland. Use two Hem-o-lok clips to close the proximal end and one clip to close the distal end, and cut off the central vein. At this time, the adrenal gland is only connected to some liver surface tissues, and there are no important blood vessels running, which can be sharply separated directly with an ultrasonic knife, and finally the surrounding connected tissues are coagulated with an ultrasonic knife. Lower the pneumoperitoneum pressure and observe whether there is bleeding at the wound.

Adrenal Surgery: Case 3 Laparoscopic Retroperitoneal Left Adrenal Tumor Removal

Dongxu Qiu

Chief Complaint

Hypertension for 20 years, left adrenal tumor found 4 months ago.

Medical History

Female, 64 years old. Hypertension was found 20 years ago, treated with antihypertensive drugs, and blood pressure was controlled at 140–150/80–90 mmHg. One year ago, the patient's physical examination revealed a blood potassium level of 2.9 mmol/L. Complete endocrine examination revealed angiotensin level of 0.22 ng/(ml·h), and abdominal and pelvic enhanced CT suggested a nodule on the lateral limb of the left adrenal gland, with a diameter of about 1.1 cm. The plain CT value is about 21 HU, showing mild enhancement, considering left adrenal nodule (primary aldosteronism is likely) (Figs. 1 and 2). The patient was given oral spironolactone 40 mg bid and potassium chloride sustained-release tablets 1 g tid. There is poor blood pressure control; blood

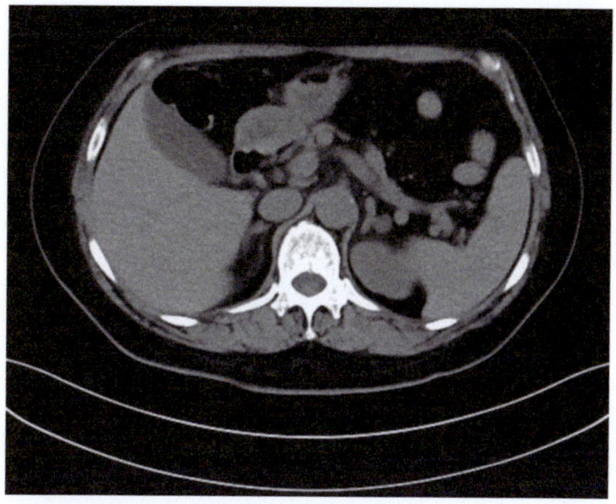

Fig. 1 Adrenal CT plain scan image

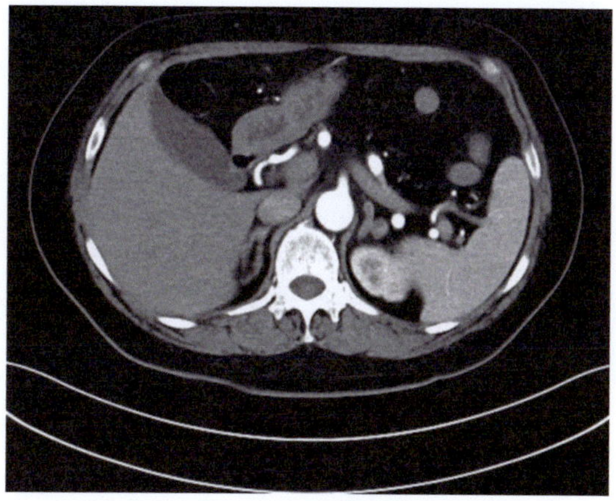

Fig. 2 Adrenal CT-enhanced image

Supplementary Information The online version contains supplementary material available at https://doi.org/10.1007/978-981-96-8598-1_5.

D. Qiu (✉)
Hunan Provincial People's Hospital the First Affiliated Hospital of Hunan Normal University, Changsha, China

Y. Zhang, X. Zhao (eds.), *Laparoscopic Surgery in Urology*,
https://doi.org/10.1007/978-981-96-8598-1_5

pressure fluctuates at 150–200/90–100 mmHg. The patient has no dizziness, headache, chest tightness, shortness of breath, back pain, periodic paralysis, etc. This time she was admitted to the hospital because of "left adrenal tumor; primary aldosteronism is likely."

Past History

Hysterectomy due to uterine fibroids, appendectomy history.

Physical Examination

No special findings in the heart and lungs; old surgical scars can be seen in the abdomen, right lower abdomen, and middle and lower abdomen. No other special findings.

Preoperative Assessment

The patient has a history of hypertension and hypokalemia, and imaging examination suggests a left adrenal nodule, with a diameter of about 1.1 cm, with mild enhancement, considering left adrenal tumor. Primary aldosteronism is likely, and the effect of drug treatment is not satisfactory; the surgical indications are clear. Further assessment of cardiopulmonary function, routine blood tests, liver and kidney function and electrolytes, coagulation function, and other preoperative related examinations did not show obvious abnormalities after admission. The planned surgical treatment is laparoscopic left adrenal tumor removal.

Surgical Process

1. Adopt the retroperitoneal upper urinary tract surgical position. Mark the surgical side in the ward before surgery. General anesthesia with endotracheal intubation is used. A urinary catheter is placed. Routine disinfection and draping.
2. After establishing pneumoperitoneum, establish the upper urinary tract surgical channel. This operation uses three holes (3 cm above the xiphoid process on the midaxillary line, below the 12th rib on the posterior axillary line, below the 12th rib on the anterior axillary line).
3. Clean the extraperitoneal fat; the nourishing blood vessels of the extraperitoneal fat can be seen during the separation process, which can be sharply cut with an ultrasonic knife.
4. Longitudinally cut the Gerota's fascia; the range is up to the diaphragm and down to the level of the pelvic brim. There is a relatively avascular space between the renal fat capsule in the upper part of the kidney and the anterior layer of the renal fascia, which can reveal the kidney along this space (Fig. 3).
5. Separate the perirenal fat along the upper pole of the kidney, suspend the dissected fat capsule using the peritoneum, open the space at the upper pole of the kidney, and dissect the plane at the junction of the adrenal gland base and the kidney (Fig. 4).
6. Combine preoperative imaging examination and surgical field to find the approximate location of the adrenal tumor (Fig. 5).
7. Along the plane between the surface of the upper pole of the kidney and the fat capsule at the base of the adrenal gland, lift the adrenal gland, and separate the sur-

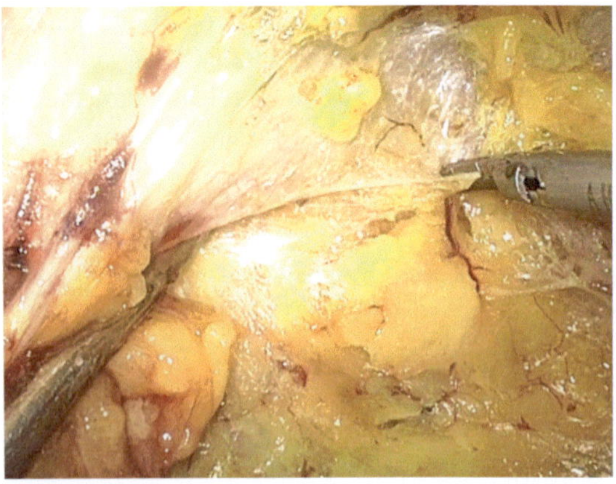

Fig. 3 Opening the renal fascia

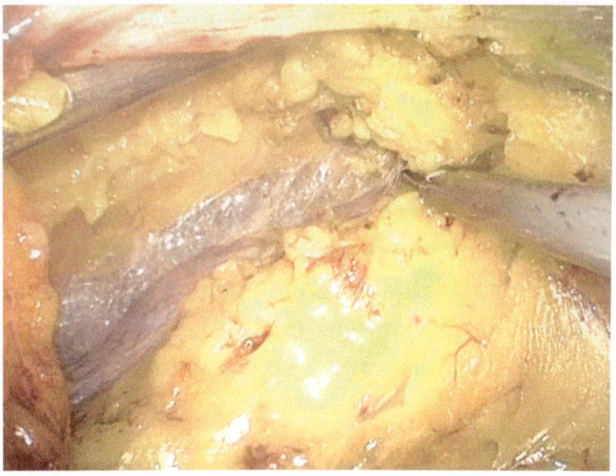

Fig. 4 Freeing upward along the ventral side of the kidney

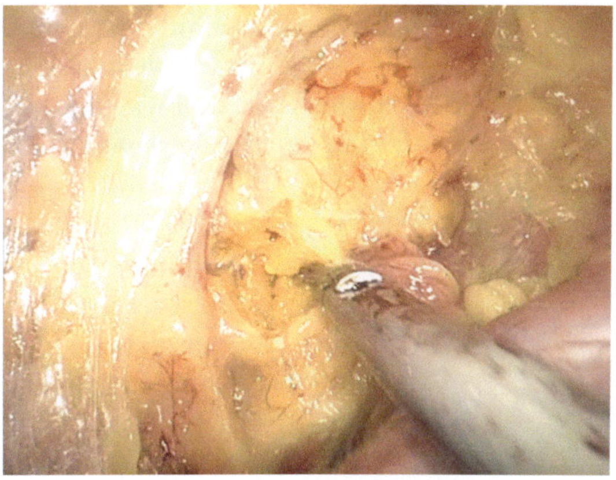

Fig. 5 Localization of the adrenal tumor

rounding tissues of the adrenal gland with a combination of blunt and sharp dissection to fully expose the adrenal tumor. During the operation, pay attention to using the ultrasonic knife to coagulate the blood vessels (Fig. 6).

8. During the operation, central vein injury was found, with a small amount of bleeding. Use a separation clamp to clamp the end of the central vein, and use Hem-o-lok to clamp the central vein (Fig. 7).
9. Completely free and remove the adrenal tumor, use Hem-o-Lok to ligate the adrenal stump for hemostasis, and put the adrenal tumor into the specimen bag. Check whether there are bleeding points on the wound surface, and take out the specimen completely through the observation hole. Place a drainage tube (Fig. 8).

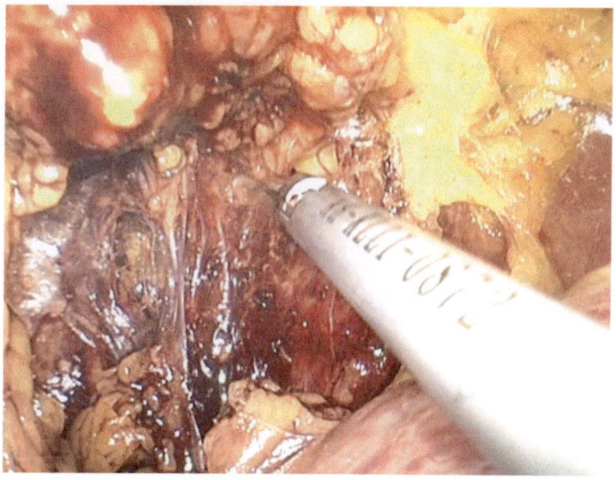

Fig. 6 Separation of the adrenal and kidney interface

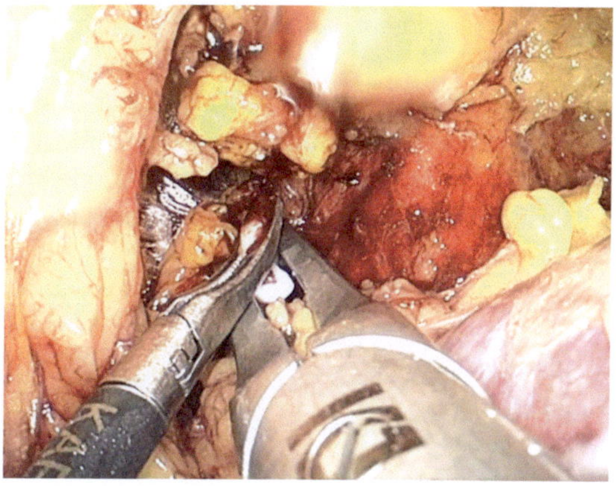

Fig. 7 Treatment of the central vein of the left adrenal gland

Expert Comments

1. The surgical indications are clear. The patient has typical symptoms of hypertension and hypokalemia, and imaging examinations suggest a

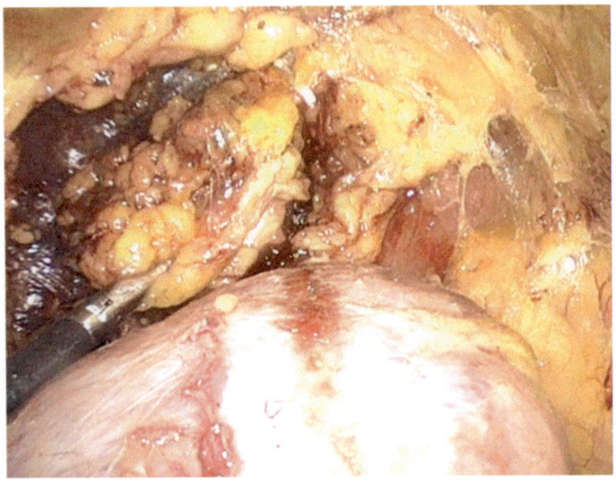

Fig. 8 Removal of the adrenal tumor

left adrenal tumor. Laboratory tests suggest a significant decrease in plasma renin activity (PRA). The diagnosis is basically clear; it is a left adrenal tumor, primary aldosteronism.

2. The basic surgical path is to free along the surface of the kidney to the upper pole of the kidney to find the adrenal gland, which is suitable for patients with less perirenal fat. Its surgical thinking is clear, especially suitable for beginners.
3. The separation and dissection of the central vein is an important step in adrenal surgery. In this case, the patient's adrenal central vein was damaged during the operation, but due to the intra-abdominal pressure, there was no excessive bleeding. The treatment method used in this case was to use a separation clamp to close the cut end and then use a Hem-o-lok to close it. A laparoscopic gauze can also be used to compress and stop the bleeding, and after the local surgical field is clear, hemostasis treatment can be performed. Of course, the safest way is to operate carefully during the operation, separate the central vein clearly, and then decide whether to deal with the central vein according to the location of the patient's tumor.

Adrenal Surgery: Case 4 Laparoscopic Transperitoneal Right Adrenal Tumor Resection

Yang Zhao

Chief Complaint

Dizziness, nausea, and excessive sweating for 1 year; right adrenal mass found during physical examination 3 months ago. Male, 58 years old. One year ago, he occasionally experienced dizziness, nausea, and excessive sweating. When the symptoms occurred, his blood pressure was 110/80 mmHg, with no palpitations or headaches, and the symptoms eased after rest. In July 2022, the patient came to our hospital for a physical examination. CT examination showed a 1.6 cm × 1.0 cm mass in the right adrenal gland. For further diagnosis and treatment, he visited our department. CTU showed a soft tissue density nodule in the junction of the right adrenal gland, about 1.6 cm × 1.3 cm in size, plain CT value 31 HU, and obvious enhancement after enhancement (Figs. 1 and 2). Complete endocrine-related tests, NMN 0.46 nmol/L and MN 0.14 nmol/L, and 24 h urinary catecholamines, NE 72.3 μg/24 h, E5.8 μg/24 h, and DA 275.8 μg/24 h. No obvious abnormalities were seen in the octreotide imaging. He was diagnozed as "right adrenal tumor", and phenoxybenzamine

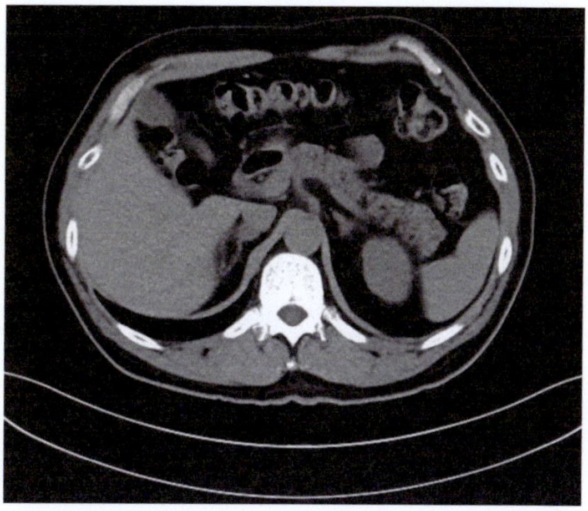

Fig. 1 Adrenal CT plain scan image

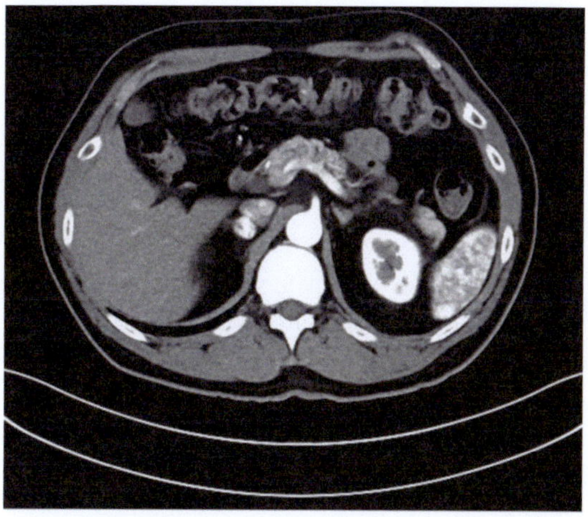

Fig. 2 Adrenal-enhanced CT image

Supplementary Information The online version contains supplementary material available at https://doi.org/10.1007/978-981-96-8598-1_6.

Y. Zhao (✉)
Beijing Union Medical College Hospital,
Beijing, China

Y. Zhang, X. Zhao (eds.), *Laparoscopic Surgery in Urology*,
https://doi.org/10.1007/978-981-96-8598-1_6

10 mg po tid was given for medication preparation. The patient has been regularly preparing medication for more than 1 month and was admitted to the hospital for surgery with the diagnosis of "right adrenal tumor."

Past History

Nothing special.

Physical Examination

Nothing special.

Imaging Data (Figs. 1 and 2)

Preoperative Assessment

The patient had previously experienced typical symptoms of pheochromocytoma such as dizziness, nausea, and excessive sweating. Outpatient endocrine and nuclear medicine examinations were performed, and blood NMN and MN were normal, and 24 h urinary catecholamines were normal. No obvious abnormalities were seen in the octreotide imaging. Phenoxybenzamine was given for preoperative preparation 1 month before admission. After admission, consultations with relevant departments were conducted.

Anesthesiology

The patient is ASA II level, with enhanced circulatory monitoring during surgery, and returns to ICU depending on the intraoperative situation. Intensive care medicine: Active respiratory function exercise before surgery. Prepare to return to ICU according to the intraoperative situation. Endocrinology: It is recommended to have a high-sodium, high-protein diet; ensure an intake greater than 3000 ml; monitor intake and output and weight; continue to give phenoxybenzamine medication preparation; closely monitor the patient's vital signs during the perioperative period; and be alert to hypertensive crisis and alternating high and low blood pressure. After admission, additional assessments of cardiopulmonary function and preoperative routine tests were performed, and no other obvious abnormalities were found. The plan is to perform surgery, and the surgical method is laparoscopic transperitoneal resection of the right adrenal tumor.

Surgical Process

1. Adopt the retroperitoneal upper urinary tract surgical approach. Mark the surgical side in the ward before surgery. Use intubation general anesthesia. Leave a catheter in place. Routine disinfection and draping.
2. Adopt the retroperitoneal upper urinary tract surgical approach; this operation uses four holes (2 cm above the axillary midline crest, below the rib edge of the axillary anterior line, below the rib edge of the axillary posterior line, and between the axillary midline and the axillary anterior line trocar).
3. Clean the extraperitoneal fat, identify the peritoneal reflection, open the renal fascia on the back of the peritoneal reflection, and expose the perirenal fat capsule (Fig. 3).
4. Dissect the perirenal fat, expose the kidney, and free upward along the renal fascia, exposing the upper pole of the kidney (Fig. 4).

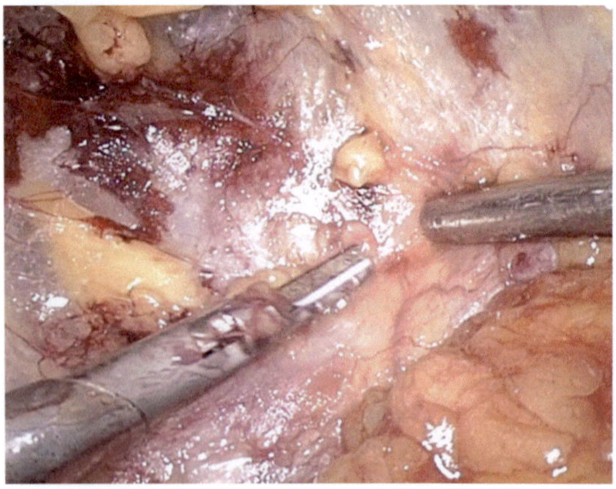

Fig. 3: (**a**) Cleaning the extraperitoneal fat. (**b**) Cleaning the retroperitoneal fat

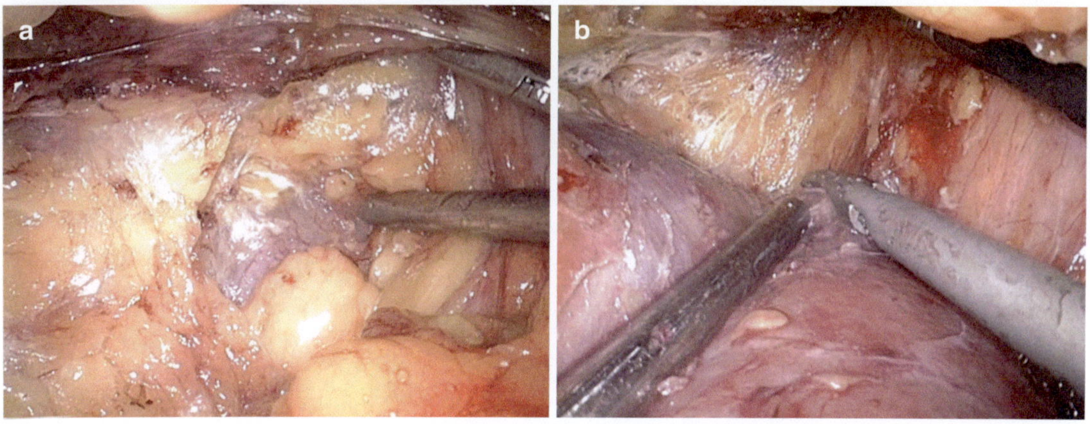

Fig. 4 (**a**, **b**) Separating along the ventral side of the kidney

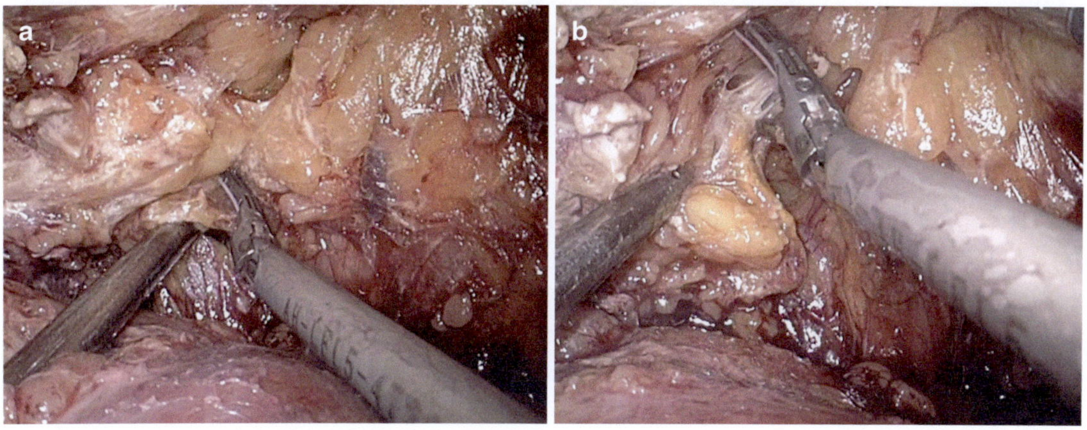

Fig. 5 (**a**, **b**) Separating the adrenal gland and the upper pole of the kidney, looking for the tumor

5. Carefully search for adrenal tissue in the fat tissue of the upper pole of the kidney (Fig. 5).
6. Free the adrenal gland along the upper pole of the kidney, Hem-o-lok clamps, and cut off the central vein of the adrenal gland (Fig. 6).
7. Continue to free the rest of the adrenal gland, cut off the tumor along the edge of the tumor, and pay attention to keep the tumor capsule intact (Fig. 7).
8. Carefully complete the hemostasis of the adrenal gland end.
9. Insert a specimen bag through the main operation hole, put the removed tissue into the bag, and take out the specimen bag from the observation hole. Re-establish pneumoperitoneum, check for bleeding, place hemostatic material and drainage tube, and the operation is over.

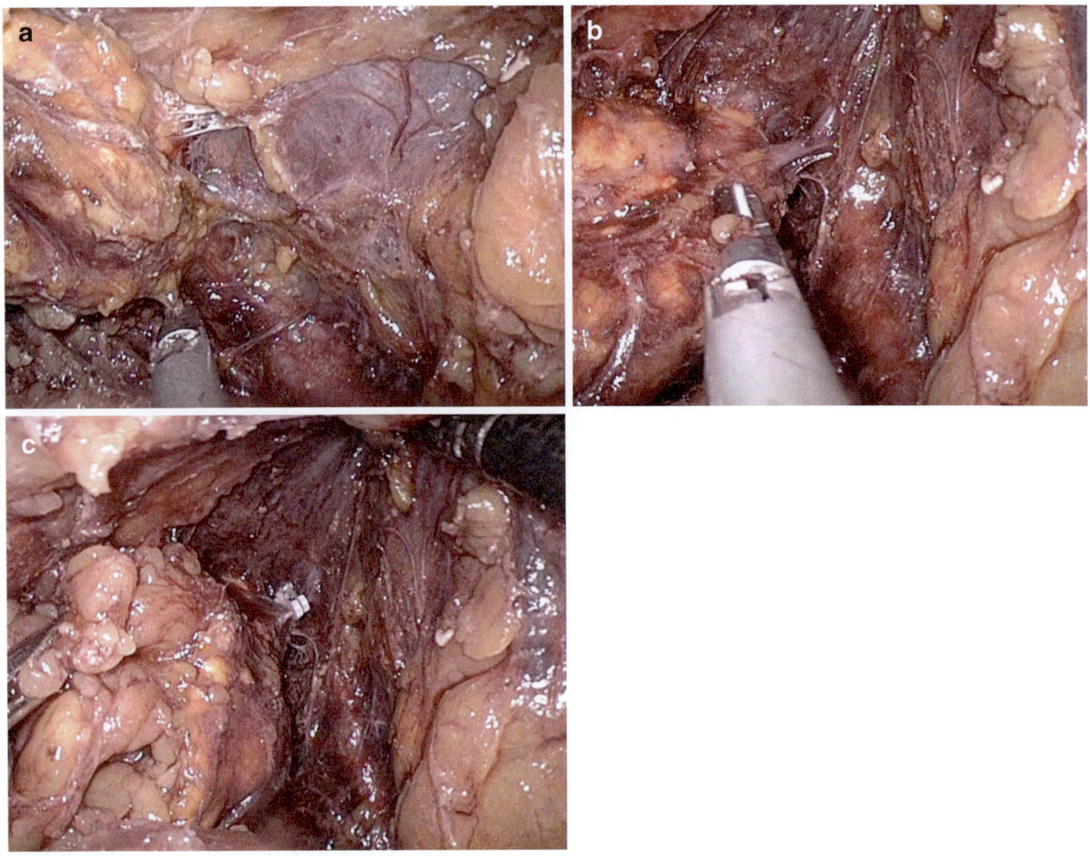

Fig. 6 (**a**–**c**) Separating and cutting off the central vein

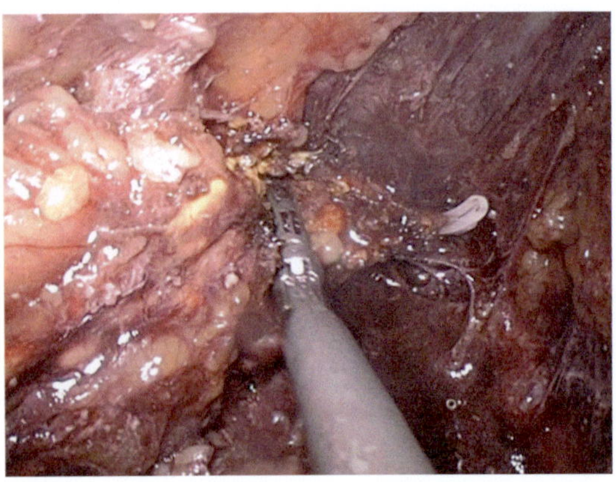

Fig. 7 Separating and removing the tumor

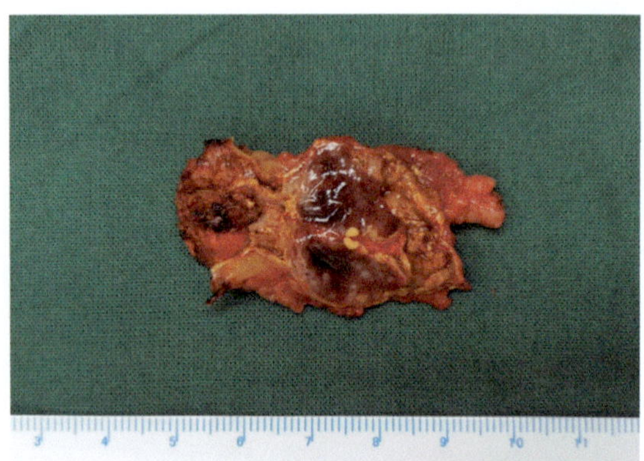

Fig. 8 Cross-sectional diagram of the right adrenal tumor

Postoperative Pathology (Fig. 8)

Immunohistochemistry results: Melan-A (−), AE1/AE3 (−), CgA (+), Ki-67 (index 3%), S-100 (supporting cells+), α-inhibin (−), SDHB (+), and MGMT (some+).

Expert Comments

1. This case is a pheochromocytoma with negative endocrine and nuclear medicine tests, clinically known as a silent pheochromocytoma. A typical pheochromocytoma requires

a complete endocrine test, octreotide imaging, and MIBG test before surgery. One month before surgery, phenoxybenzamine should be administered. Preoperative multidisciplinary consultation, assessment of surgical risk and patient's surgical tolerance, blood preparation, ICU preparation, and sufficient preoperative preparation are necessary to prevent perioperative blood pressure fluctuations. In this case, the patient only had mild clinical symptoms, low frequency of onset, and normal blood pressure when the disease occurred. Both endocrine and nuclear medicine tests were negative. However, the patient's enhanced CT showed significant enhancement, so pheochromocytoma could not be completely ruled out. Despite the lack of clear evidence of pheochromocytoma, the patient was still advised to prepare adequately for surgery in line with the principle of surgical safety first, to ensure stable blood pressure during the perioperative period.

Adrenal Surgery: Case 5 Laparoscopic Retroperitoneal Recurrence of Left Adrenal Tumor and Second Surgery Removal

Yang Zhao

Chief Complaint

Recurrence of left adrenal tumor 11 years after removal, discovered 5 years ago. Female, 54 years old. The patient developed hypertension 13 years ago without any obvious cause, with a maximum of 160/90 mmHg, treated with nifedipine controlled-release tablets 30 mg qd; blood pressure was controlled at around 150/80 mmHg. Eleven years ago, a nodular lesion was found in the lateral limb of the left adrenal gland in our hospital, with a diameter of about 1.7 cm. Blood potassium 3.0 mmol/L. Endocrine-related tests: renin 0.1 ng/(ml·h) and aldosterone 363.42 pmol/L. The diagnosis was considered primary hyperaldosteronism, and laparoscopic left adrenal tumor removal was performed. Postoperative pathology report: adrenal cortical nodular hyperplasia. After surgery, blood pressure partially relieved, regular oral nifedipine controlled-release tablets were continued, blood pressure was controlled at around 130/80 mmHg, and blood potassium returned to normal. Five years ago, blood pressure rose again, with a maximum of 160–170/100–110 mmHg. She visited our outpatient clinic; rechecked blood potassium 3.1 mmol/L. Renin 0.17 ng/(ml·h) and aldosterone 358.44 pmol/L. Captopril test: aldosterone 274.23 pmol/L before medication and aldosterone 254.01 pmol/L after medication. Abdominal enhanced CT showed: left adrenal occupation, diameter about 1.6 cm, considering adenoma possibility (Figs. 1 and 2). Treated with spironolactone 20 mg tid, blood pressure control was not good, and the patient stopped medication on her own. Two months ago, the patient had hand numbness and weakness; outpatient rechecked blood potassium 2.9 mmol/L. After oral potassium supplementation and spironolactone treatment, rechecked blood potassium 3.7 mmol/L. Now admitted for surgery.

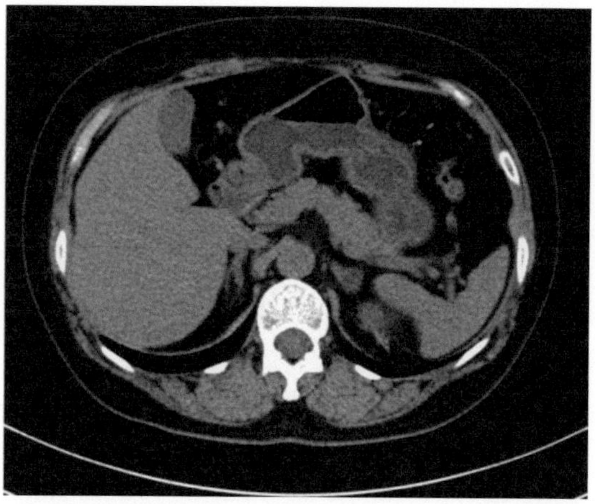

Fig. 1 Adrenal CT plain scan image

Supplementary Information The online version contains supplementary material available at https://doi.org/10.1007/978-981-96-8598-1_7.

Y. Zhao (✉)
Beijing Union Medical College Hospital,
Beijing, China

Y. Zhang, X. Zhao (eds.), *Laparoscopic Surgery in Urology*,
https://doi.org/10.1007/978-981-96-8598-1_7

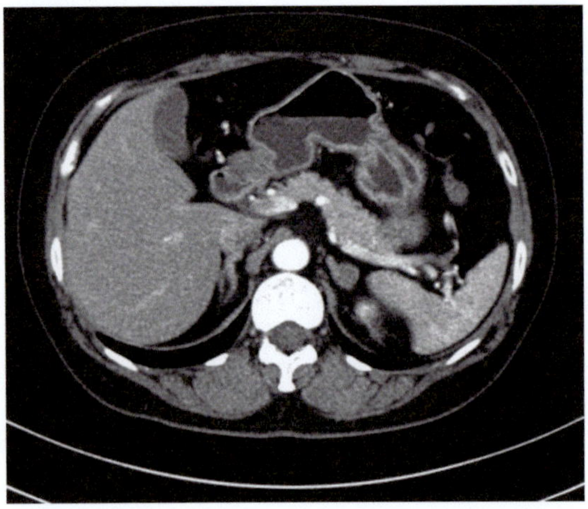

Fig. 2 Adrenal enhanced CT image

Past History

Surgical history as per present illness, nothing else special.

Physical Examination

Old surgical scar can be seen on the left waist. Nothing else special.

Imaging Data (Figs. 1 and 2)

Preoperative Assessment

The patient developed hypertension and hypokalemia 13 years ago, with endocrine examination indicating low renin activity and an ARR of 131.2. Imaging examination revealed a mass in the left adrenal gland. After the adrenal mass was surgically removed, the hypertension and hypokalemia improved. Hypertension and hypokalemia reappeared 5 years ago. Endocrine-related examinations suggested an ARR of 76.1, and the aldosterone level was not suppressed in the captopril test. A follow-up imaging examination found a mass about 1.6 cm in diameter in the left adrenal gland. It was considered to be a recurrence of the left adrenal tumor and primary hyperaldosteronism. The patient has hypertension and hypokalemia. The effect of internal medicine treatment is not good, and the surgical indications are clear. After admission, further supplementary assessments of cardiopulmonary function and preoperative routine tests were carried out, with no obvious abnormalities found. The surgical method is laparoscopic transperitoneal total left adrenalectomy.

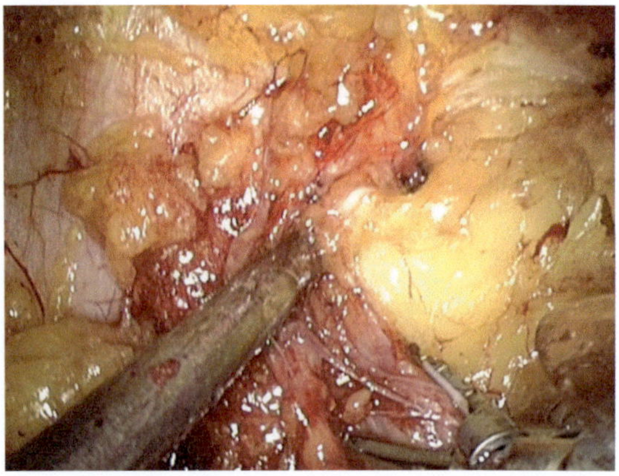

Fig. 3 Clean the fat and open the renal fascia

Surgical Process

1. The surgical side is marked in the ward before the operation. Intubation anesthesia is used. A urinary catheter is placed.
2. The transperitoneal upper urinary tract surgical approach is used, and this operation uses three holes (2 cm above the midaxillary line, below the rib edge of the anterior axillary line, and below the rib edge of the posterior axillary line).
3. After cleaning the extraperitoneal fat and recognizing the peritoneal fold, the renal fascia is opened on the back side of the peritoneal fold, revealing the perirenal fat capsule (Fig. 3).
4. Dissect the perirenal fat, expose the kidney, and separate upward along the renal fascia to expose the upper pole of the kidney (Fig. 4).
5. Carefully search for adrenal tissue in the fatty tissue of the upper pole of the kidney (Fig. 5).

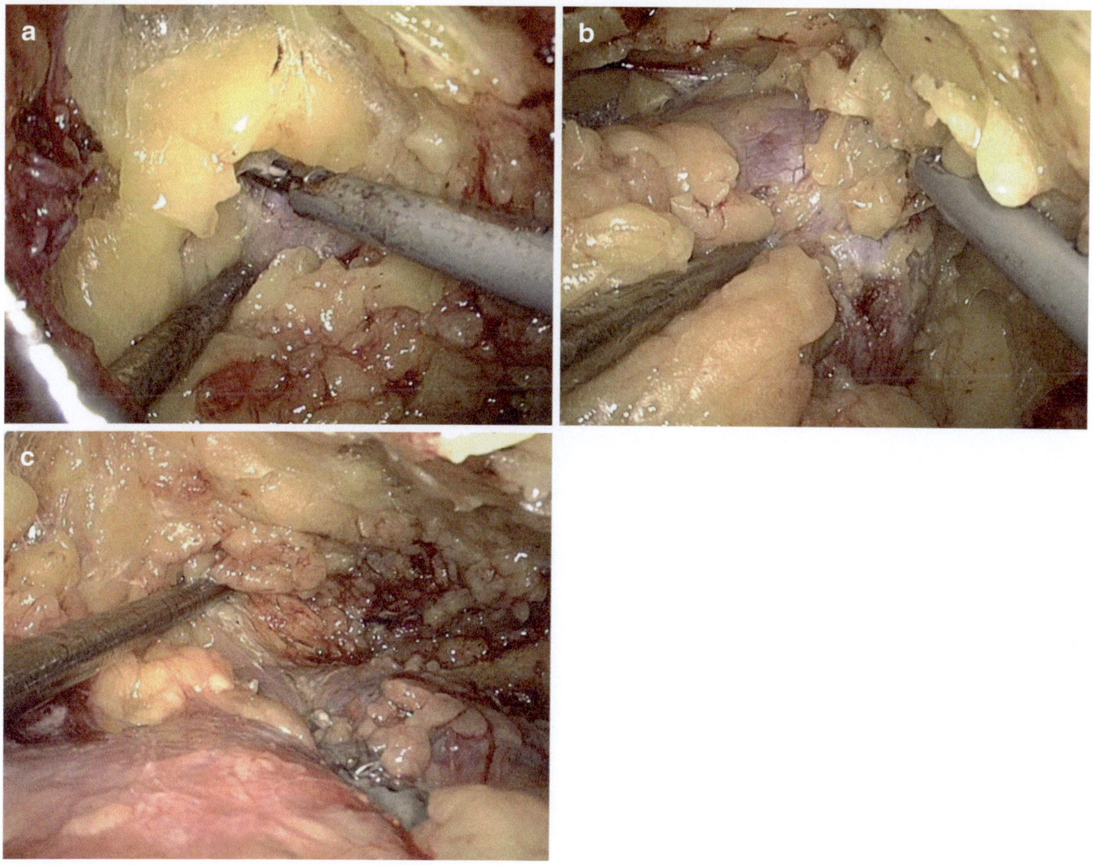

Fig. 4 (**a–c**) Locate the kidney and separate along the ventral side of the kidney

6. Dissect the adrenal gland along the upper pole of the kidney, and clamp and cut off the central vein of the adrenal gland with a Hem-o-lok (Fig. 6).
7. Continue to free the remaining surface of the adrenal gland until the left adrenal gland is completely removed (Fig. 7).
8. Carefully check the surgical area and stop the bleeding carefully (Fig. 8).
9. The specimen is completely removed, a drainage tube is placed, and the operation is over.

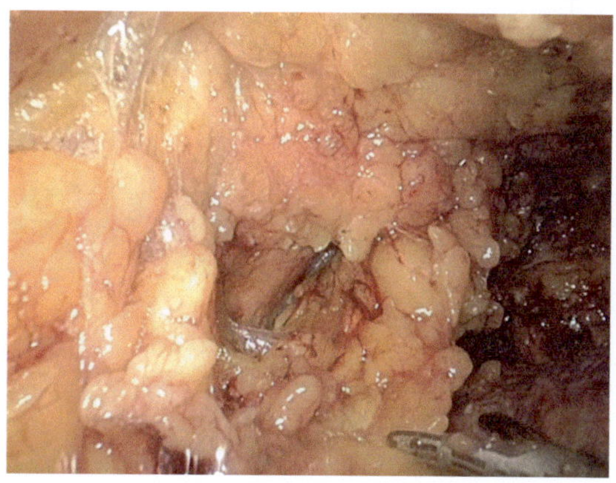

Fig. 5 Separate the upper pole of the kidney and locate the adrenal tumor

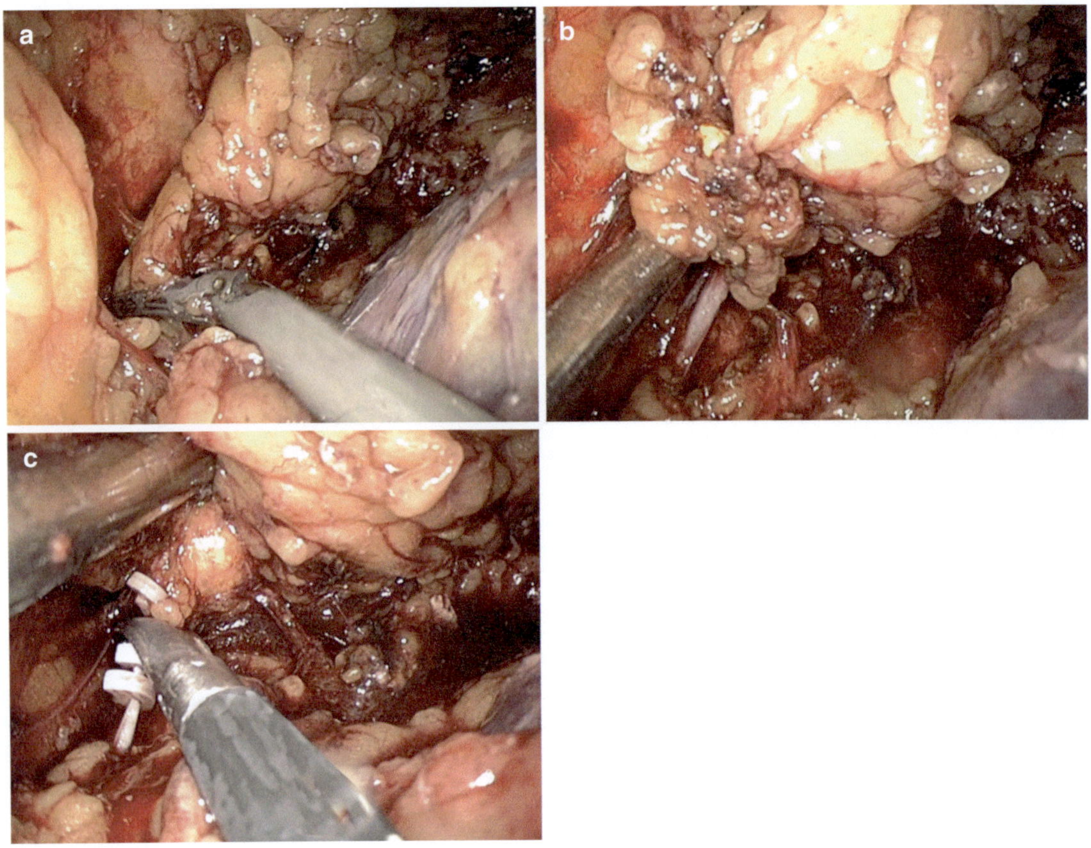

Fig. 6 (**a**–**c**) Dissect the adrenal gland and deal with the central vein

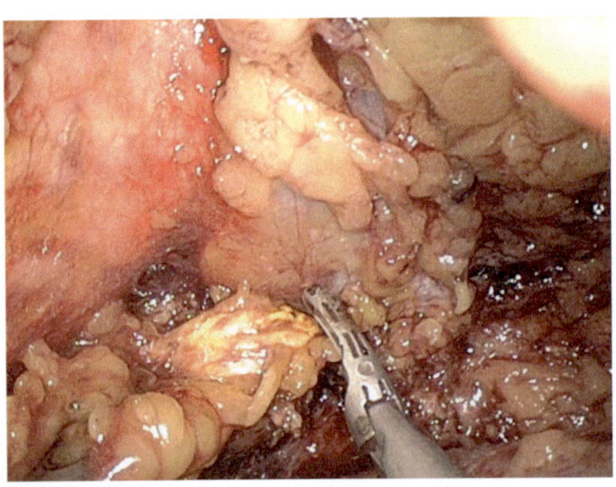

Fig. 7 Completely remove the adrenal gland

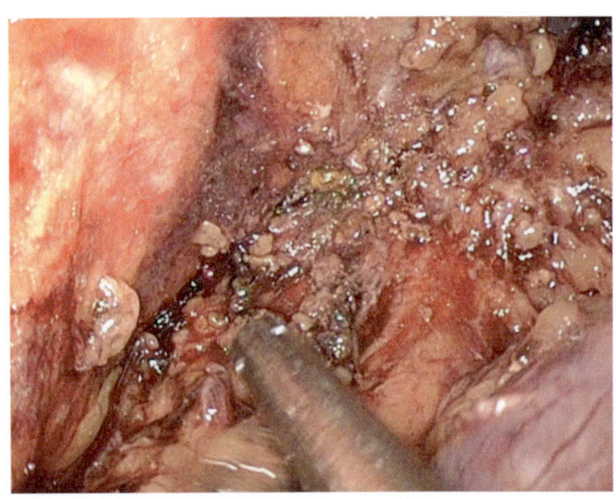

Fig. 8 Hemostasis of the surgical wound

Expert Review

1. Adhesion in the surgical area: The patient underwent a left adrenal tumor removal surgery 11 years ago, and this surgery is a second operation after the recurrence of the adrenal tumor. Adhesion in the surgical area is the main difficulty of this operation, which makes it difficult to locate the adrenal gland and increases the risk of damaging the kidney, pancreas, and other tissues. The risk of damaging large blood vessels and important organs in adrenal surgery through the retroperitoneal approach is relatively small, but careful dissection, proper hemostasis in the surgical area, and careful identification of adrenal structures should still be observed to avoid damaging the pancreas and other adjacent organs.
2. Choice of surgical method for adrenal tumors: A simple adrenal tumor removal can be performed, preserving part of the normal adrenal gland, or a total adrenalectomy can be performed. Some researchers have advocated for a total adrenalectomy on the affected side to avoid a second operation, but clinical studies have shown that the recurrence rate of tumors is not high after preserving part of the normal adrenal tissue. The specific surgical method should be chosen based on the tumor's location, size, the relationship between the central vein of the adrenal gland and the tumor, whether there are suspicious changes in the adrenal gland on the opposite side, the patient's age, general condition, and other factors. The choice of surgical method for adrenal tumors should consider the benefits of preserving the adrenal gland and the risk of tumor recurrence.

Adrenal Surgery: Case 6 Laparoscopic Retroperitoneal Bilateral Total Adrenalectomy—Target Gland Removal Surgery for Ectopic ACTH Tumor

Yi Zhao

Chief Complaint

Face becoming round and red, high blood pressure discovered for over a year.

Medical History

Male, 39 years old. In January 2019, the patient's face became round and red, with swelling under both jaws; high blood pressure was measured, with the highest blood pressure being 170/110 mmHg. No headache or dizziness. Later, symptoms such as "chest bone fracture," edema in both lower limbs, acne on the head, neck, and chest, purple striae on the inner thighs, and decreased libido appeared. No treatment was sought during this period. In September 2019, the above symptoms worsened, accompanied by dry mouth, polydipsia, fatigue, and increased appetite. ACTH 258 pg/ml and 24-h UFC 1778 nmol were found at an outside hospital. Both large and small doses of dexamethasone suppression tests were not suppressed. Adrenal CT: bilateral adrenal thickening (Fig. 1); PET-CT: slightly increased metabolic activity in the slightly thickened bilateral adrenal glands, suggesting possible hyperplasia; no obvious abnormalities were seen in the pituitary MRI. On November 7, 2019, the cortisol rhythm disappeared, ACTH (8 o'clock) 122.0 pg/ml; LDDST was not suppressed, and HDDST was not suppressed. IPSS+DDAVP stimulation test showed no obvious gradient. Pituitary MRI: an abnormal enhancement shadow of 8 mm × 4 mm on the right wing of the pituitary; pituitary microadenoma cannot be ruled out. No abnormalities were seen in the octreotide imaging. Ga-DOTATATE-PET-CT: A slightly high-density shadow can be seen on the right wing of the pituitary, and the radioactive uptake is slightly lower than normal pituitary tissue, bilateral adrenal thickening, highly suggestive of hyperplasia. Chest and abdominal enhanced CT: bilateral adrenal thickening. Ga-DOTA JR11PET-CT: No clear pituitary lesions or ectopic lesions were seen. Thoracic spine MRI: T11–12 and L2 pathological compression fracture of the vertebral body and osteoporosis of the lumbar vertebral body. The endocrinology team considered a definitive diagnosis of periodic Cushing's syndrome during their ward rounds, with no gradient in IPSS, a high likelihood of ectopic ACTH syndrome, and considered it consistent with the possibility of periodic Cushing's syndrome. Due to the difficulty in locating the lesion, bilateral adrenalectomy is planned to alleviate the state of hypercortisolism.

Supplementary Information The online version contains supplementary material available at https://doi.org/10.1007/978-981-96-8598-1_8.

Y. Zhao (✉)
Beijing Union Medical College Hospital,
Beijing, China

Y. Zhang, X. Zhao (eds.), *Laparoscopic Surgery in Urology*,
https://doi.org/10.1007/978-981-96-8598-1_8

Past History

Denies the use of exogenous glucocorticoids. History of hepatitis, presently cured.

Physical Examination

Centripetal obesity; purple striae can be seen on both axillae, inner thighs, and abdominal wall. Skin is slightly thin; supraclavicular fat pad; buffalo hump (+); face is round and red; scattered acne-like rash can be seen on the head, face, neck, chest, and back; and upper eyelid is red and swollen. Abdomen is distended.

Imaging Data (Fig. 1)

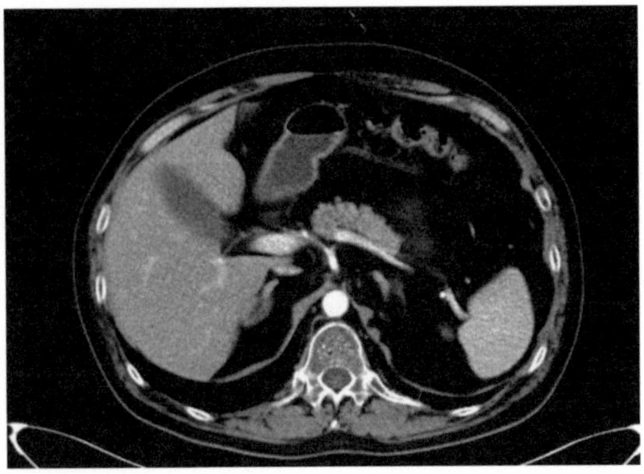

Fig. 1 Adrenal CT enhancement image

Preoperative Assessment

The patient's imaging examination suggests bilateral adrenal thickening. Combined with the patient's clinical data, the patient's present diagnosis of periodic Cushing's syndrome is confirmed. The patient's present general condition is stable, and the anesthesiology department assesses that the patient's cardiopulmonary function can tolerate surgery. After fully explaining the condition to the patient and family, it was decided to perform laparoscopic bilateral adrenalectomy.

Surgical Procedure

Left Adrenal Gland

1. The surgical approach is through the retroperitoneal space. The surgical side was marked in the ward before surgery. General anesthesia with endotracheal intubation was used. A urinary catheter was placed. Routine disinfection and draping.
2. Establish pneumoperitoneum. Use four holes (3 cm above the iliac crest on the midaxillary line, below the 12th rib on the posterior axillary line, below the 12th rib on the anterior axillary line, and between the first and third holes).

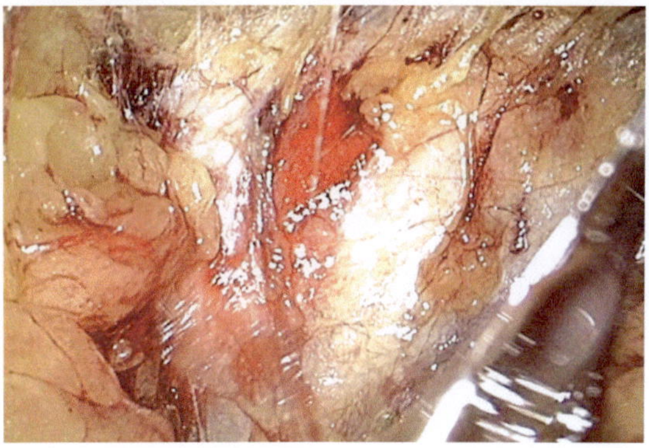

Fig. 2 Clean the extraperitoneal fat, and open the renal fascia

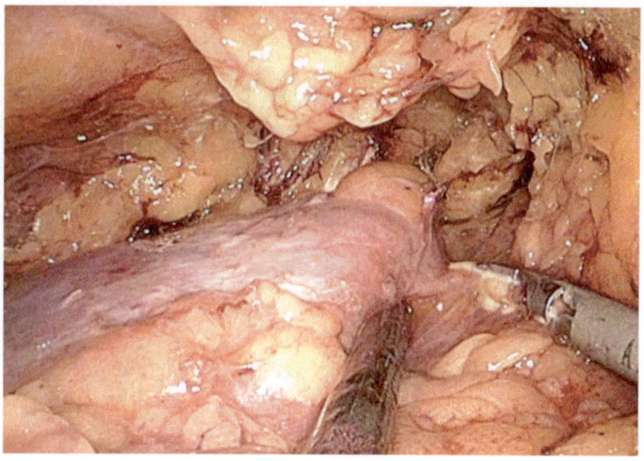

Fig. 4 Free the plane between the upper pole of the kidney and the adrenal gland

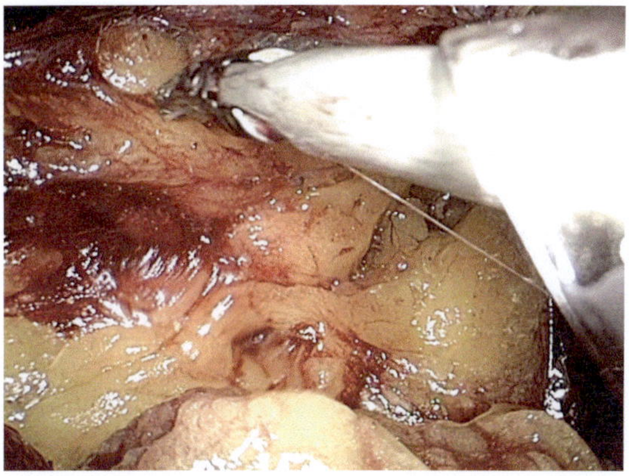

Fig. 3 Free the ventral side of the kidney, and expand the space

3. Clean the left extraperitoneal fat, and open the renal fascia longitudinally on the back of the peritoneal fold, revealing the psoas major muscle and perirenal fat pad (Fig. 2).
4. The left perirenal adhesion is relatively light, so it is loosened to further expand the retroperitoneal space (Fig. 3).
5. The upper pole of the left kidney is fully freed, and then the left adrenal gland is completely separated from the upper pole of the left kidney (Fig. 4).
6. Free the adrenal fat pad along the peritoneum, gradually revealing the back of the adrenal gland, which is a bloodless area of the adrenal gland that can be quickly separated by electrocautery. Lift the adrenal fat pad. Carefully free along the gap between the upper pole of the kidney and the adrenal fat pad. Gradually lift the left adrenal gland. There will be some small blood vessel branches here. Pay attention to reduce blunt separation. Try to separate by electrocoagulation. Carefully free and expose the adrenal tissue (Fig. 5).
7. Further expose the central vein of the left adrenal gland, fully free it, clamp it with Hem-o-lok, and cut it off (Fig. 6). Use an ultrasonic knife to cut off the blood supply around the adrenal gland until the left adrenal gland is completely removed (Fig. 7).
8. Carefully inspect the wound, stop the bleeding thoroughly, remove the excised adrenal gland specimen, leave a drainage tube, and close the incision.

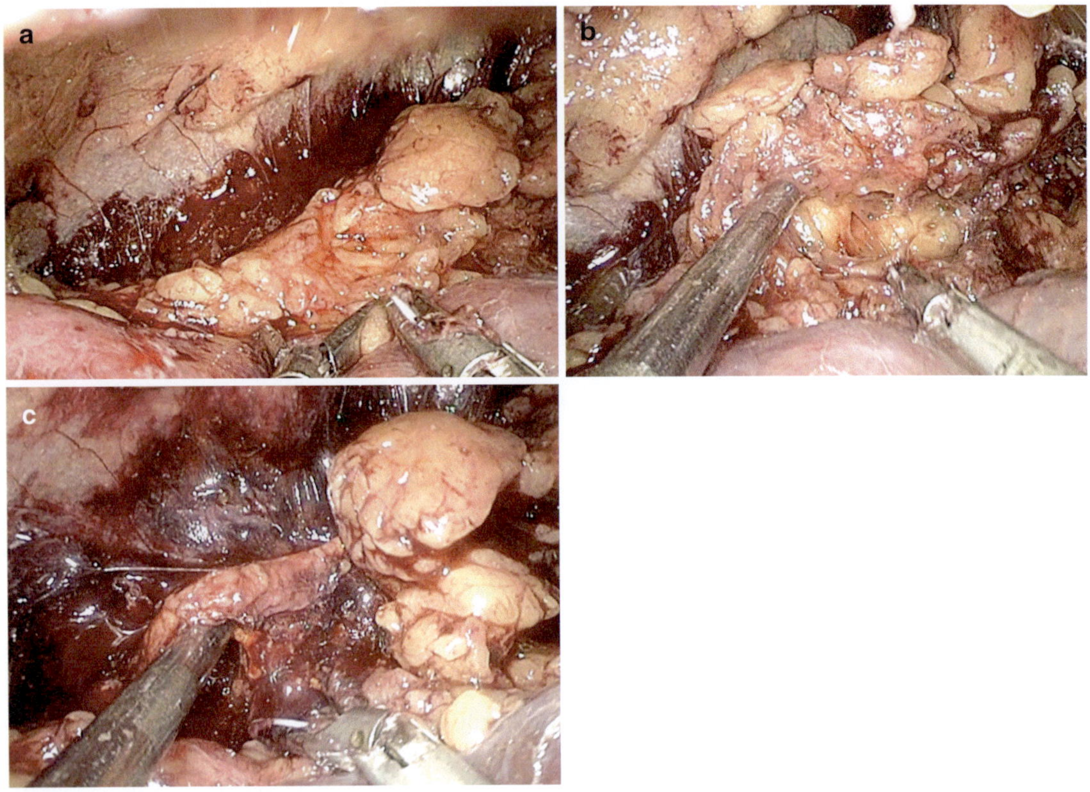

Fig. 5 (**a–c**) Various surfaces of the free adrenal gland

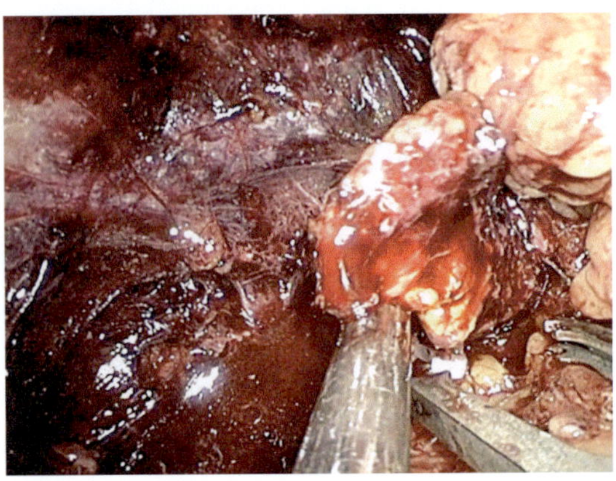

Fig. 6 Cutting off the central vein of the adrenal gland

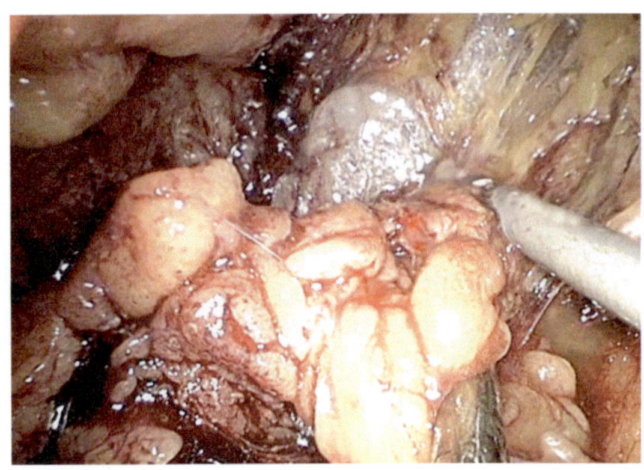

Fig. 7 Complete removal of the left adrenal gland

Surgical Procedure

Right Adrenal Gland

1. The surgical approach is through the retroperitoneal cavity. Routine disinfection and draping.
2. Establish pneumoperitoneum. Use four holes (3 cm above the iliac crest on the midaxillary line, below the 12th rib on the posterior axillary line, below the 12th rib on the anterior axillary line, and between the first and third holes).
3. Clean the right extraperitoneal fat, open the renal fascia longitudinally on the back side of the peritoneal fold, expose the perirenal fat capsule, and free the perirenal fat capsule to further expose the kidney (Fig. 8).
4. The right perirenal adhesion is relatively light, so it is loosened to further expand the retroperitoneal space (Fig. 9).
5. Fully free the upper pole of the right kidney, and then completely separate the right adrenal gland from the upper pole of the right kidney (Fig. 10). Free the right adrenal gland fat capsule along the peritoneum, gradually exposing the venous side of the lower cavity of the right adrenal gland (Fig. 11).
6. Slowly pull the right adrenal gland toward the head side, exposing the right central vein. Clamp and cut off with Hem-o-lok (Fig. 12).
7. Use an ultrasonic knife to cut off the blood supply around the adrenal gland until the right adrenal gland is completely removed (Fig. 13).
8. Carefully inspect the wound, stop the bleeding thoroughly, remove the excised adrenal gland specimen, leave a drainage tube, and close the incision.

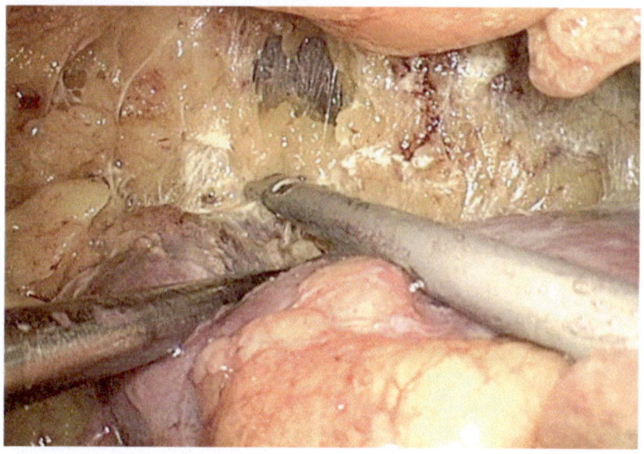

Fig. 9 Free along the kidney surface, and expand the space

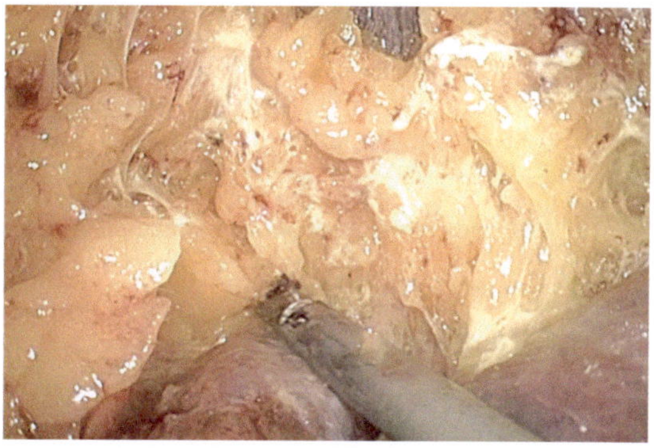

Fig. 10 Separate the adrenal gland from the kidney surface

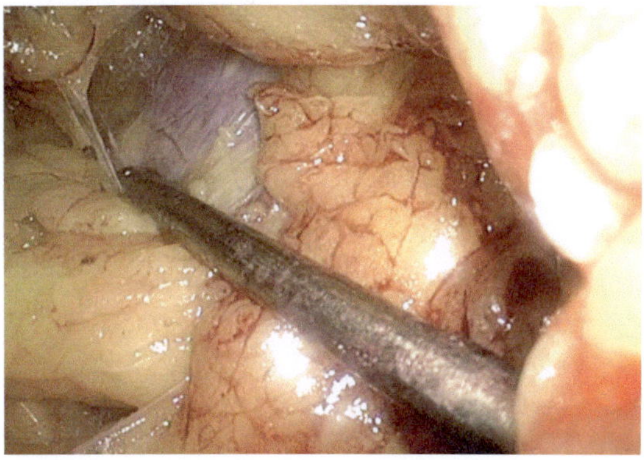

Fig. 8 Open the renal fascia, and free the perirenal fat capsule

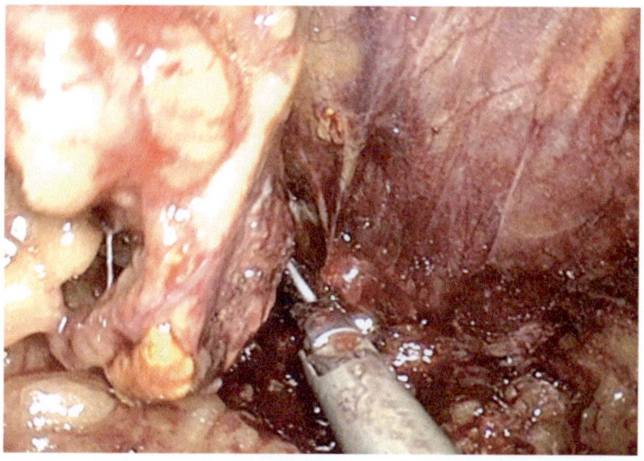

Fig. 11 Separate the adrenal gland along the ventral surface of the adrenal gland

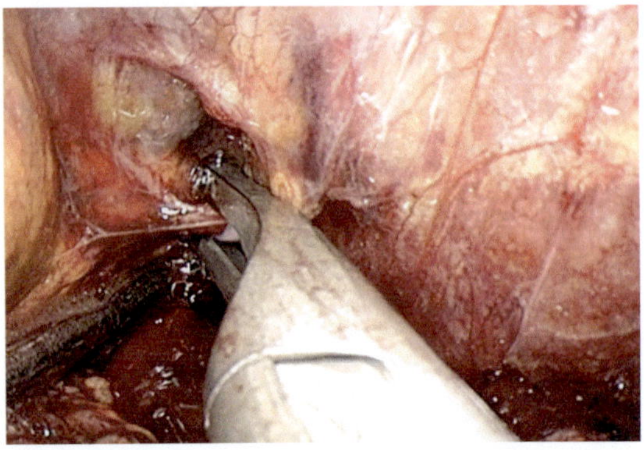

Fig. 12 Separate and cut off the central vein

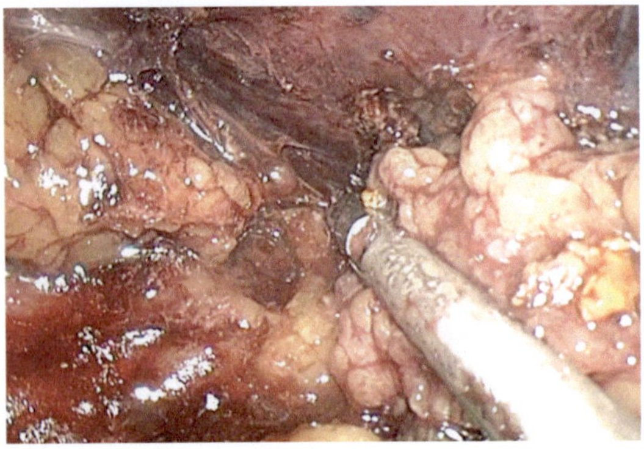

Fig. 13 Free and completely remove the adrenal gland

Expert Review

Choice of Surgical Approach for Patients with Cushing's Syndrome: For patients with Cushing's syndrome, the tissue structure is relatively "friable" and prone to bleeding, so the operation must be handled with extra care. In terms of the choice of surgical approach, especially for cases that require the removal of both adrenal glands, there are generally two options: the transabdominal approach and the retroperitoneal approach. The transabdominal approach can avoid the need to change the patient's position when removing the other adrenal gland, but because patients are generally overweight and the liver needs to be moved aside during the right-side removal, the operation is relatively difficult. It is recommended to perform the removal separately on both sides via the retroperitoneal approach.

Principles of Adrenal Central Vein Management: When dealing with the central veins of both adrenal glands, the anatomical position of the central vein must first be clarified. During the dissection of the ventral vascular area of the adrenal gland, dissection should be performed with hemostatic coagulation layer by layer until the central vein is exposed and then clamped with a Hem-o-lok. Special attention should be paid to the occasional variations of the central vein.

Adrenal Surgery: Case 7 Laparoscopic Retroperitoneal Left Pheochromocytoma Resection

Jingmin Zhou

Chief Complaint

Hypertension for 2 years, palpitations, chest tightness, and a mass in the left retroperitoneal space found 5 months ago. Female, 35 years old. The patient reported that her blood pressure was found to be high 2 years ago, reaching a maximum of 220/180 mmHg, accompanied by excessive sweating, occasional dizziness, headaches, and palpitations but no fever, no cold extremities, and no fatigue. The patient was treated with oral medication for primary hypertension at a local hospital, but the blood pressure control was not satisfactory. In November 2020, the patient suddenly experienced palpitations and chest tightness without any obvious cause. She went to a local hospital for a checkup, and after completing CT, MRI, and other imaging examinations, a mass about 7 cm in size was found in the left retroperitoneal space, with uneven enhancement seen in the enhanced scan (Figs. 1, 2, and 3). The patient came to our outpatient clinic for further diagnosis and treatment and completed related endocrine tests, and 24-hour urinary catecholamines showed norepinephrine

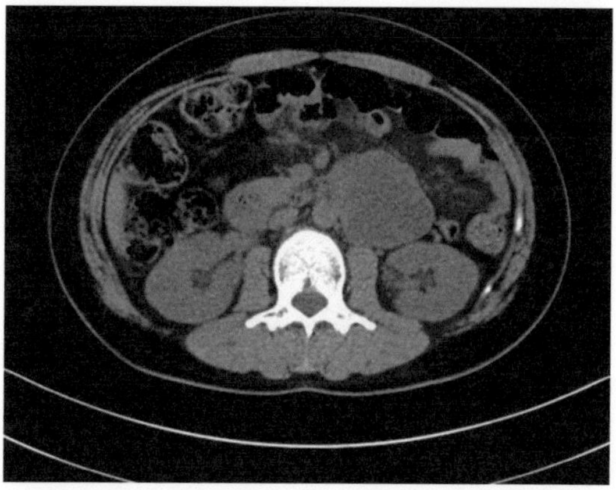

Fig. 1 Adrenal CT plain scan image (transverse section)

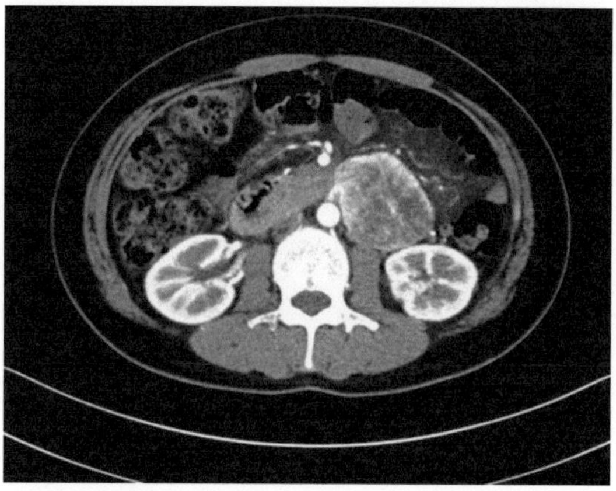

Fig. 2 Adrenal CT-enhanced image (transverse section)

Supplementary Information The online version contains supplementary material available at https://doi.org/10.1007/978-981-96-8598-1_9.

J. Zhou (✉)
Beijing Union Medical College Hospital,
Beijing, China
e-mail: zhoujm@pumch.cn

Y. Zhang, X. Zhao (eds.), *Laparoscopic Surgery in Urology*,
https://doi.org/10.1007/978-981-96-8598-1_9

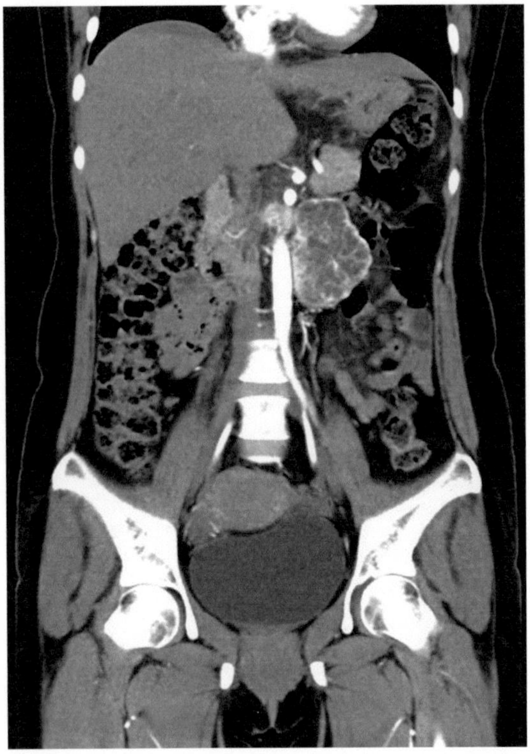

Fig. 3 Adrenal CT-enhanced image (coronal section)

(NE) 2113.15 μg/24 h, epinephrine (E) 26.10 μg/24 h, dopamine (DA) 580.08 μg/24 h; normetanephrine (NMN) 58.54 nmol/L. Considering the high possibility of pheochromocytoma, the patient was started on oral phenoxybenzamine 30 mg q 8 h at the end of November 2020. During the medication period, the patient's general condition was good, and her blood pressure and heart rate were well controlled.

Past History

Type 2 diabetes for 2 years, presently subcutaneously injecting insulin glargine, with good blood sugar control; underwent cesarean section in 2019.

Physical Examination

No special findings in the heart and lungs, cesarean section scar visible on the lower abdomen.

Imaging Data (Figs. 1, 2, and 3)

Preoperative Assessment

The patient's imaging examination suggested a left adrenal mass, approximately 7 cm × 6 cm in size, with significant enhancement. Combined with the patient's clinical symptoms of hypertension and palpitations, as well as endocrine examination, 24-h urinary catecholamine NE, E, and DA and NMN levels were significantly elevated, suggesting a clear diagnosis of left adrenal pheochromocytoma, with clear indications for surgery. Outpatient assessment of cardiopulmonary function showed no significant abnormalities, and there was no evidence of paraganglioma in other parts of the body. The patient has been taking phenobarbital for over 4 months, and preoperative medication preparation is sufficient. The plan is to perform surgery, specifically a laparoscopic left adrenal pheochromocytoma resection.

Surgical Procedure

1. The retroperitoneal upper urinary tract surgical position was adopted. The surgical side was marked in the ward before surgery. General anesthesia with endotracheal intubation was used. A urinary catheter was placed. Routine disinfection and draping were performed.
2. After establishing the retroperitoneal cavity, an upper urinary tract surgical pathway was placed. This surgery used four ports.
3. After cleaning the extraperitoneal fat and identifying the peritoneal fold, the Gerota's fascia was longitudinally opened on the dorsal side of the peritoneal fold, revealing the psoas major muscle and the perirenal fat capsule (Fig. 4).
4. At a position close to the peritoneum, the renal fat capsule was longitudinally opened, and the left kidney was fully freed (Fig. 5).
5. Continue to free the medial and deep parts of the upper pole of the kidney, gradually exposing the tumor, and the corresponding tumor capsule can be seen (Fig. 6).

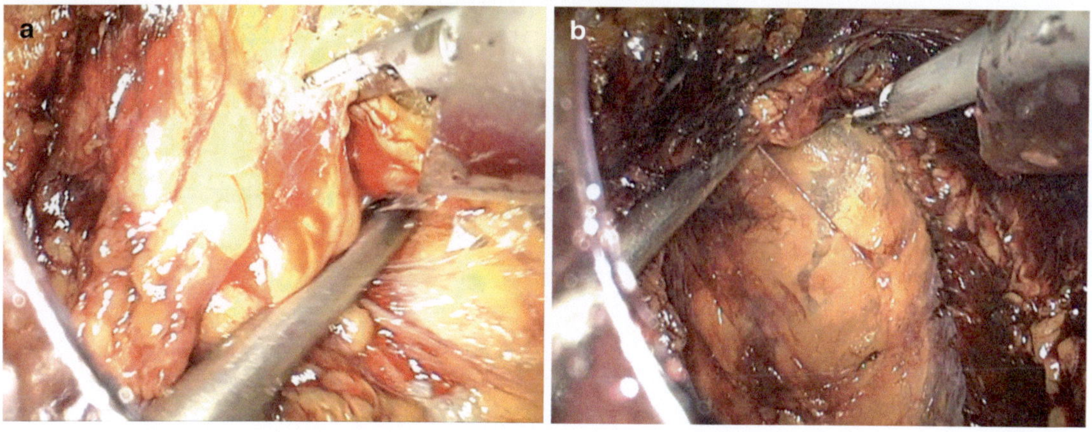

Fig. 4 (**a**, **b**) Cleaning the extraperitoneal fat, opening the renal fascia

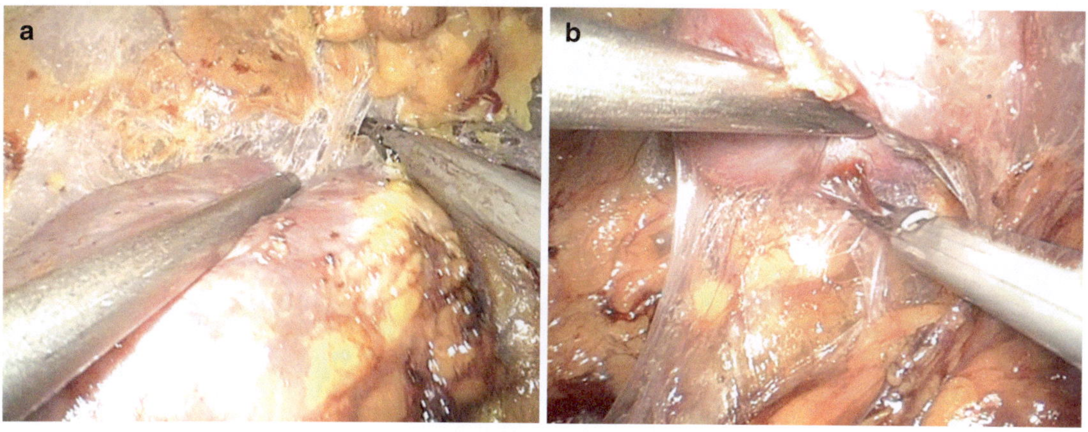

Fig. 5 (**a**, **b**) Opening the perirenal fat capsule, freeing the ventral side of the kidney upward

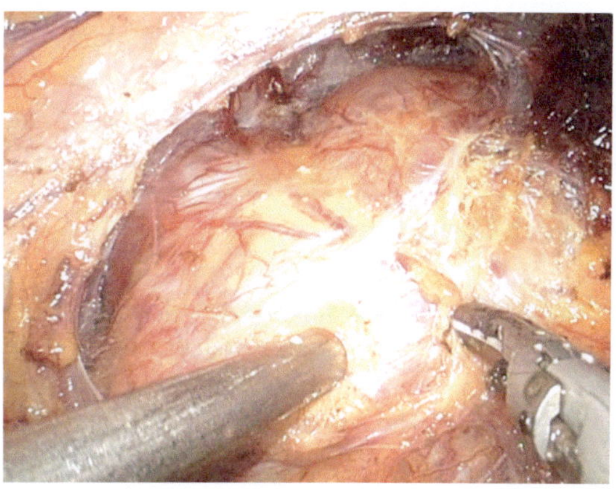

Fig. 6 Separating and locating the tumor

6. Close to the tumor capsule; the tumor was dissected using a combination of blunt and sharp techniques on its surface. There were fewer neovascularizations on the ventral side of the tumor, and the interface was generally clear (Fig. 7).
7. There were many supplying blood vessels and reflux veins on the tumor surface, which were carefully disconnected to reduce bleeding (Fig. 8).
8. There were many neovascularizations on the dorsal side of the tumor, which were clamped and disconnected with Hem-o-lok, and the tumor was gradually lifted (Fig. 9).
9. The upper pole of the tumor was separated, and the tumor was separated from the adrenal gland (Fig. 10).
10. Continue to fully free until the tumor is completely removed (Fig. 11).
11. After careful hemostasis, a specimen bag was placed through the auxiliary hole, and

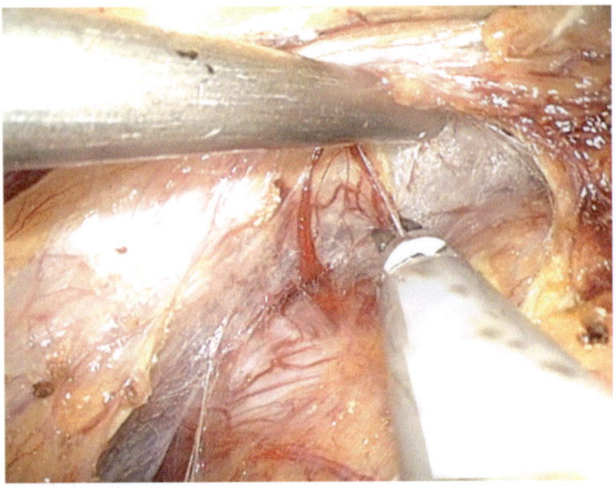

Fig. 7 Separating the tumor along the ventral side

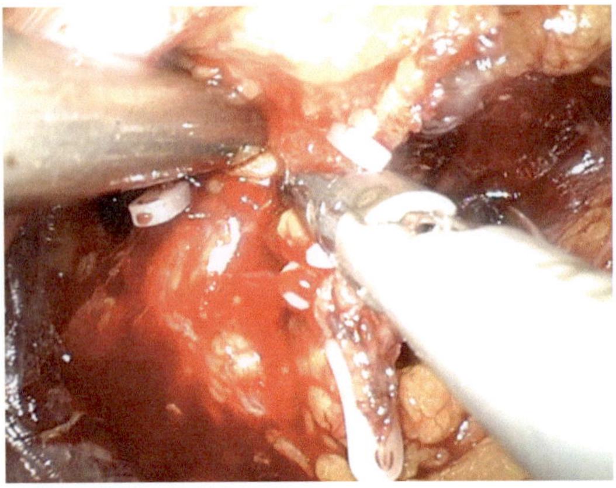

Fig. 8 Separating the tumor while hemostasis

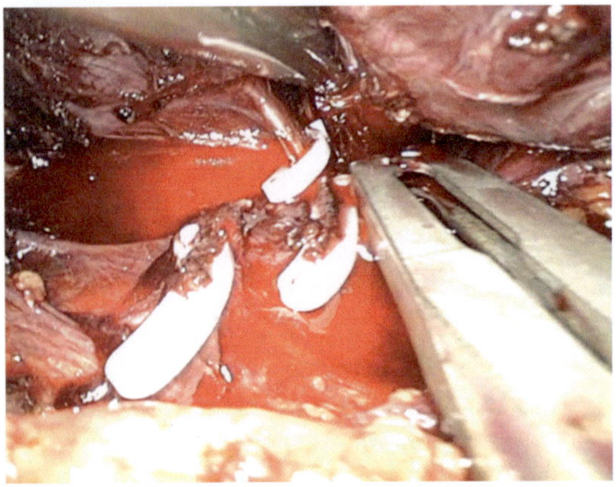

Fig. 9 Separating the dorsal side of the tumor

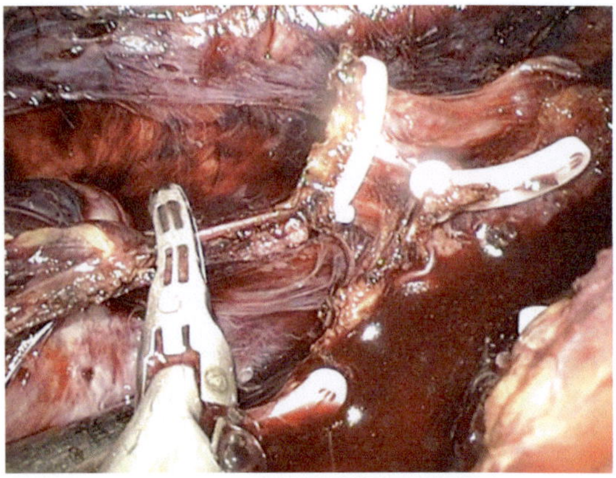

Fig. 10 Separating the upper pole of the tumor

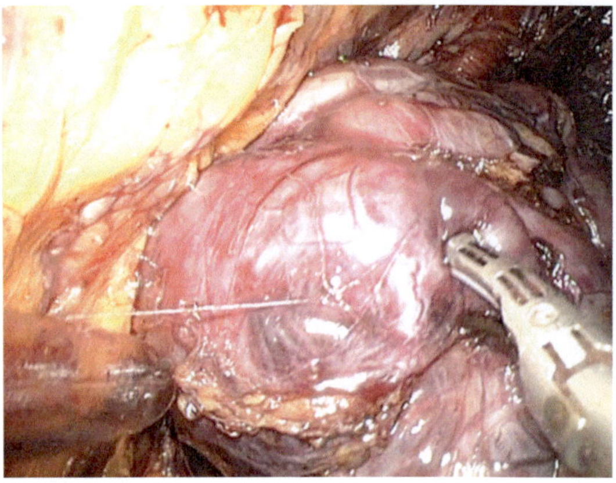

Fig. 11 Completely removing the tumor

the tumor was placed in the bag. A drainage tube was placed. Finally, after enlarging the auxiliary hole incision, the specimen was completely removed.

Expert Comments

Choice of Surgical Approach: Laparoscopic adrenalectomy for pheochromocytoma can be performed via the transperitoneal or retroperitoneal approach. The choice should be based on the surgeon's preference, tumor location, tumor size, left or right side, and the relationship with surrounding organs and blood vessels. The transperitoneal approach provides a more spacious operating field and more anatomical landmarks, making it more convenient and safer for beginners. For those who are proficient in laparoscopic surgery, or those with less experience in the transperitoneal approach, the retroperitoneal approach for pheochromocytoma removal is also feasible. The advantages of the retroperitoneal approach include avoiding interference from the intestines, less influence from surrounding organs, and simpler anatomical structure.

Adequate Mobilization of the Kidney: In the retroperitoneal approach, adequate mobilization of the kidney plays an important role in the removal of pheochromocytoma, especially for larger tumors. After the kidney is fully mobilized, there is better space and surgical field for tumor exposure, separation, and ligation of neovascularization, as well as hemostasis after local bleeding. Adequate mobilization of the kidney is an important step in the removal of pheochromocytoma.

Blood Supply of Pheochromocytoma: Pheochromocytomas generally have a rich blood supply, with many and varied neovascularization, especially on the dorsal side and the lower pole of the tumor. During surgery, careful dissection is required, and most of the slightly thicker blood vessels should be clamped and cut off with Hem-o-lok. Minor local bleeding should not be overly concerned, as pheochromocytomas often bleed more locally during removal, and local bleeding naturally decreases after the entire tumor is removed.

Preservation of the Adrenal Gland: Whether to preserve the adrenal gland in adrenal pheochromocytoma should be determined based on preoperative imaging and intraoperative anatomy of the adrenal gland. If the adrenal gland is small and difficult to separate from the tumor, it can be removed together; if the tumor is small, relatively lightly adhered, or bilateral, the adrenal tissue should be preserved as much as possible.

Adrenal Surgery: Case 8 Laparoscopic Transperitoneal Right Paraganglioma Resection

Xin Zhao

Chief Complaint

Intermittent palpitations, chest pain, high blood pressure for 4 months, and a retroperitoneal tumor found for over 2 months.

Medical History

Female, 40 years old. The patient experienced palpitations and chest pain after fatigue in March 2022, with no headache or excessive sweating. She was treated at a community hospital where an ECG showed sinus tachycardia, heart rate > 120 beats/min, and blood pressure > 150/100 mmHg. After taking metoprolol, her blood pressure returned to normal, heart rate was 110 beats/min, and symptoms of palpitations and chest pain were relieved. Further examination at Fuwai Hospital of the Chinese Academy of Medical Sciences showed elevated blood catecholamines, NE 2.092 ng/ml (normal value <0.548) and NMN 0.886 ng/ml (normal value 0.01–0.168), and urine catecholamines, NMN 3291.02 μg/24 h (normal value 28–615). A CTA of the abdomen in May 2022 showed a mass near the right renal hilum, approximately 40 mm × 42 mm in size, with uneven enhancement and necrotic cystic changes inside, suggesting a high possibility of paraganglioma. In June 2022, she was treated in our hospital's endocrinology department, blood MN 0.11 nmol/L, NMN 8.16 nmol/L, 24-h urinary catecholamines: NE 756.8 μg/24 h. CTU suggests a cystic and solid mass in the retroperitoneal space and right side of the inferior vena cava, approximately 4.4 cm × 4.2 cm × 5.0 cm in size, with significantly uneven enhancement at the edges and non-enhancing cystic necrosis in the center, considering the possibility of a paraganglioma (Figs. 1, 2, 3, and 4). Octreotide, MIBG, and PET-CT all suggest a high likelihood of paraganglioma. The patient denies numbness and weak-

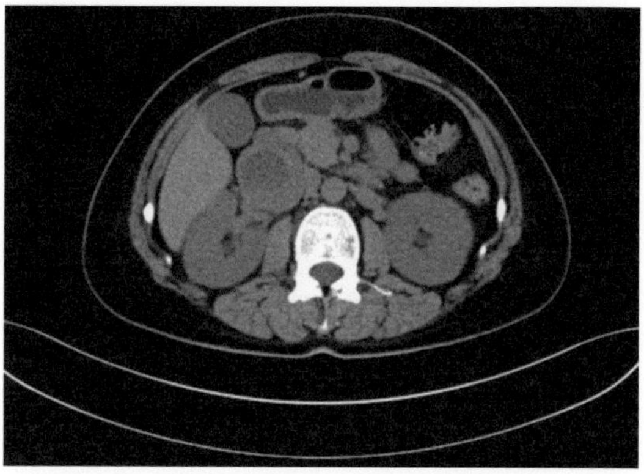

Fig. 1 Abdominal CT imaging (non-contrast)

Supplementary Information The online version contains supplementary material available at https://doi.org/10.1007/978-981-96-8598-1_10.

X. Zhao (✉)
Beijing Union Medical College Hospital,
Beijing, China

Y. Zhang, X. Zhao (eds.), *Laparoscopic Surgery in Urology*,
https://doi.org/10.1007/978-981-96-8598-1_10

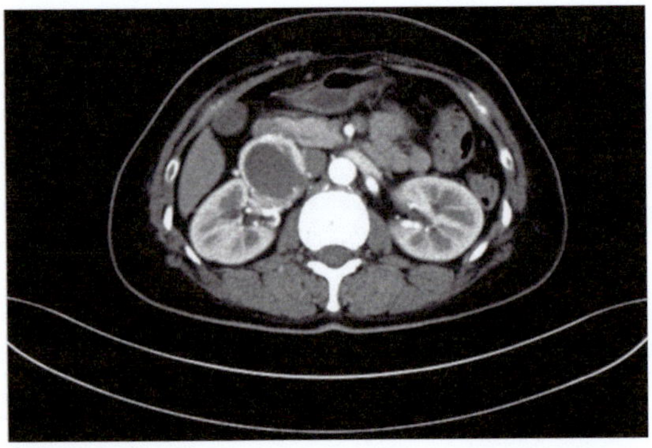

Fig. 2 Abdominal CT imaging (contrast-enhanced)

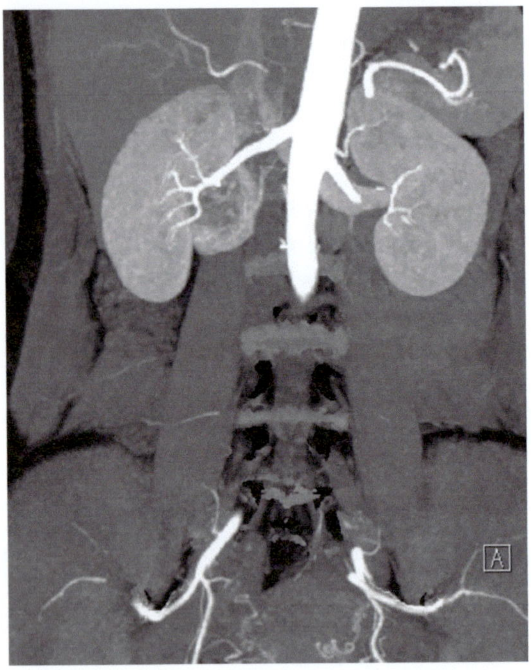

Fig. 3 Abdominal CT imaging (reconstructed)

ness in the limbs, moon face, central obesity, and abdominal striae. Considering the overall diagnosis, there is a high possibility of paraganglioma, and surgical treatment is recommended. The patient is prepared for surgery with oral phenoxybenzamine: 7.5 mg tid (2022-6-10) → 10 mg tid (2022-6-20) → 15 mg + 15 mg + 10 mg (2022-7-1) → 15 mg tid (2022-7-8). Since taking the medication, the patient's weight has increased by approximately 1.5 kg, presently with mild nasal congestion and slightly cool and moist extremities. The patient is now admitted to our department for surgical treatment. The patient's recent

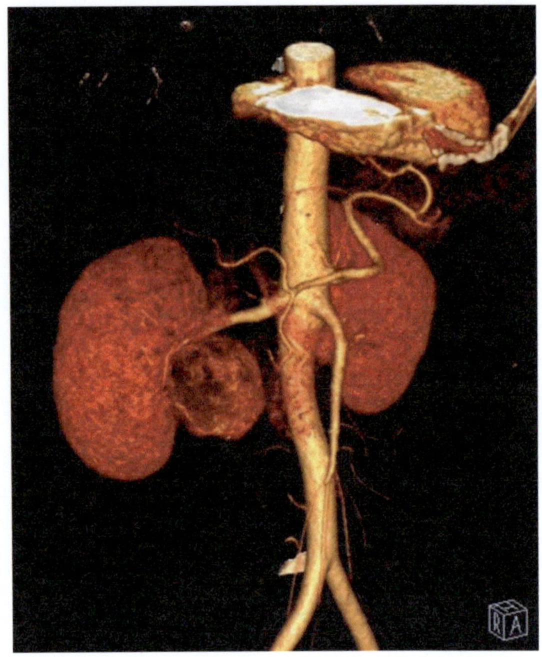

Fig. 4 Abdominal CT imaging (three-dimensional reconstruction)

mental state, sleep, and appetite are good, urination is normal, constipation is present, there is long-term use of lactulose to assist bowel movements, and weight has increased by approximately 1.5 kg in the past 2 months.

Past Medical History

Three years of thyroid nodules, 3 years of elevated platelets, 2 years of multiple uterine fibroids, 2 years of ovarian cysts, and 2 years of breast nodules with hyperplasia.

Physical Examination

Slightly cool and moist extremities. No other special abnormalities.

Preoperative Preparation

After admission, a complete preoperative assessment was performed; the patient had no paroxysmal symptoms, blood pressure was stable at

120/70 mmHg, heart rate was 70–90 beats/minute, and weight increased by 1.5 kg. Complete blood cell analysis: HCT 38.8%. No other special abnormalities. According to the patient's condition, a laparoscopic right paraganglioma resection was planned.

Surgical Procedure

1. Adopt the transabdominal upper urinary tract surgical position. The surgical side is marked in the ward before surgery. Intubation general anesthesia is used. A urinary catheter is placed. Routine disinfection and draping.
2. Semi-lateral position, right side at 45° to the horizontal plane. Establish a transabdominal upper urinary tract surgical channel. This operation uses five ports (0.5 cm above the navel, 4 cm below the 12th rib on the right anterior axillary line, 10 cm above the navel and 1 cm to the left, right clavicle midline 5 cm below the navel to the right, and 2 cm below the xiphoid process, respectively).
3. It was found that the right ascending colon was widely adherent to the right abdominal wall, which was carefully freed (Fig. 5).
4. Open the right peritoneum, free the ascending colon and duodenum downward, and use a needle holder to block the part of the right lobe of the liver covering the surgical area (Fig. 6).
5. The visible tumor is located below the right lobe of the liver; below the right kidney; on the lateral side of the vena cava, closely adhering to the surface of the vena cava; and in front of the right renal arteries and veins, tightly compressing the right renal arteries and veins. There is one tumor, measuring 5–8 cm in size, with abundant blood supply, intact capsule, and severe local adhesion (Fig. 7).

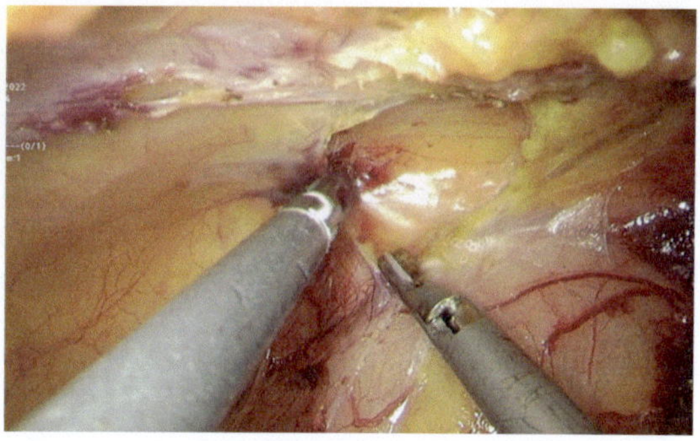

Fig. 5 Separation of the right colonic gutter

6. Open the mesentery along the surface of the tumor, taking care not to damage the mesenteric vessels (Fig. 8).
7. First, separate the base of the tumor and lift the tumor (Fig. 9). The tumor has a rich blood supply, with the surface densely covered with distended blood vessels. Adhere closely to the surface of the tumor; completely free the tumor; use Hem-o-lok to clamp multiple vessels originating from the abdominal aorta (Fig. 10); take care to protect the inferior vena cava, right renal arteries and veins, ascending colon, and duodenum; and completely remove the tumor (Fig. 11).
8. Completely remove the tumor. Place local hemostatic material. Leave a perirenal drainage tube. The operation is over. The gross

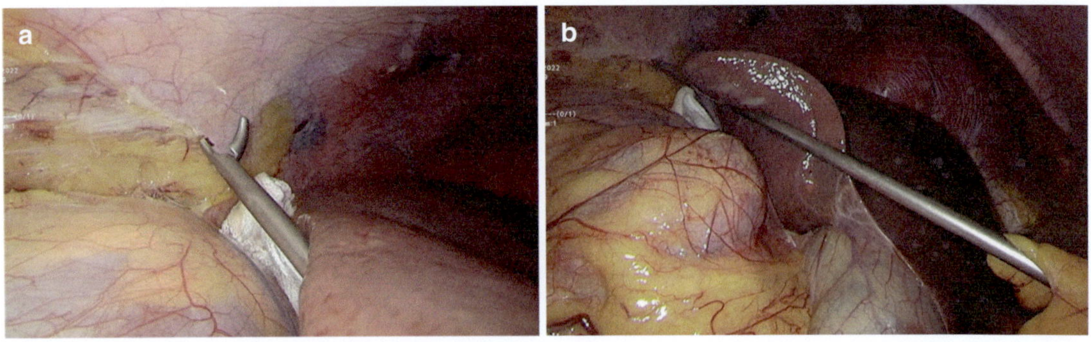

Fig. 6 (**a**, **b**) Open the right peritoneum, and retract the right liver lobe

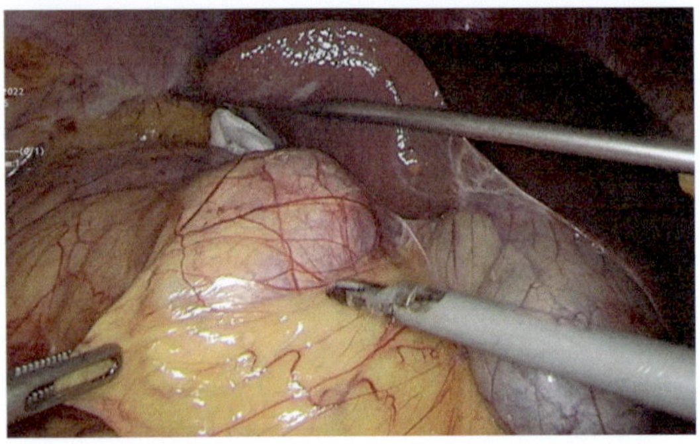

Fig. 7 Expose the tumor, and observe its overall shape

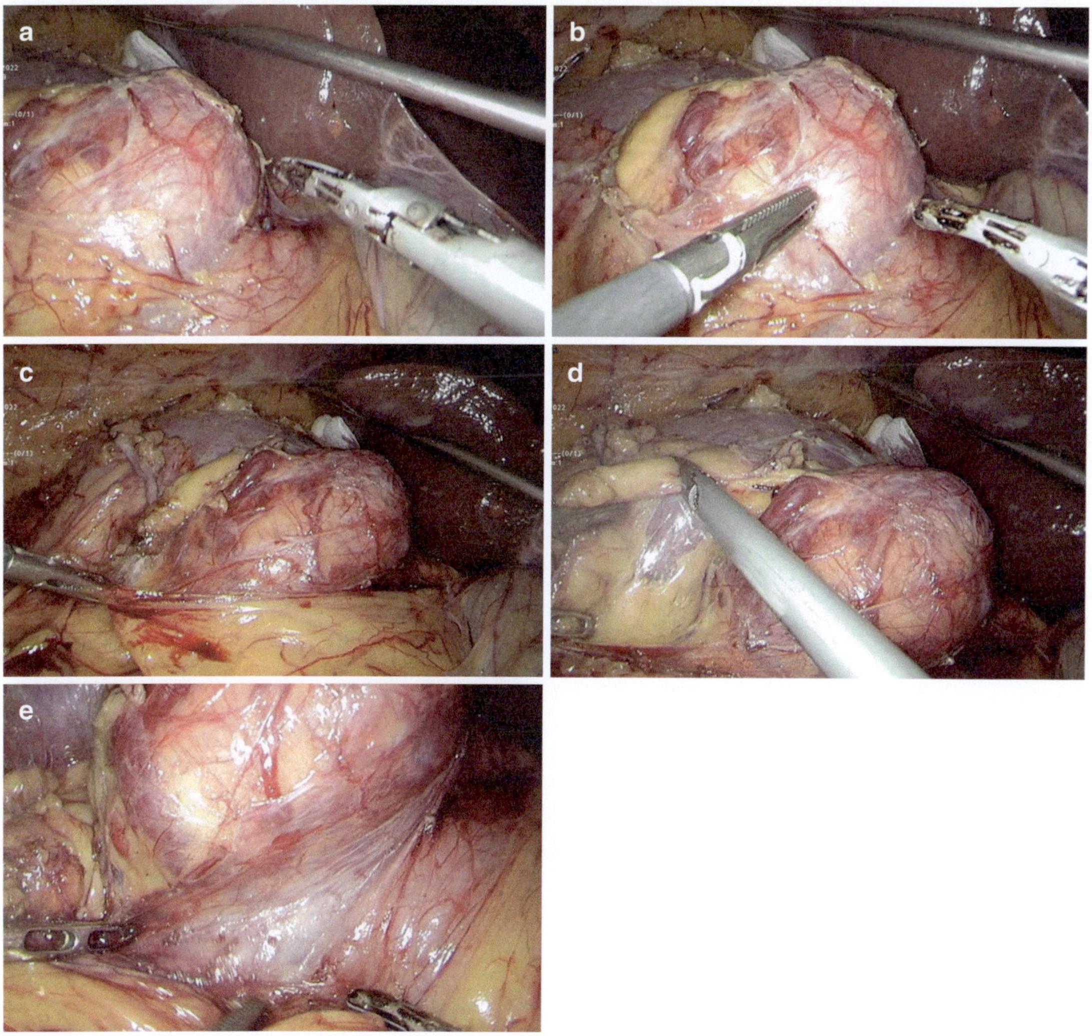

Fig. 8 (**a**–**e**) Open the mesentery on the surface of the tumor

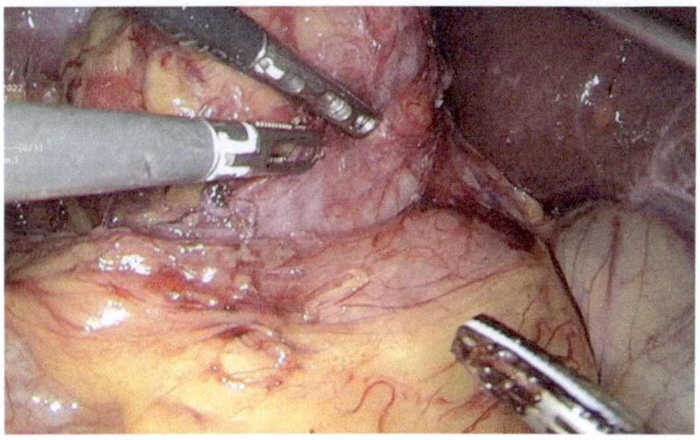

Fig. 9. Lift the base of the tumor

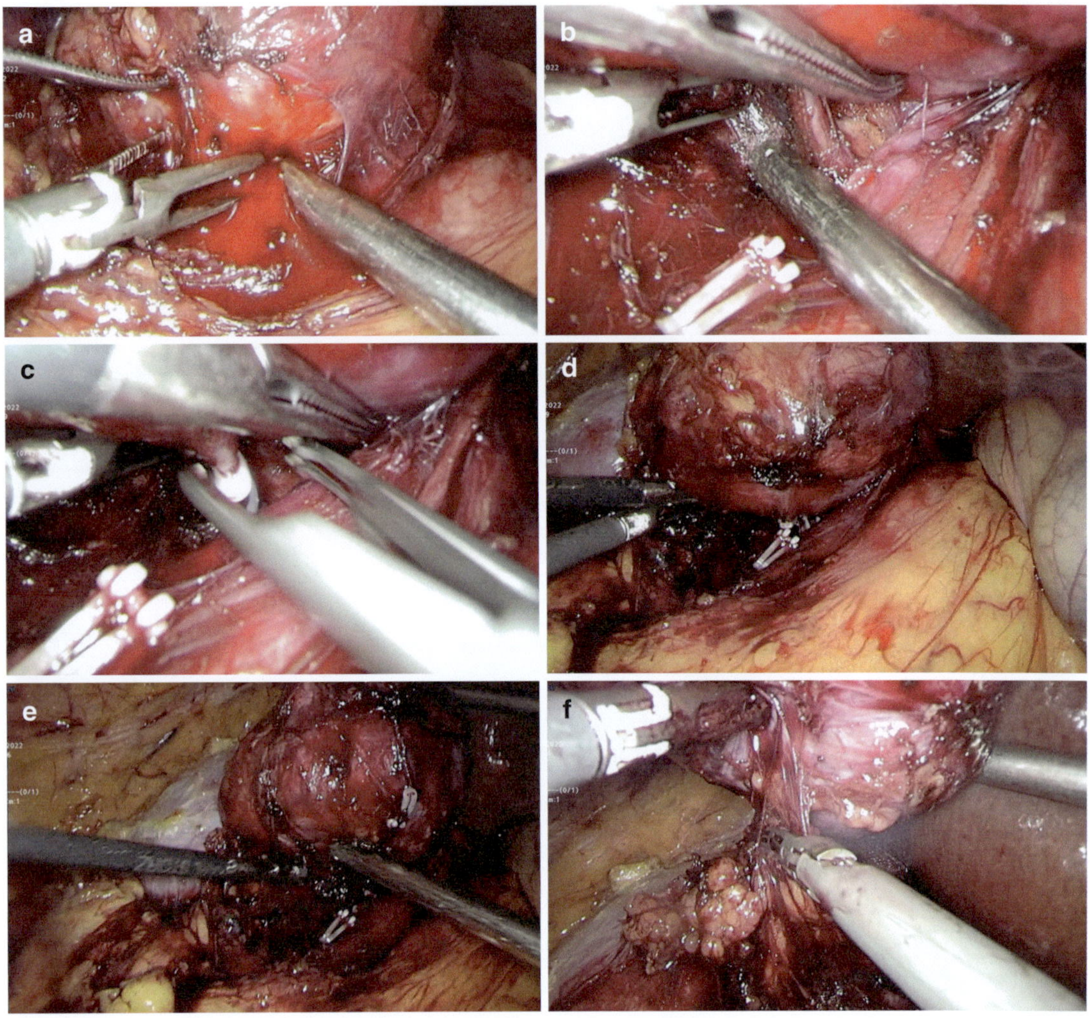

Fig. 10. (**a**–**f**) Separate and cut off the blood supply at the base of the tumor

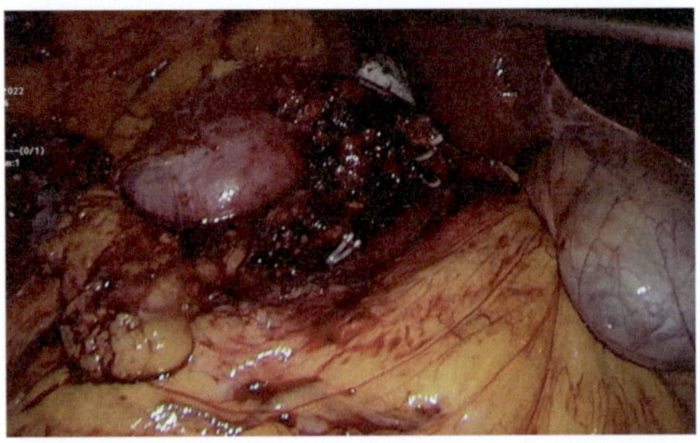

Fig. 11 Completely remove the tumor

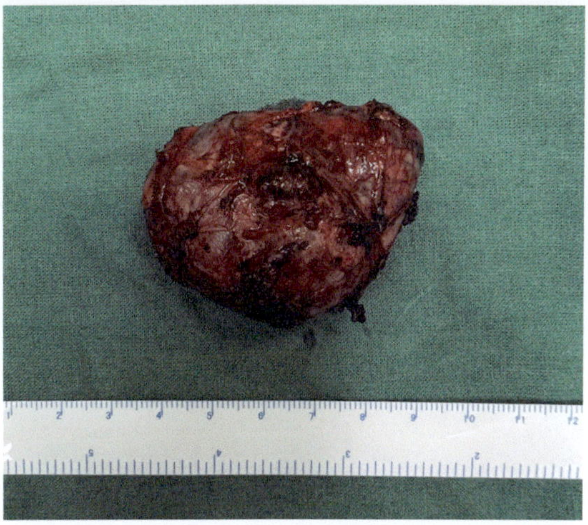

Fig. 12 Gross specimen of the tumor

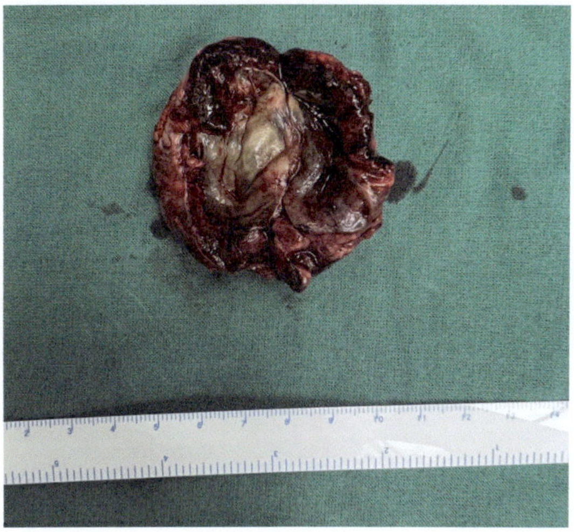

Fig. 13 Cross-sectional view of the gross tumor specimen

specimen of the tumor is shown in Figs. 12 and 13.

Expert Commentary

This case surgery allows us to understand the characteristics and treatment of paragangliomas. Paragangliomas have a rich blood supply, and adjacent blood vessels can supply blood to them. Blood vessels are often distributed on the surface of the tumor, and they are prone to damage and bleeding during separation. When handling during surgery, the tumor should be exposed first, and the position, size, and relationship with surrounding organs of the tumor should be observed. Then, carefully separate along the tumor, and clamp and cut off the blood supply while separating. Before cutting, you can use a separation clamp to clamp first, and then cut. If there is bleeding, you can use Hem-o-lok to clamp. Paragangliomas are mainly located within the distribution range of sympathetic ganglia. This tumor can release catecholamines, affecting the patient's cardiovascular system. Therefore, after a clear diagnosis, use phenoxybenzamine for preoperative preparation; wait for the patient's blood pressure and heart rate to stabilize, weight to increase, and microcirculation to dilate before performing surgical treatment.

Adrenal Surgery: Case 9 Laparoscopic Transperitoneal Radical Adrenalectomy for Right Adrenal Cortical Carcinoma (Central Venous Tumor Thrombus Treatment)

Xin Zhao

Chief Complaint

Right adrenal tumor found during physical examination for 3 months.

Medical History

Female, 54 years old. The patient went to a local hospital for abdominal pain 3 months ago. Enhanced CT showed a right adrenal tumor, about 3.4 cm × 2.5 cm, with uneven enhancement in the arterial phase and slightly reduced enhancement in the venous phase; irregular non-enhanced areas within the lesion (Fig. 1). Pain relief was achieved with analgesic and symptomatic treatment. The patient had no symptoms such as hypertension, periodic fatigue, moon face, headache, palpitations, etc. The patient came to our hospital for further diagnosis and treatment. PET-CT showed: a soft tissue density nodule in the right adrenal gland with increased metabolism (SUVmax 6.2), considered a malignant lesion; multiple nodules with increased metabolism in both lungs (SUVmax 4.5), all considered tumor metastases. Diagnosed with "right adrenal tumor, high possibility of adrenal cortical carcinoma, and high possibility of bilateral lung metastasis" and admitted to the hospital for further treatment.

Past History

Gallstones found 3 months ago.

Physical Examination

No special abnormalities were seen.

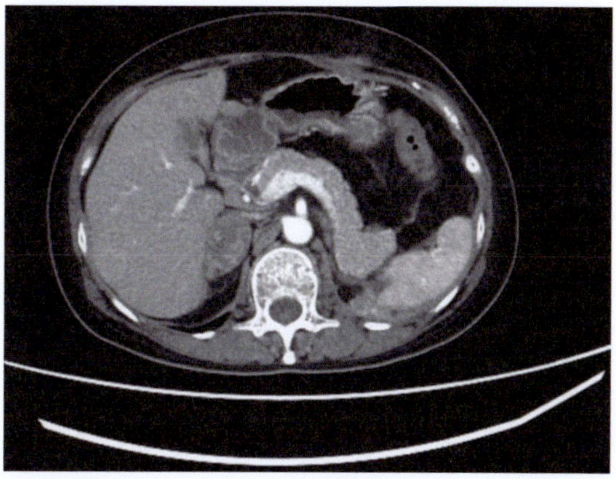

Fig. 1 Abdominal enhanced CT image

Supplementary Information The online version contains supplementary material available at https://doi.org/10.1007/978-981-96-8598-1_11.

X. Zhao (✉)
Beijing Union Medical College Hospital,
Beijing, China

Y. Zhang, X. Zhao (eds.), *Laparoscopic Surgery in Urology*,
https://doi.org/10.1007/978-981-96-8598-1_11

Preoperative Preparation

After admission, a complete preoperative assessment was performed; no special abnormalities were seen. According to the patient's condition, a transperitoneal total adrenalectomy of the right adrenal gland was planned. Preoperative film reading showed that the right adrenal tumor was closely related to the inferior vena cava, and the possibility of tumor thrombus could not be ruled out.

Surgical Procedure

1. Adopt the transperitoneal upper urinary tract surgical position. The surgical site was marked in the ward before surgery. General endotracheal anesthesia was used. A urinary catheter was placed. Routine disinfection and draping.
2. Establish the transperitoneal upper urinary tract surgical channel. This surgery used a four-port approach, and the exposure was clearer with the assistant's auxiliary traction.
3. Clean the retroperitoneal fat. The patient was thin, and care should be taken not to damage the peritoneum when cleaning the extraperitoneal fat (Fig. 2).
4. Open the perirenal fascia (Fig. 3).
5. The patient had less perirenal fat, so the approach was along the surface of the kidney (Fig. 4).

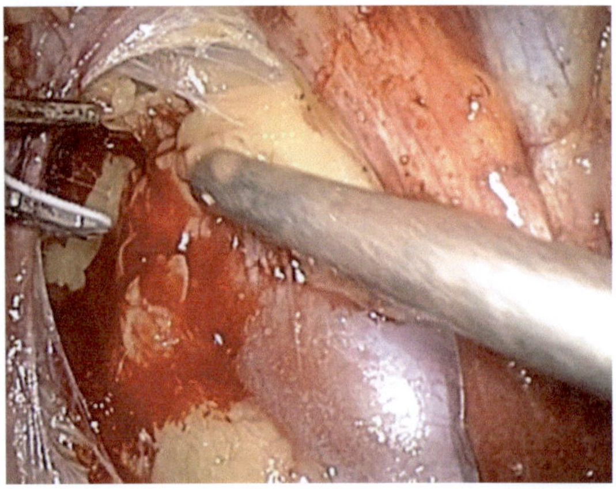

Fig. 3 Opening the perirenal fascia to expose the kidney

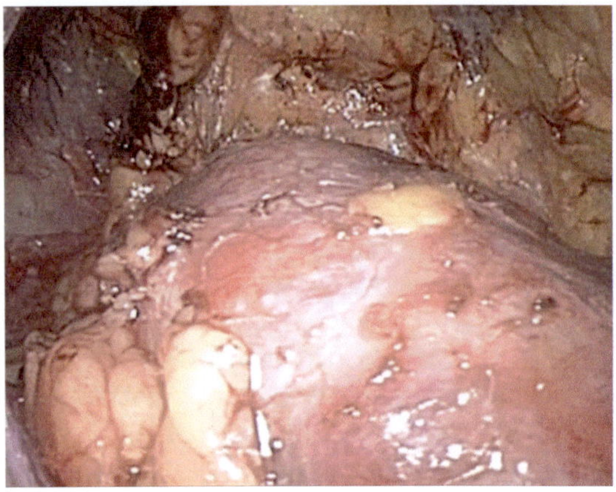

Fig. 4 Separating along the ventral side of the kidney toward the diaphragm

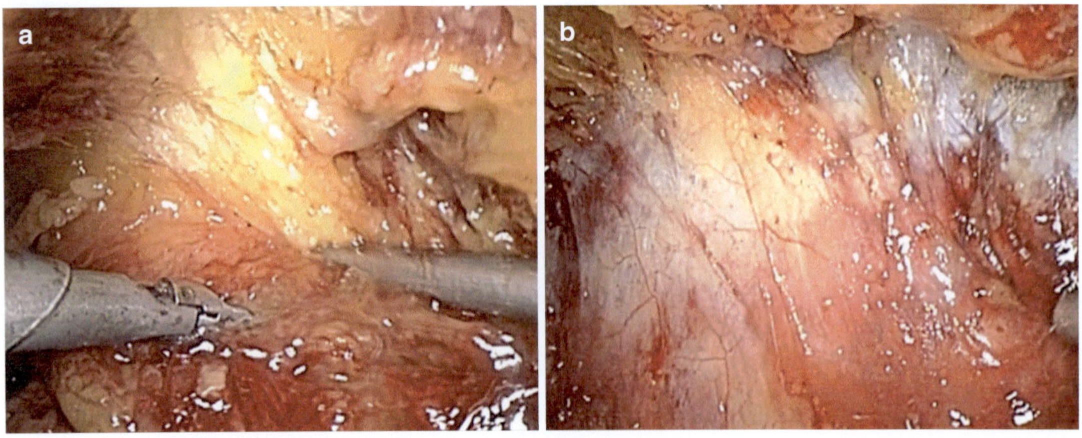

Fig. 2 (**a**, **b**) Cleaning the extraperitoneal fat

6. Along the surface of the kidney, free it upward to the base of the adrenal gland (Fig. 5).
7. Fully expose the right adrenal tissue. Use the reverse separation method: First, separate the base of the right adrenal gland, lift the adrenal gland, separate it upward in reverse, then separate the plane of the psoas major muscle, and lift the adrenal gland by pulling the peritoneum. Then separate the ventral side. This prevents the adrenal gland from sagging and affecting the operation. Remove the surrounding fat of the adrenal gland in one piece to achieve the R0 resection standard for cortical carcinoma (Fig. 6).

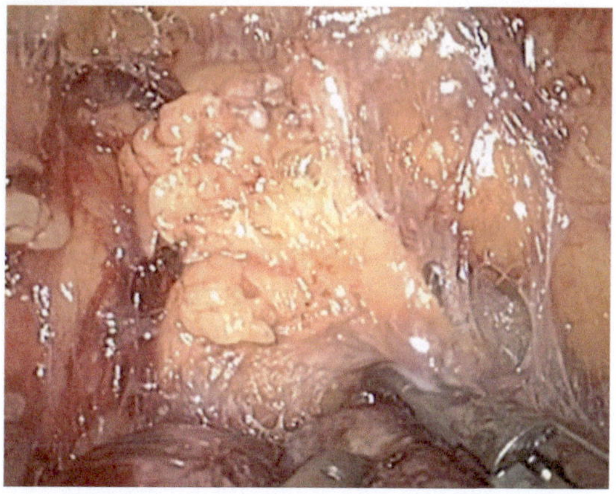

Fig. 5 Separating the kidney surface of the adrenal gland

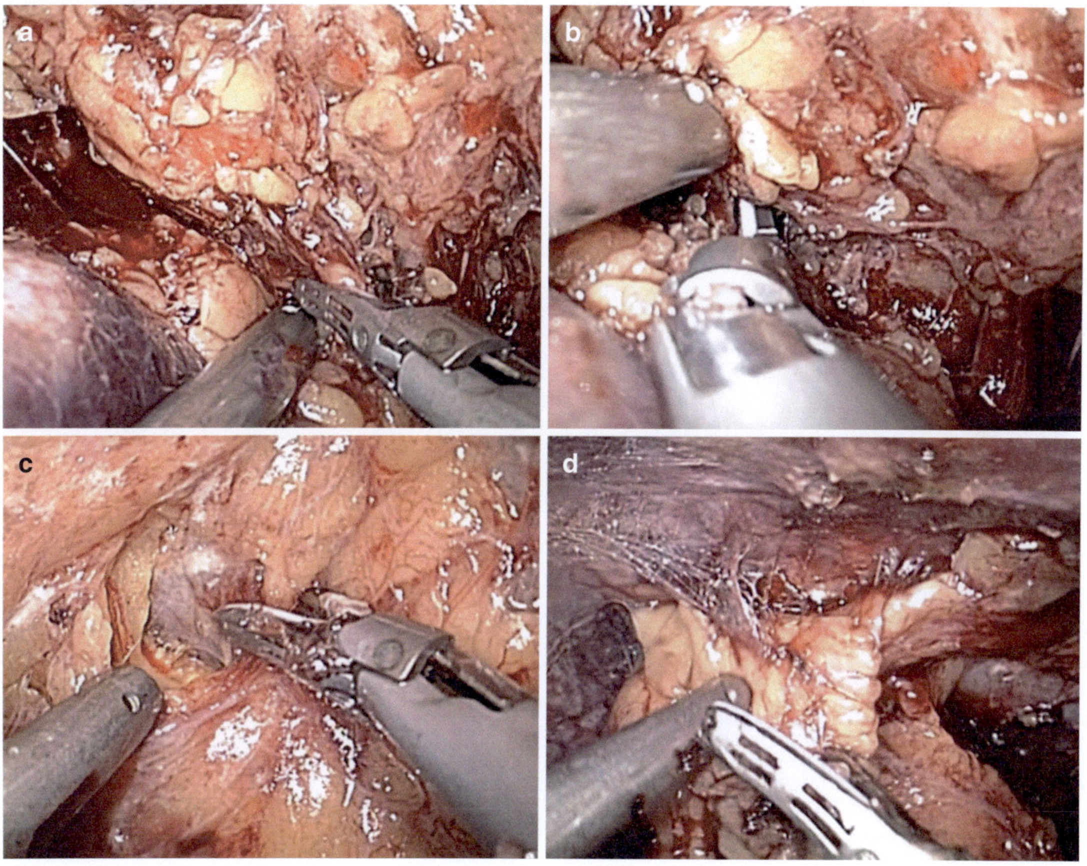

Fig. 6 (**a–d**) Separating adrenal tissue

8. Finally, separate the medial side of the right adrenal gland. Separate the central vein on the right side, pull the right adrenal gland laterally, and you can see solid material in the central vein, some of which is located in the inferior vena cava (Fig. 7).
9. Pull the right adrenal gland laterally, and use a curved hemostat to clamp the distal part of the tumor in the inferior vena cava. Pulling the right adrenal gland laterally, you can see the range of the tumor thrombus, and clamp the part of the inferior vena cava wall outside the tumor thrombus (Fig. 8). Remove part of the inferior vena cava wall, the right adrenal gland, and the tumor thrombus (Fig. 9).
10. Suture the inferior vena cava wall (Fig. 10).
11. Release the blockage and observe if there is active bleeding at the suture site (Fig. 11).
12. Completely remove the tumor (Fig. 12).
13. Place local hemostatic material and leave a perirenal drainage tube. The operation is completed.

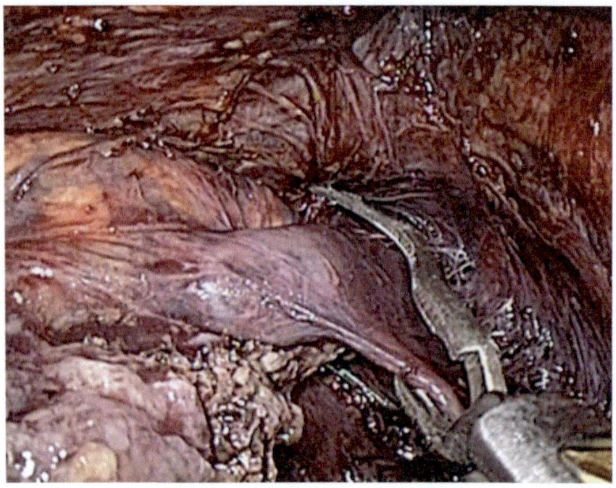

Fig. 8 Pulling and clamping the central vein

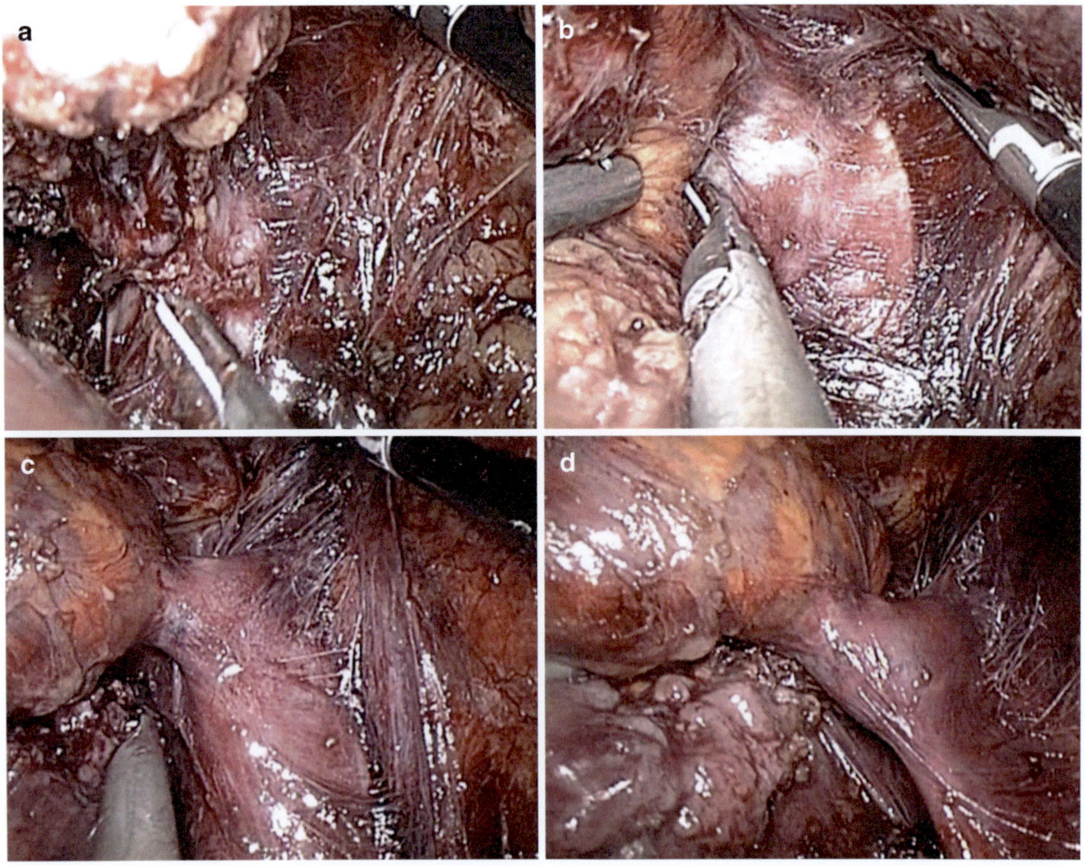

Fig. 7 (**a–d**) Exposing and separating the central vein

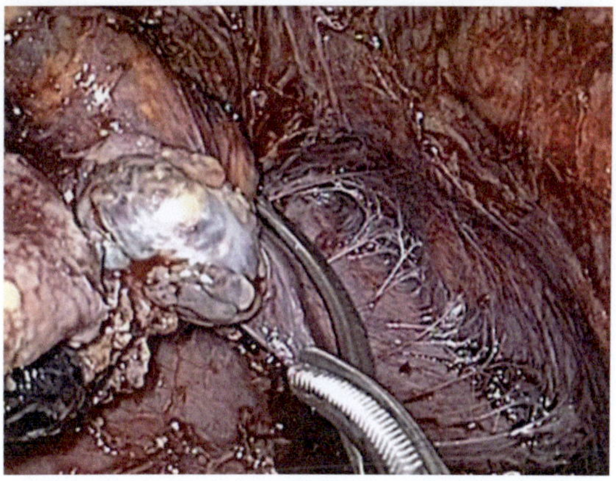

Fig. 9 Removing part of the inferior vena cava wall, the right adrenal gland, and the tumor thrombus

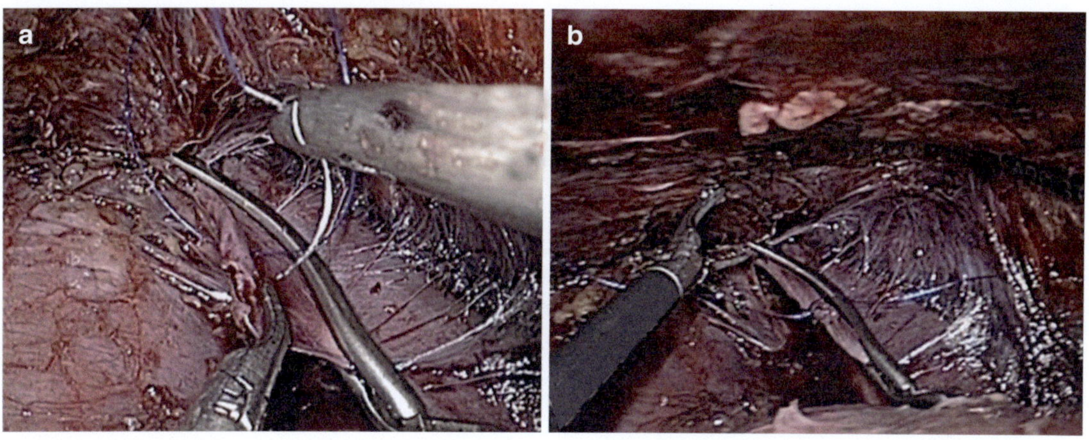

Fig. 10 (**a**, **b**) Suturing the inferior vena cava wall

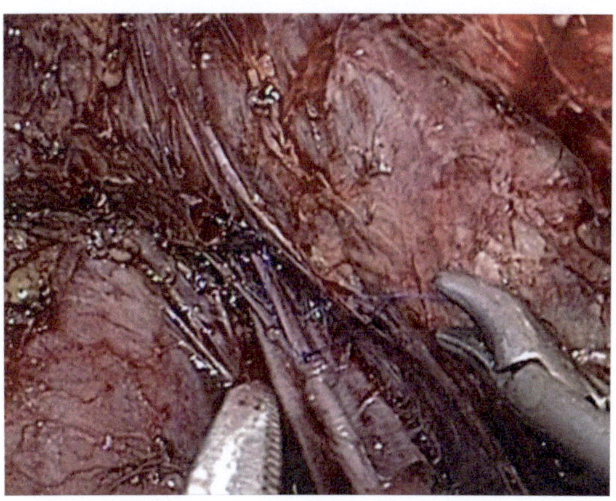

Fig. 11 Release the blockage and check for bleeding

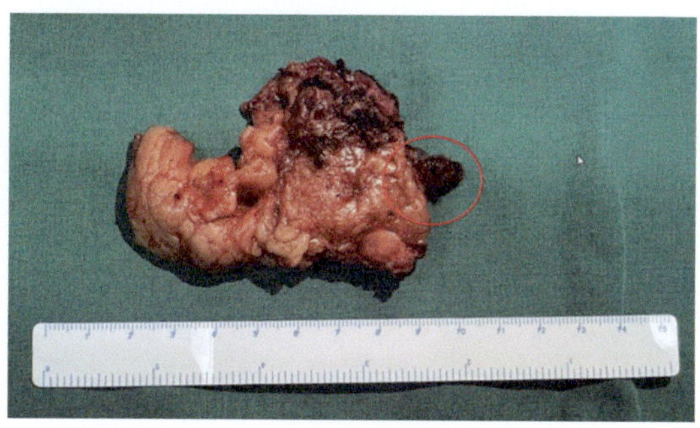

Fig. 12 Gross specimen of the tumor

Expert Comment

The characteristics of this operation are the R0 resection of cortical carcinoma and the handling of tumor thrombus. The basic approach is the same as the handling of renal carcinoma thrombus, pulling the adrenal gland to clarify the range of the thrombus, blocking, cutting, and suturing the blood vessels near the thrombus. The central vein is shorter and thinner, so a curved hemostat is used for blocking. The curvature of the hemostat just plays the role of a heart ear forceps. Preoperative reading of the film found that there might be a tumor thrombus in the adrenal central vein, so full preparation was made before the operation, and the operation was successfully completed as planned.

MRI has a better diagnostic effect on tumor thrombus. If a tumor thrombus is considered possible, an MRI can be added before the operation to make the diagnosis clearer, which is beneficial for the formulation of surgical strategies.

Adrenal Surgery: Case 10 Laparoscopic Transperitoneal Adrenalectomy for Right Adrenal Cyst

Guoyang Zheng

Medical Record Summary

Chief Complaint: Physical examination revealed a cystic mass in the right adrenal gland for 2 months.

History of Present Illness

Female, 41 years old. The patient went to a local hospital for intermittent dull pain in the right lumbar and abdominal region 2 months ago. A CT scan of the abdomen and pelvis revealed two round low-density shadows in the right adrenal region, with diameters of 6.7 cm and 4.2 cm respectively. To further diagnose and treat, the patient came to our department of urology outpatient clinic. Enhanced CT of the abdomen and pelvis suggested: Two round slightly low-density shadows without obvious enhancement can be seen in the right adrenal gland, the larger one is about 6.3 cm in diameter, the CT value is about 20.1 HU, and calcification can be seen at the edge; it is considered to be a right adrenal cyst with cyst wall calcification (Fig. 1). Endocrine-related test results suggested: ALD 2610.8 pmol/L (22.05 ng/dl), PRA 20.06 ng/(ml·h), plasma ACTH 5.9 pg/ml, and blood cortisol (8 am) 201.48 nmol/L (7.3 μg/dl). Octreotide imaging results suggested: Two cystic low-density shadows can be seen in the right adrenal region, with sizes of 6.6 cm × 5.9 cm and 4.6 cm × 4.3 cm, respectively, calcification can be seen at the edge of the larger one, and no increased radioactive uptake was seen. For surgical treatment, the outpatient clinic admitted her with the diagnosis of "right adrenal cyst."

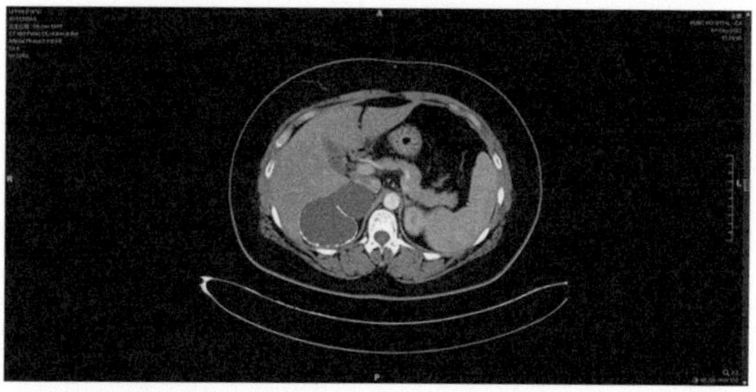

Fig. 1 Enhanced abdominal CT image

Past Medical History

Five years after cesarean section; history of chronic cholecystitis.

Supplementary Information The online version contains supplementary material available at https://doi.org/10.1007/978-981-96-8598-1_12.

G. Zheng (✉)
Beijing Union Medical College Hospital, Beijing, China

Y. Zhang, X. Zhao (eds.), *Laparoscopic Surgery in Urology*, https://doi.org/10.1007/978-981-96-8598-1_12

Physical Examination

The patient is conscious; no special findings on heart, lung, and abdominal examination, no moon face, no buffalo hump, no centripetal obesity signs, no striae or ecchymosis on the skin, no mass or percussion pain in both renal areas, no tenderness in the course of both ureters, and no full bladder palpable above the pubis.

Imaging Data (Fig. 1)

Preoperative Assessment

The patient's abdominal and pelvic enhanced CT scan suggests: Two round-like, slightly low-density shadows with no obvious enhancement are visible in the right adrenal gland, the larger one with a diameter of about 6.3 cm, and a CT value of 20.1 HU. Calcification can be seen at the edge; it is considered to be a right adrenal cyst with cyst wall calcification. The results of the octreotide SPECT/CT imaging examination were negative. Combined with the patient's symptoms, signs, and endocrine test results, the diagnosis of right adrenal cyst is basically clear. The cyst is large and calcified, and the patient actively requests surgical treatment, and the surgical indications are clear. The outpatient clinic further supplemented the assessment of cardiopulmonary function, and no obvious abnormalities were found.

The planned surgical procedure is laparoscopic right adrenal cystectomy.

Surgical Process

1. The patient's position is the retroperitoneal laparoscopic upper urinary tract surgical position. The surgical side is marked in the ward before the operation. General anesthesia is used, a urinary catheter is placed, and routine disinfection and draping are performed.
2. Establish the retroperitoneal cavity; this operation uses four holes.
3. Clean the extraperitoneal fat, identify the peritoneal reflection, and open the renal fascia longitudinally on the back side of the peritoneal reflection to reveal the psoas major muscle and the perirenal fat capsule (Fig. 2).
4. Using a suction device and an ultrasonic knife, using a combination of blunt and sharp separation methods, the fat capsule is separated upward along the perirenal fat capsule and the psoas major muscle, and the perirenal fat capsule and the peritoneum, revealing the adrenal gland and the cyst (Fig. 3).
5. Free the surrounding adipose tissue along the surface of the adrenal gland and cyst, coagulate the surrounding small blood vessels with an ultrasonic knife, and fully free the adrenal

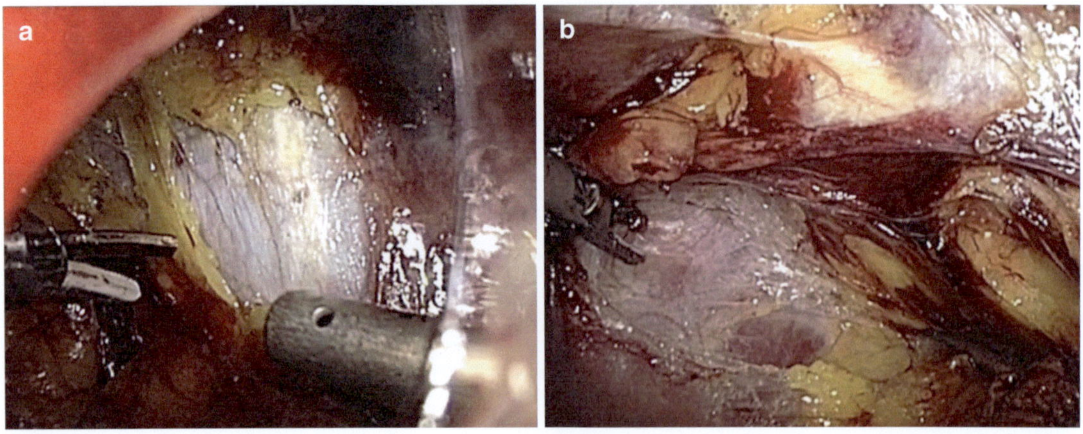

Fig. 2 Remove the extraperitoneal fat and open the renal fascia (one and two)

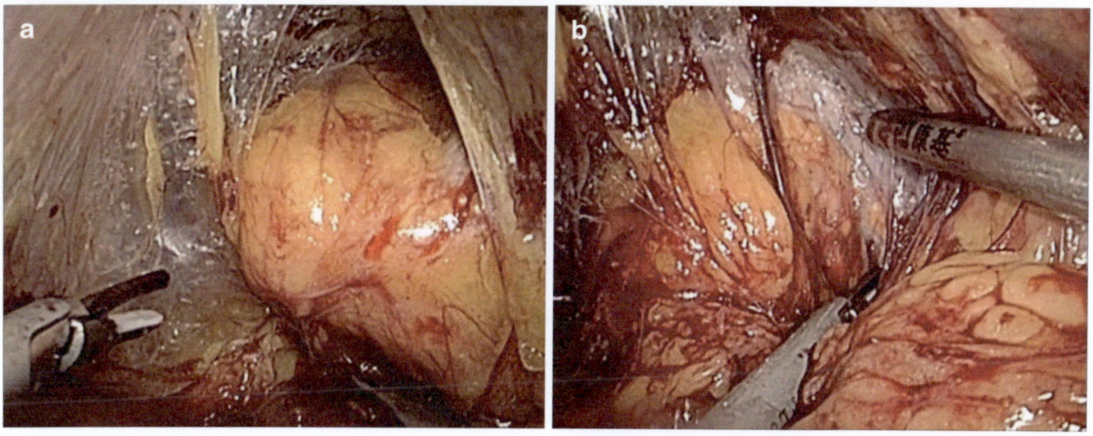

Fig. 3 Separate and expose the tumor from the dorsal and ventral sides (one and two)

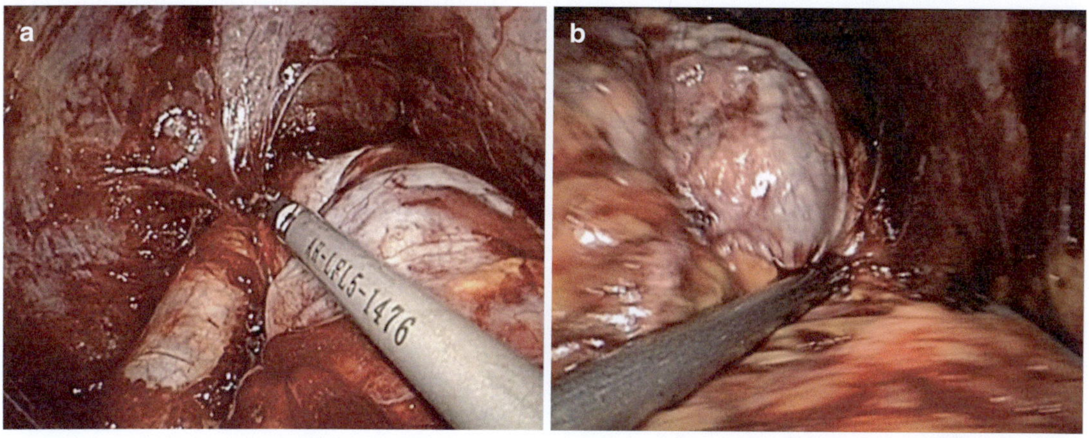

Fig. 4 Free along the surface of the tumor (one and two)

cyst from the surface of the psoas major muscle and the peritoneum (Fig. 4).

6. The ultrasonic knife opens the upper pole fat capsule of the kidney, reveals the surface of the upper pole of the kidney, lifts the adrenal cyst and the gland body upward, combines blunt and sharp separation, fully separates it from the upper pole of the kidney, and coagulates small blood vessels with an ultrasonic knife (Fig. 5).
7. After the adrenal gland and cyst are mostly freed, find the central vein of the right adrenal gland between the inner edge of the adrenal gland and the inferior vena cava, and clamp and cut off the central vein with Hem-o-lok. Finally, cut off the surrounding tissues and completely remove the adrenal cyst (Fig. 6).

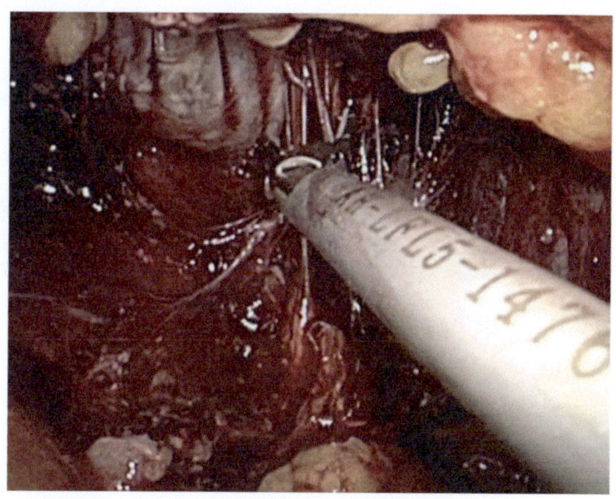

Fig. 5 Separation of the adrenal kidney surface

8. Check the wound surface for active bleeding, carefully stop the bleeding, insert the specimen bag through the auxiliary hole, put the specimen into the bag, and take it out (Fig. 7). Place a drainage tube, and the operation is over.

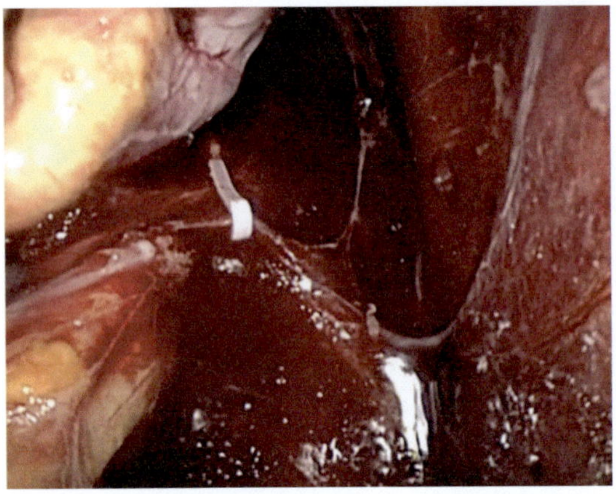

Fig. 6 Separation and severance of the central vein

Expert Commentary

1. Choice of surgical approach: Both the abdominal and retroperitoneal approaches are possible, and a comprehensive judgment should be made based on the patient's own conditions and the doctor's experience. Since the retroperitoneal approach is more direct and has less impact on the intestinal tract in the abdomen, patients recover faster after surgery, and our department more often uses the retroperitoneal approach for adrenal cystectomy. However, because the retroperitoneal space is a potential gap with a small space, for larger cysts, the extraperitoneal fat should be fully freed, and the peritoneum should be pushed as far as possible to obtain a wider surgical field and operating space.
2. Treatment of the adrenal gland: Since the adrenal cyst is a benign lesion, it is possible to only completely free and remove the cyst

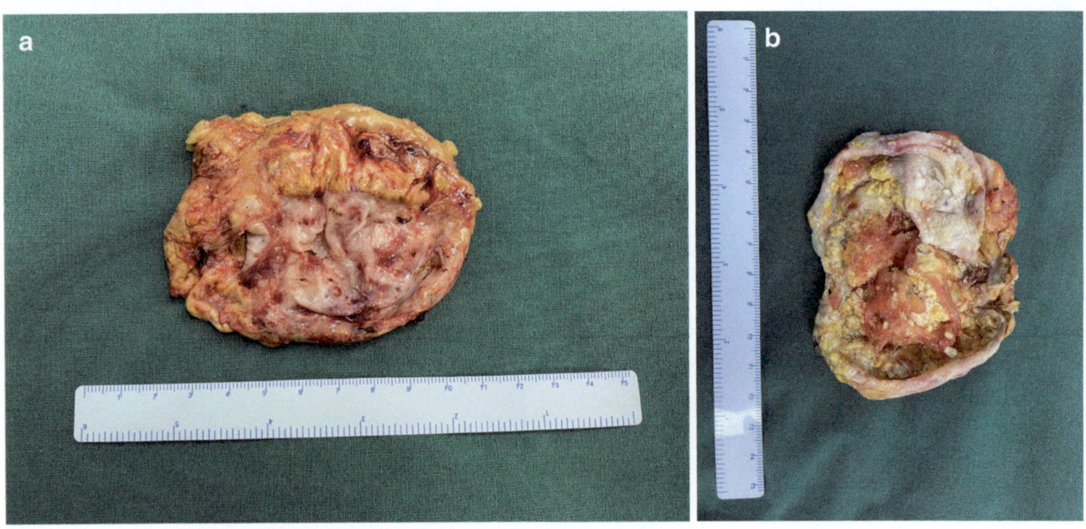

Fig. 7 Gross specimen of adrenal cyst (I and II)

while preserving the normal adrenal tissue. Because the patient in this case had a large adrenal cyst, the normal shape and structure of the gland disappeared, and there was little residual normal adrenal tissue, the surgery completely removed the adrenal cyst and all glandular tissue. For smaller cysts, it is recommended to retain part of the gland.

3. Treatment of the cyst: The adrenal cyst is a benign lesion, and the cyst wall is usually thin, so it is difficult to avoid rupture of the cyst during surgery. Especially for larger adrenal cysts, in order to obtain a wide surgical operating space and field, the cyst wall can be actively cut open to decompress and reduce the volume of the cyst, which helps to reduce the risk of damaging surrounding tissues. In this case, the cyst fluid should be promptly sucked clean, and the cyst wall and the boundary of the cyst should be carefully identified to ensure the complete removal of the cyst and avoid residual cyst wall.
4. Treatment of blood vessels: For patients who need to completely remove the adrenal gland, the central vein of the adrenal gland should be carefully found and definitively clamped and severed. Especially for the right adrenal gland, the central vein is short and thick and directly drains into the inferior vena cava, so it should be handled carefully to avoid damaging the inferior vena cava. When freeing the tissue between the lower pole of the adrenal gland and the upper pole of the kidney, it is necessary to ensure the definitive coagulation of the blood vessels below the adrenal gland to avoid damaging the renal pedicle vessels. The adrenal tissue should be lifted upward to maintain tension and obtain sufficient operable space, and a combination of blunt and sharp dissection should be used.

Kidney Surgery: Case 11 Laparoscopic Retroperitoneal Radical Nephrectomy for Right Renal Carcinoma

Yihong Liu

Chief Complaint

Right renal tumor found during physical examination for over a year. Present illness: Male, 42 years old. A right renal tumor was suggested by ultrasound during a physical examination a year ago, with a diameter of about 4 cm, considered to be a hamartoma. No special diagnosis and treatment. Follow-up urinary system color Doppler ultrasound showed: moderate echo in the middle of the right kidney, size 6.0 cm × 5.4 cm × 3.6 cm, morphological rules. Chest-abdomen-pelvis enhanced CT: A soft tissue density tumor protruding from the middle of the right kidney, with a maximum cross section of about 5.1 cm × 4.1 cm, considering the possibility of malignant lesions (Figs. 1, 2, 3, and 4). Further improvement with PET/CT: shows a right kidney mass and high CAIX expression, considering the possibility of clear cell carcinoma. Surgery is recommended. During the course of the disease, the patient denied high blood pressure and had no fever, abdominal pain, diarrhea, back pain, hematuria, etc. Admitted to our department for further surgical treatment.

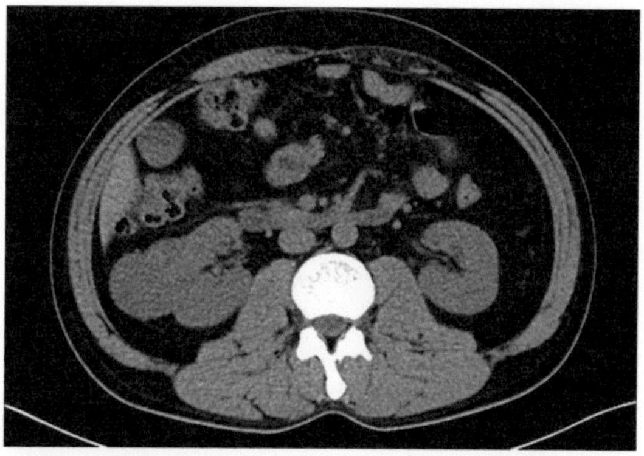

Fig. 1 Abdominal CT imaging (non-contrast)

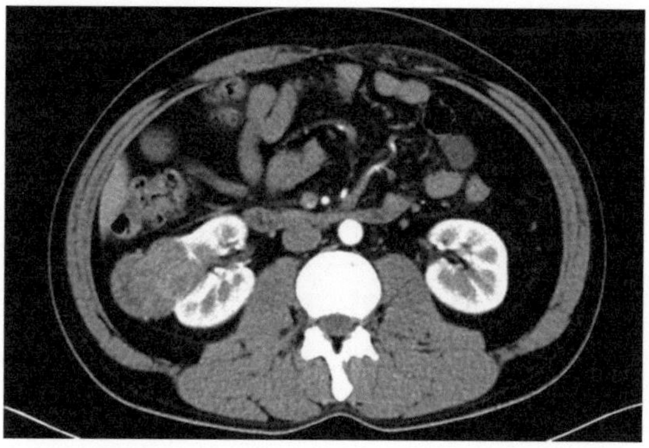

Fig. 2 Contrast-enhanced abdominal CT imaging (arterial phase)

Supplementary Information The online version contains supplementary material available at https://doi.org/10.1007/978-981-96-8598-1_13.

Y. Liu (✉)
The 7th People's Hospital of Zhengzhou,
Henan, China

Y. Zhang, X. Zhao (eds.), *Laparoscopic Surgery in Urology*,
https://doi.org/10.1007/978-981-96-8598-1_13

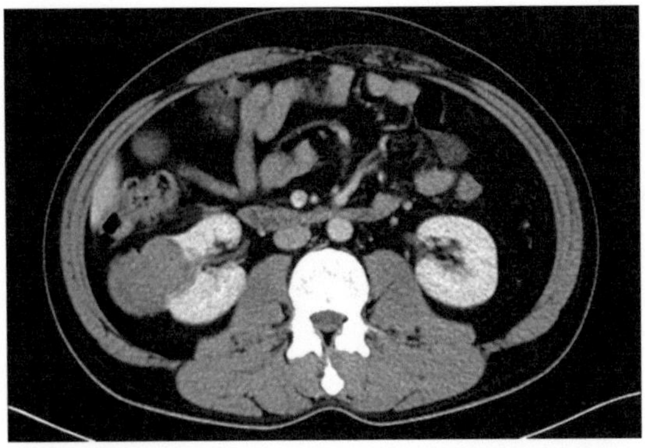

Fig. 3 Contrast-enhanced abdominal CT imaging (parenchymal phase)

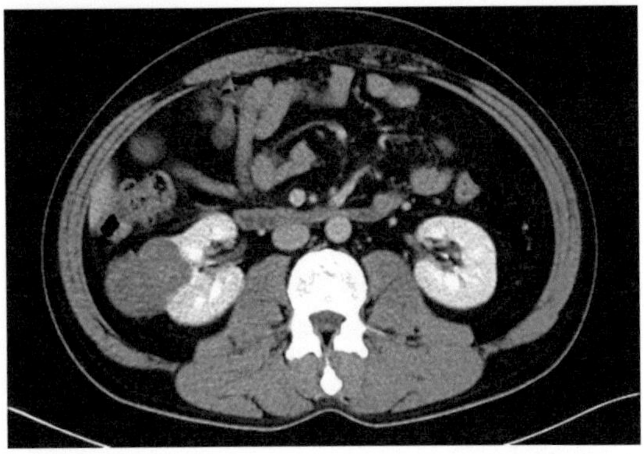

Fig. 4 Contrast-enhanced abdominal CT imaging (excretory phase)

Past History

Nothing special in the past.

Physical Examination

No special findings in the heart, lungs, and abdomen and no percussion pain in both renal areas.

Auxiliary Examination

Routine blood test: Hemoglobin 158 g/L, white blood cells 5.0 × 10^9\L; blood creatinine 79 μmol/L; ALT 23 U/L.

Preoperative Assessment

The patient's imaging examination suggests a right kidney tumor, with a diameter of about 6.0 cm, and the possibility of malignancy is high. Combined with the patient's clinical data, the diagnosis of right kidney tumor is basically clear, and renal cell carcinoma is possible, clinical stage cT1bN0M0. The indications for surgery are clear. In further outpatient assessment of cardiopulmonary function, no obvious abnormalities were found. Lung CT showed no evidence of distant metastasis. Renal blood flow imaging suggests normal perfusion and function of both kidneys. The total GFR is 106.51 ml/(min·1.73 m^2), with the left kidney GFR being 52.30 ml/(min·1.73 m^2) and the right kidney GFR being 54.21 ml/(min·1.73 m^2). Considering the above clinical data, the planned surgical method is laparoscopic radical nephrectomy of the right kidney.

Surgical Process

1. Adopt the retroperitoneal upper urinary tract surgical position. The surgical side was marked in the ward before surgery. Intubation general anesthesia was used. A catheter was placed. Routine disinfection and draping.
2. Establish the retroperitoneal cavity and insert the upper urinary tract surgical channel. This operation uses four holes.
3. Clean the extraperitoneal fat and recognize the peritoneal reflection (Fig. 5).
4. Open the renal fascia longitudinally on the dorsal side of the peritoneal reflection, revealing the psoas major and the perirenal fat capsule (Fig. 6).
5. Free the perirenal fat capsule along the surface of the psoas major, and push the perirenal fat capsule to the ventral side. Find the medial arcuate ligament on the surface of the psoas major, and free it deeply between the ligament and the medial edge of the psoas

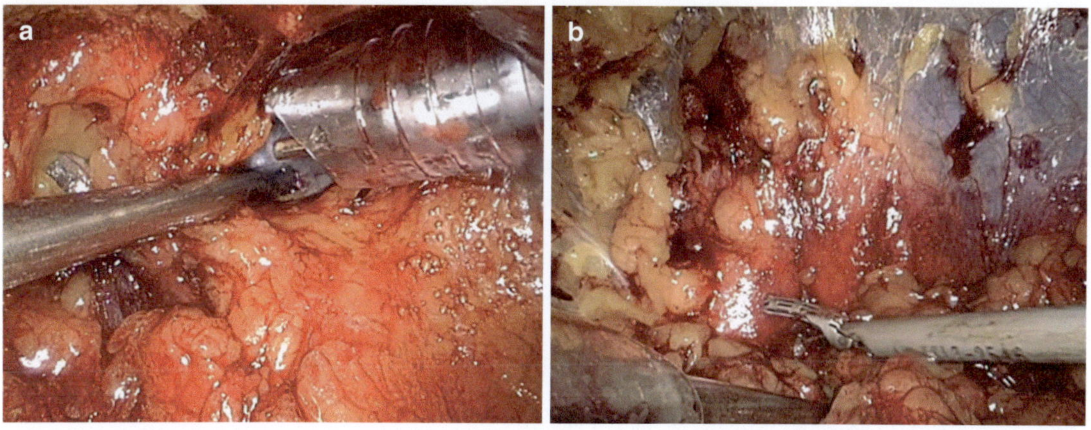

Fig. 5 Dissection of extraperitoneal fat (parts 1 and 2)

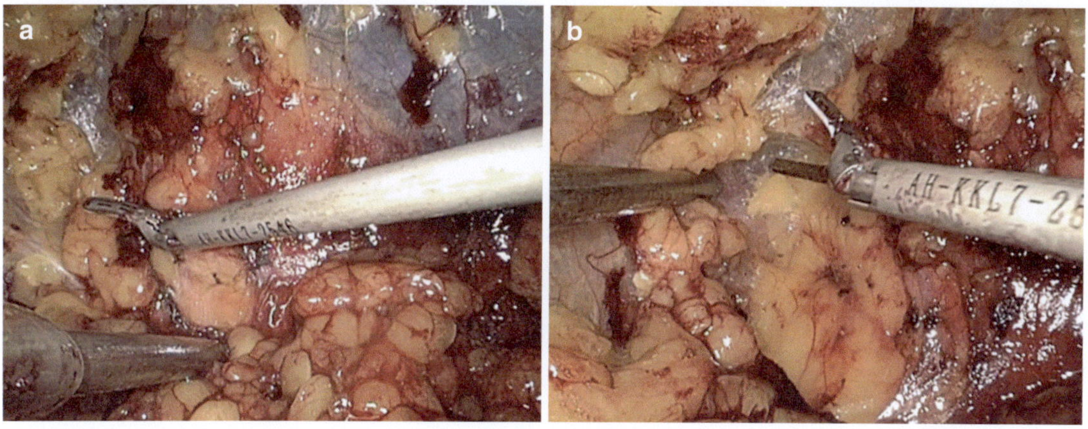

Fig. 6 Incision of the renal fascia to expose the perirenal fat (parts 1 and 2)

major. The inferior vena cava is often exposed first on the right side (Fig. 7).

6. In the middle of the kidney, that is, at the renal hilum, arterial pulsation can often be seen. The ultrasonic knife opens the vascular sheath, and the separation forceps free the renal artery. Hem-o-lok in the "2 + 1" mode (two for the proximal end + one for the distal end) is used to clamp the renal artery, which is then cut with scissors at the distal end of the two proximal Hem-o-loks (Fig. 8).
7. Free upward along the inferior vena cava; the renal vein can be exposed, and its angle with the inferior vena cava can be exposed. Hem-o-lok in the "2 + 1" mode (two for the proximal end + one for the distal end) is applied to clamp the renal vein, which is subsequently cut with the scissors (Fig. 9) (this patient has two renal veins).
8. Free between the renal fascia and the peritoneum toward the deep surface, expose the prerenal space, and expand toward the abdominal side and lower pole (Fig. 10).
9. First free the lower pole of the kidney, and separate the ureter. Hem-o-lok clamps the ureter, and cut it off with scissors or an ultrasonic knife (Fig. 11).
10. Free the upper pole of the kidney, preserving the adrenal gland. The ultrasonic knife completely frees the remaining tissue on the dorsal, ventral, upper, and lower poles of the kidney, and the kidney is completely removed (Fig. 12).

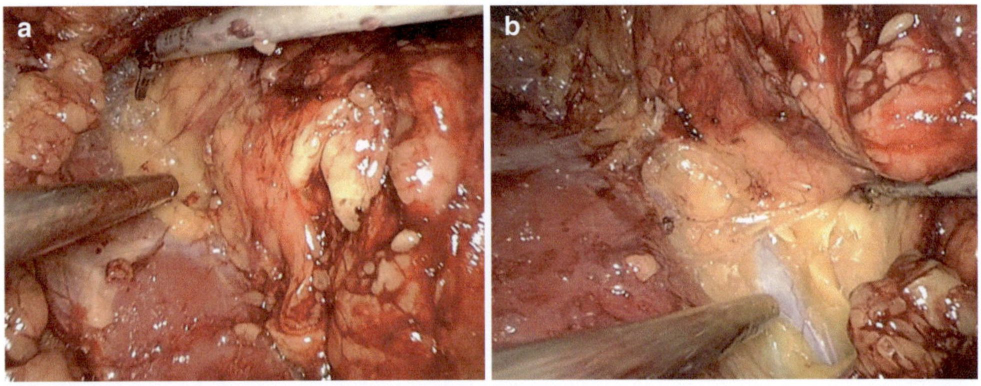

Fig. 7 Mobilization of the dorsal perirenal fat (parts 1 and 2)

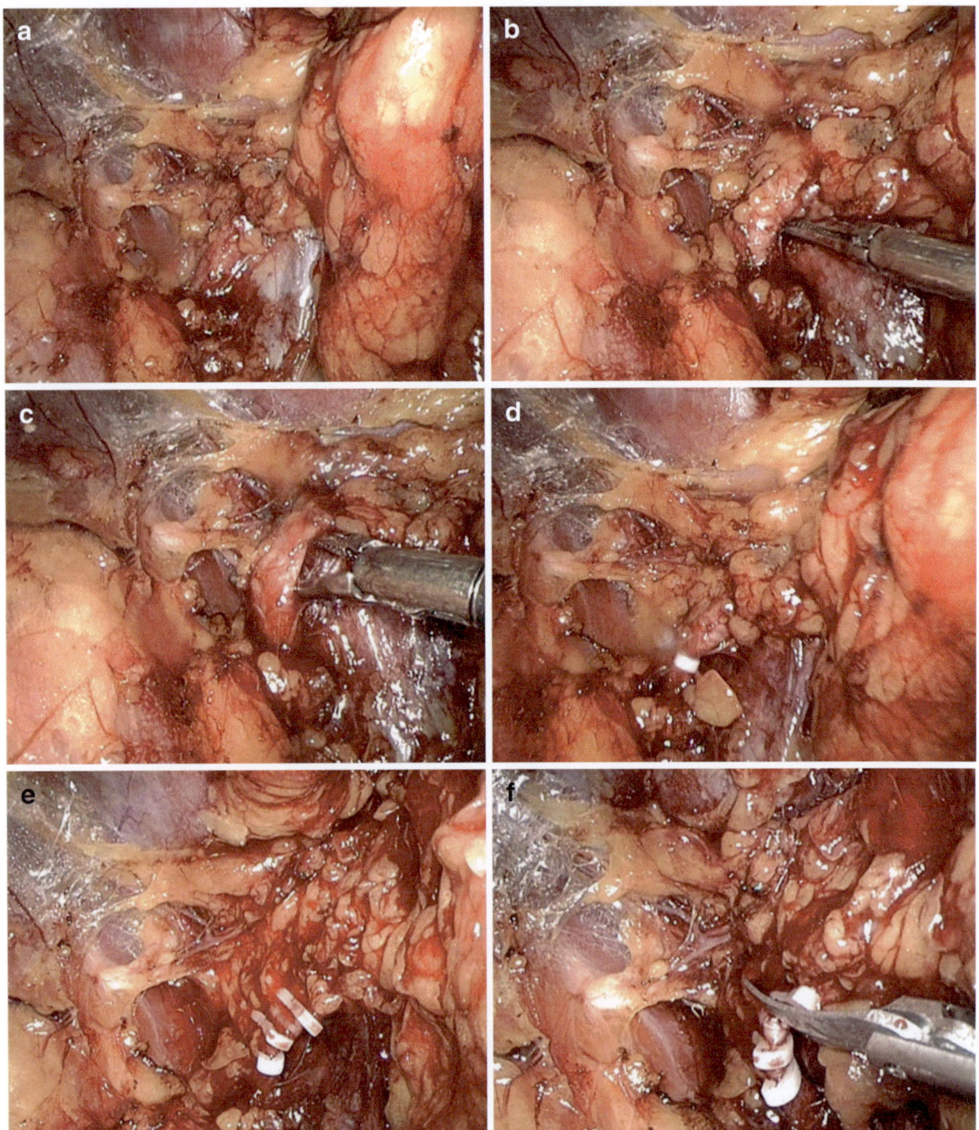

Fig. 8 Mobilization and management of the renal artery (parts 1–6)

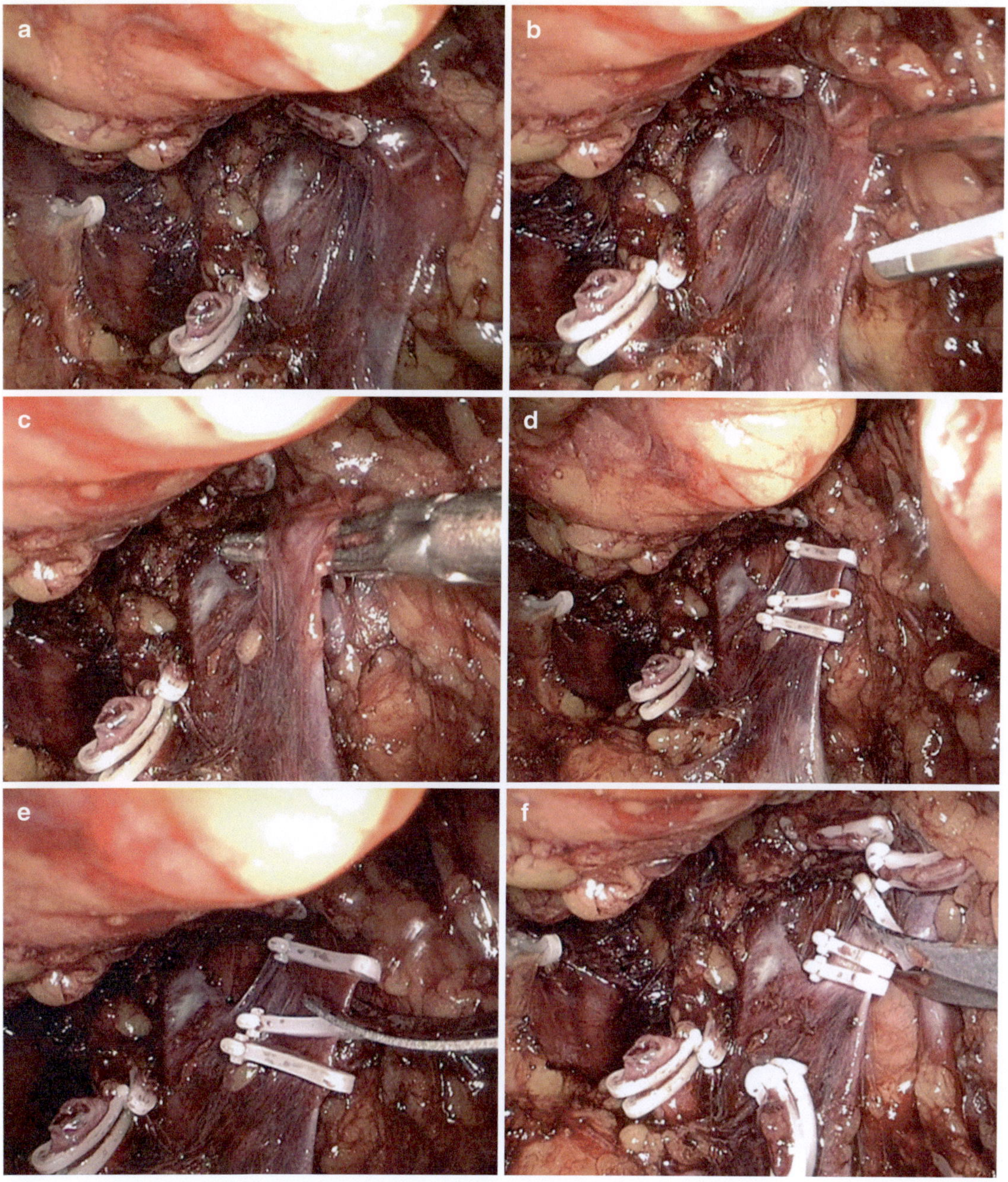

Fig. 9 Mobilization and management of the renal vein (parts 1–6)

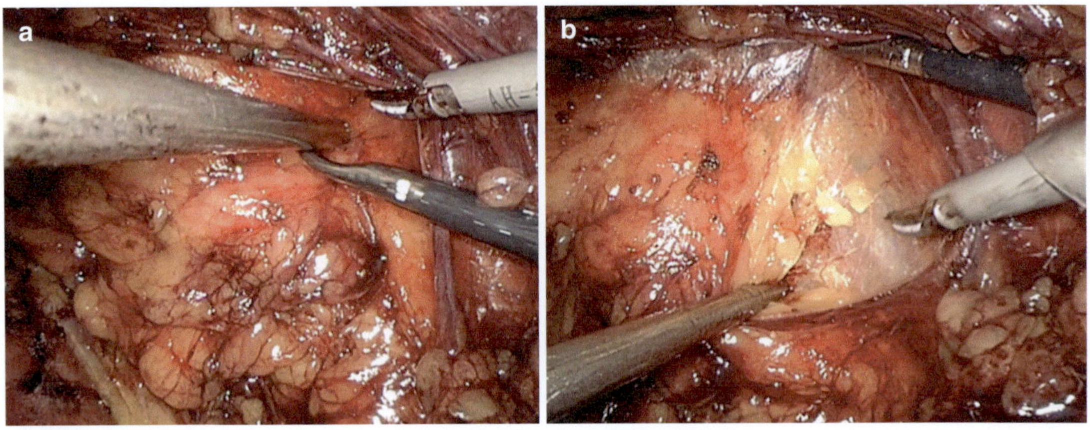

Fig. 10 Ventral renal mobilization external to the fatty capsule (parts 1 and 2)

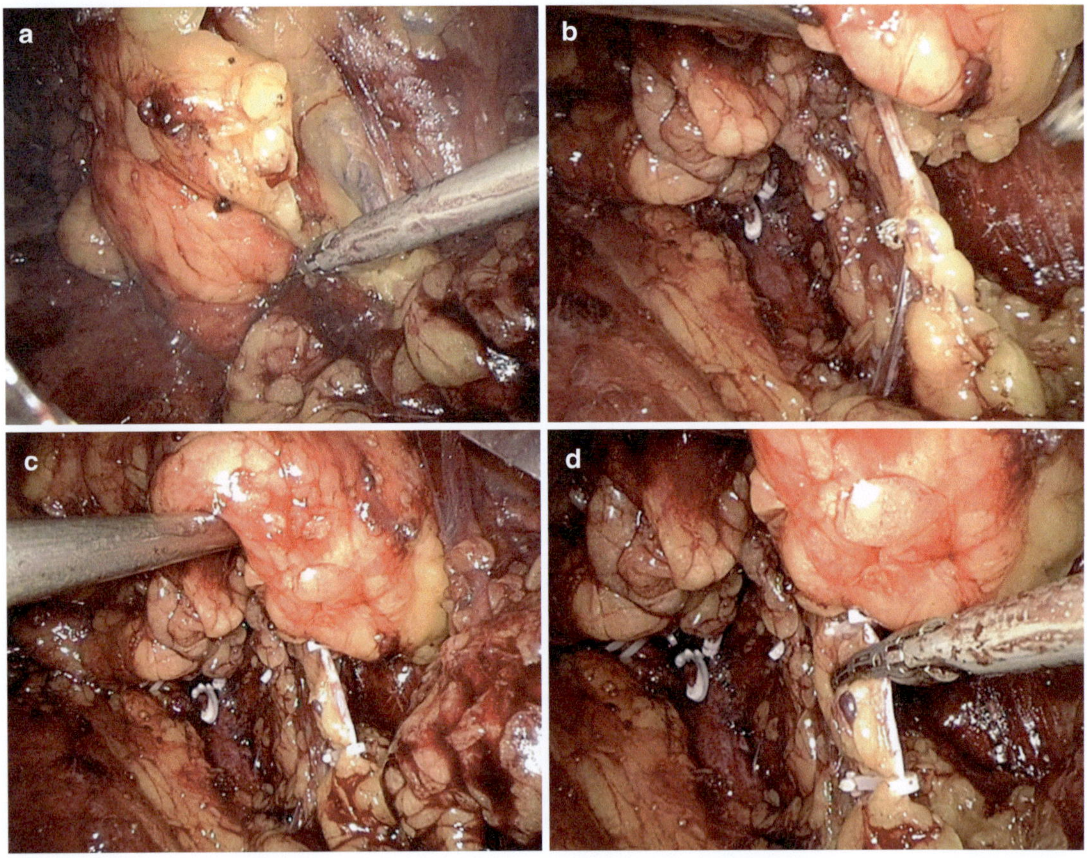

Fig. 11 Mobilization of the renal lower pole and ureter with ureteral transection (parts 1–4)

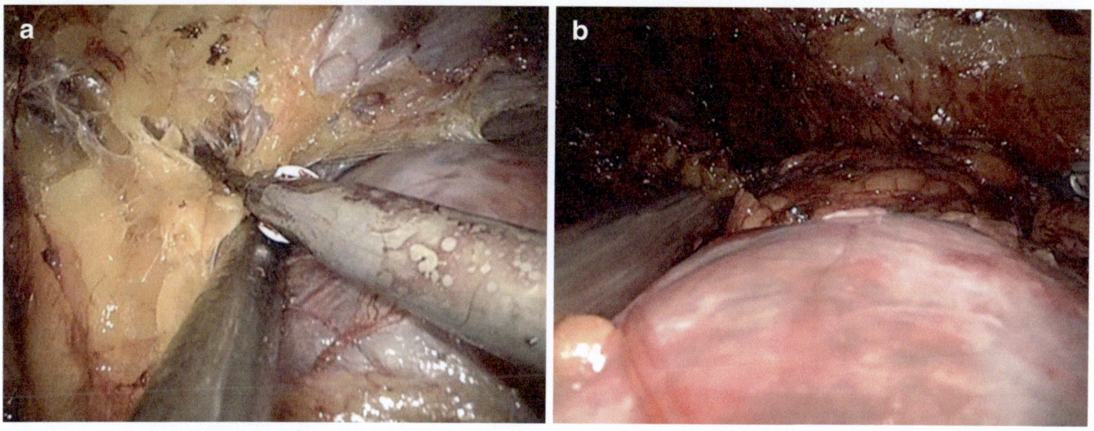

Fig. 12 Mobilization of the renal upper pole with complete nephrectomy (parts 1 and 2)

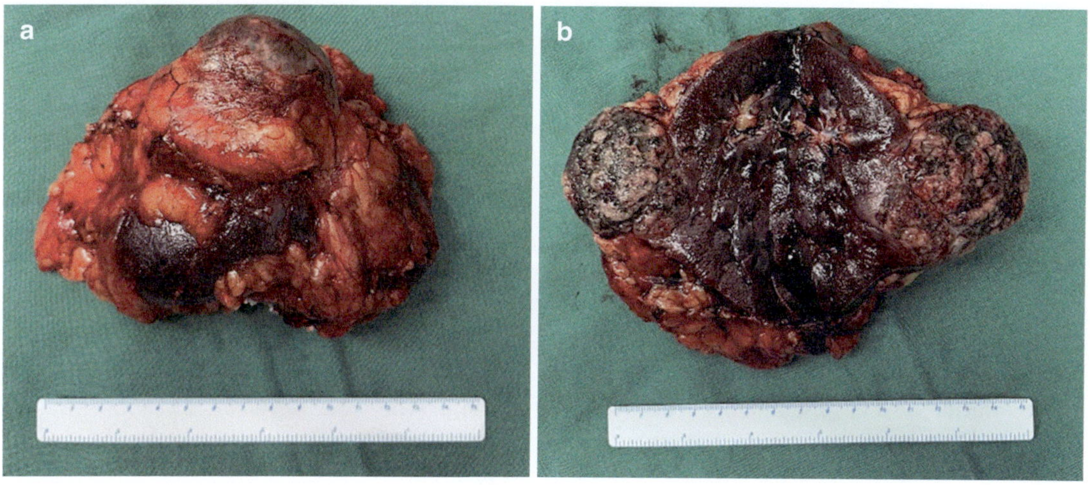

Fig. 13 Gross specimen of renal tumor (parts 1 and 2)

11. Extend the abdominal incision, and remove the specimen. Check for active bleeding, leave a drainage tube, and close and suture each incision (Fig. 13).

Expert Comments

1. Placement of the trocar: Because the space in the retroperitoneal cavity is small, for patients with more fat, the expansion of space and the auxiliary hole are very important when placing the trocar. In this case, the patient places the fourth hole on the basis of three holes as an auxiliary hole, which can assist the surgeon in exposing the surgical field and providing tension for pulling tissues. This can make the surgeon's operation more convenient and the surgical process smoother.
2. Choice of surgical approach: The retroperitoneal approach is more direct than the abdominal approach. With the auxiliary hole pushing open the peritoneum and providing tension, it can maximize the distance between the perirenal tissue and the abdominal organs (such as the liver, duodenum, etc.). And it has less impact on the intestines in the abdomen, and the patient recovers faster after surgery. Our department often uses the retroperitoneal approach for radical nephrectomy. Of course,

the choice of surgical approach also needs to be comprehensively judged based on the patient's own conditions and the doctor's experience.

3. Handling of renal pedicle vessels: During the radical nephrectomy of the right kidney, the handling of renal vessels is particularly important. The handling order is usually to deal with the renal artery first and then the renal vein. The renal vein is usually located in the front and upper part of the renal artery, so the retroperitoneal approach usually sees the renal artery first when separating along the psoas major. When Hem-o-lok blocks the renal vessels, our department usually uses the "2 + 1" mode, that is, two proximal + one distal. For special cases, the "3 + 1" mode can also be used. The right renal artery is longer than the left renal artery. Some patients have early branches of the renal artery or multiple renal arteries, which may cause the main surgeon to mistake the freed branch or one of the renal arteries for the main trunk of the renal artery, resulting in incomplete clamping of the renal artery and increasing the risk of bleeding. The right renal vein is relatively short and may have multiple tributaries that drain into the inferior vena cava separately. This patient has two renal veins, and attention should be paid to identification during surgery.
4. Freeing the kidney: First, free the lower pole of the kidney, which can be facilitated by the traction of the upper pole of the kidney and the peritoneum, making the freeing more convenient. After freeing the lower pole of the kidney, lift the kidney to see the ureter, clamp and cut off the ureter, and continue to free the kidney along the inferior vena cava upward until it crosses the renal hilum vessels. During the process of freeing the kidney, sometimes undivided accessory renal arteries and renal vein branches can be found, which can be clamped and cut off together in a "2 + 1" mode. During the freeing process, the kidney can be freed from multiple directions and angles according to the situation during the operation.
5. Specimen removal: In radical nephrectomy, the specimen is usually large in volume. It is time-consuming and laborious to put the specimen into the specimen bag under laparoscopy. In the process of dragging the specimen out of the wound, the specimen bag rope increases the risk of injury, especially the risk of Hem-o-lok falling off after hooking near the renal pedicle and dragging. The incision can be appropriately extended to remove the specimen without tension.

Kidney Surgery: Case 12 Laparoscopic Retroperitoneal Radical Nephrectomy for Left Renal Cell Carcinoma (Management of Involved Left Adrenal Gland)

Jiaquan Zhou

Chief Complaint

Left renal tumor found during physical examination for 6 years.

History of Present Illness

Male, 60 years old. The patient was found to have a cystic lesion in the left kidney with a diameter of about 5.1 cm during a color Doppler ultrasound examination 6 years ago, with no symptoms of back pain, hematuria, dysuria, frequent urination, urgency, abdominal pain, or bloating. The local hospital considered it a cyst and suggested the patient to follow up closely. A reexamination of the color Doppler ultrasound 6 months ago showed that the volume of the left renal cyst had increased, with a size of about 8.1 cm × 6.5 cm × 6.0 cm, and an enhanced CT showed a lesion in the upper middle pole of the left kidney, with a size of about 6.5 cm × 6.1 cm × 7.9 cm, with a complete capsule. Both adrenal glands were irregular, with multiple nodules of varying sizes, the larger one on the left, with a diameter of about 1.9 cm (Fig. 1).

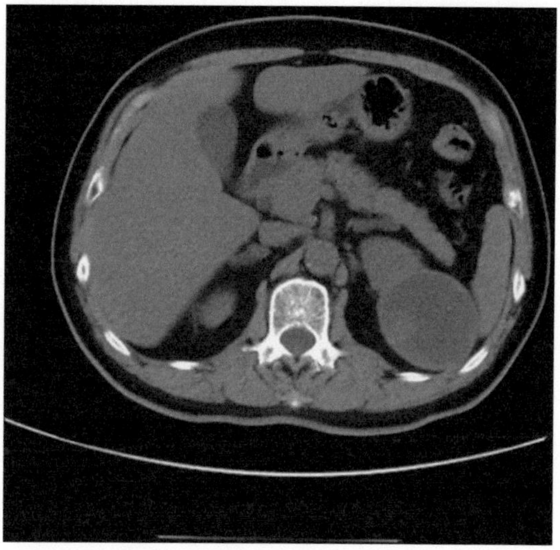

Fig. 1 Abdominal CT scan image

Past Medical History

Diabetes for over 20 years, presently taking metformin hydrochloride and pioglitazone tablets; blood sugar control is acceptable. He has a history of hypertension for over 10 years, presently tak-

Supplementary Information The online version contains supplementary material available at https://doi.org/10.1007/978-981-96-8598-1_14.

J. Zhou (✉)
Hainan Affiliated Hospital of Hainan Medical University, Hainan, China

Y. Zhang, X. Zhao (eds.), *Laparoscopic Surgery in Urology*, https://doi.org/10.1007/978-981-96-8598-1_14

ing nifedipine controlled-release tablets and metoprolol; blood pressure can be controlled at 130–140/80–90 mmHg. Hepatitis B for over 20 years, no special treatment; no other special conditions.

Personal History

Smoking for over 20 years, 20 cigarettes/day; social drinking.

Physical Examination

Vital signs stable, no special findings on heart and lung auscultation, no bulging in both renal areas, no percussion pain, no tenderness along the course of both ureters, and no bladder filling. Anus and external genitalia were not examined.

Imaging Data (Fig. 1)

Auxiliary Examination

1. Abdominal Enhanced CT: A lesion is observed in the upper-middle pole of the left kidney, with multiple enhanced nodules visible during the arterial and venous phases. The density slightly decreases during the delay phase. The lesion measures approximately 6.5 cm × 6.1 cm × 7.9 cm, with clear edges and a visible capsule, which is intact. The adrenal glands on both sides are irregular, with multiple nodules of varying sizes visible. These nodules are enhanced during the arterial and venous phases of the enhanced scan and delay in washout. The larger one is located on the left side, with a diameter of about 1.9 cm.
2. Abdominal Plain CT: There is a lesion in the left adrenal gland, with a diameter of about 1.9 cm, likely an adenoma. There is a cystic lesion in the left kidney, with a diameter of about 6.5 cm, and slightly higher density shadows within it.
3. Renal Blood Flow Imaging: The total glomerular filtration rate (GFR) is 81.2 ml/(min•1.73 m^2), the right kidney GFR is 51.9 ml/(min•1.73 m^2), and the left kidney GFR is 29.3 ml/(min•1.73 m^2).

   Indications: There may be a lesion in the upper-middle part of the left kidney with poor blood supply. The perfusion and function of the remaining kidney tissue are slightly poor; the perfusion and function of the right kidney are normal.
4. 18F-FDG PET/CT Trunk + Head Tomography: Multiple low-density nodules are seen in both adrenal glands, with no obvious increase in radioactive uptake. The larger one is located on the left side, measuring 1.7 cm × 2.1 cm, with a SUVmax of 1.6. A cystic-solid mass is seen in the upper part of the left kidney, with mostly cystic components, local thickening of the cyst wall, and slightly increased radioactive uptake, measuring 6.3 cm × 6.3 cm, with a SUVmax of 1.9. Considerations: Cystic-solid mass in the upper part of the left kidney, local thickening of the cyst wall, and slightly increased metabolism. Malignancy cannot be ruled out; adrenal nodules on both kidneys, no increased metabolism, likely benign lesions, possibly adenomas.

Preoperative Assessment

The patient sought medical attention due to a cystic lesion in the left kidney found during a physical examination. There are no obvious clinical symptoms. Combined with enhanced CT and PET/CT examinations, the possibility of cystic renal carcinoma in the left kidney is considered. The tumor's largest diameter is about 8 cm, and there is also a nodule in the left adrenal gland. Preoperative assessment shows normal creatinine; renal blood flow imaging indicates normal right kidney function and impaired left kidney function. Preoperative assessment of cardiopulmonary function shows no obvious abnormalities. The plan is to perform a laparoscopic radical nephrectomy on the left kidney, with routine preoperative preparation.

Surgical Procedure

1. General anesthesia with endotracheal intubation, placement of a urinary catheter, right lateral position, routine disinfection, and draping.
2. The first incision is made 2 cm above the midaxillary line, about 2 cm long, successively cutting through the skin, subcutaneous tissue, and fat. The muscle layer is expanded with a curved clamp, and the retroperitoneal space is entered.
3. The retroperitoneal fat is bluntly dissected with the index or middle finger closely adhering to the inner wall of the muscle layer, establishing the retroperitoneal space. This operation uses four ports.
4. A 10 cm trocar is placed in the first incision as an observation port, pneumoperitoneum is established, and surgical instruments are introduced.
5. The retroperitoneal fat is freed, revealing the posterior peritoneum. Care is taken to avoid damaging the peritoneum during the freeing process. If there is a tear in the peritoneum, it is recommended to close it before proceeding to the next step of the operation (Fig. 2).
6. The peritoneal reflection is identified, Gerota's fascia is opened, and the perirenal fat is revealed (Fig. 3).
7. Free the kidney from the dorsal perirenal fat along the psoas major muscle, identify the arcuate ligament, find the renal artery on the inner edge of the arcuate ligament, and after clamping two Hem-o-loks at the proximal end of the renal artery and one Hem-o-lok at the distal end, sever the renal artery (Fig. 4).
8. Free the renal pedicle fat on the ventral side slightly below the renal artery, and find the renal vein and central vein (Fig. 5, Fig. 6). The transection method is the same as that for the renal artery, but be careful to confirm that there are no branch arteries in the affected kidney when clamping the renal vein.
9. Closely adhere to the peritoneum, bluntly free the middle and lower part of the kidney outside the fat capsule, find the ureter, and after clamping with Hem-o-lok, sever the ureter (Fig. 7).
10. Continue to adhere closely to the peritoneum, and bluntly and sharply free the upper pole of the kidney and adrenal tissue outside the fat capsule, until the tissue specimen is completely free (Fig. 8).
11. Place the tissue specimen in the specimen bag, remove it, and examine the tissue specimen (Fig. 9).
12. Leave a drainage tube in place, and suture the incision.

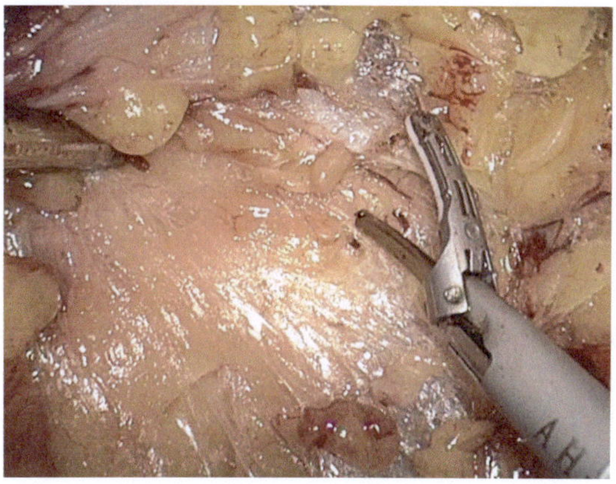

Fig. 2 Cleaning the retroperitoneal fat

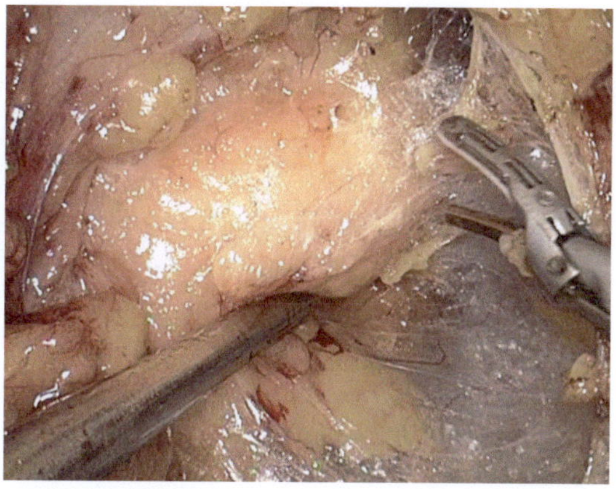

Fig. 3 Opening Gerota's fascia

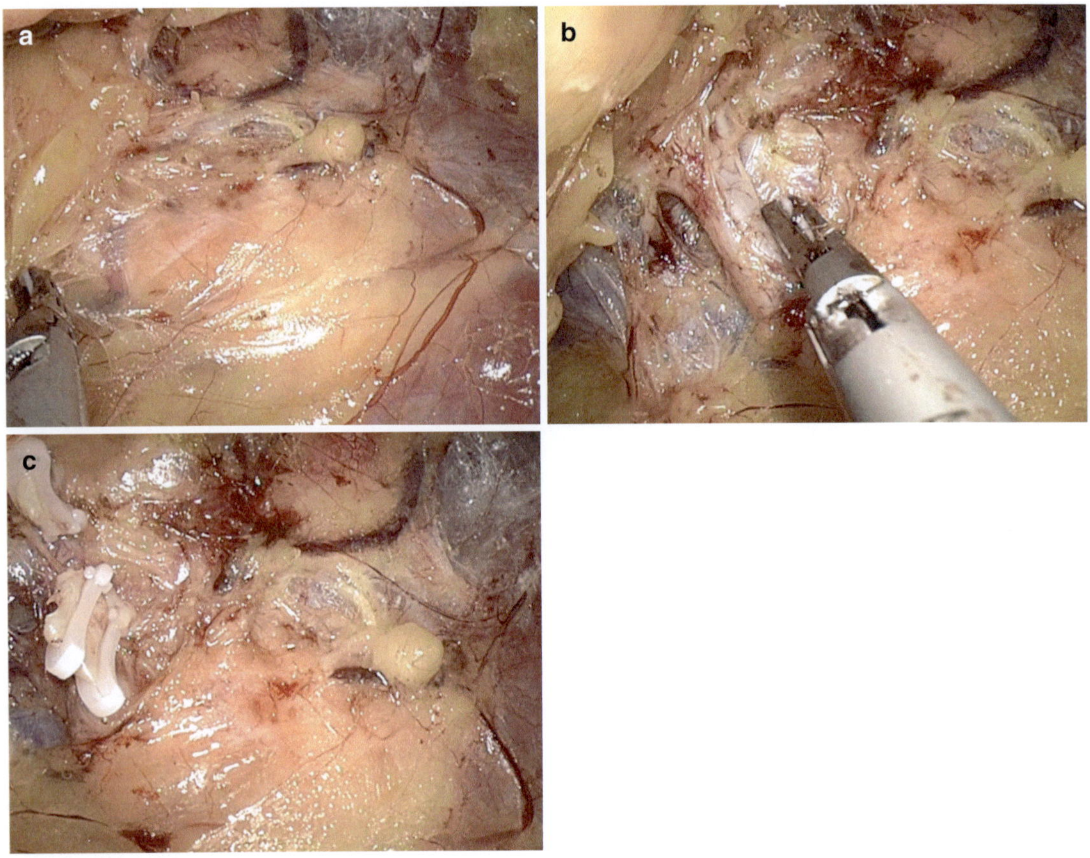

Fig. 4 Handling the renal artery (I–III)

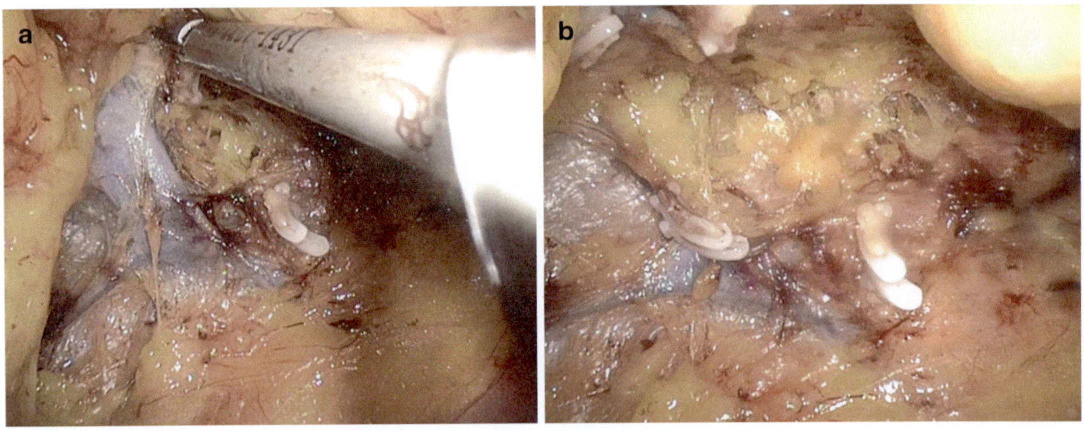

Fig. 5 Handling the renal vein (I and II)

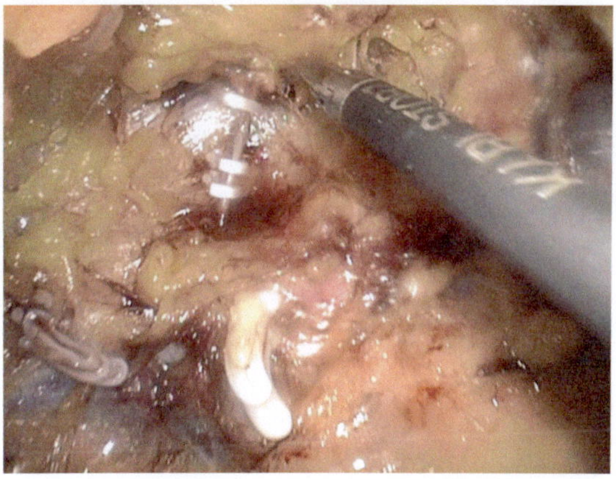

Fig. 6 Handling the central vein of the left adrenal gland

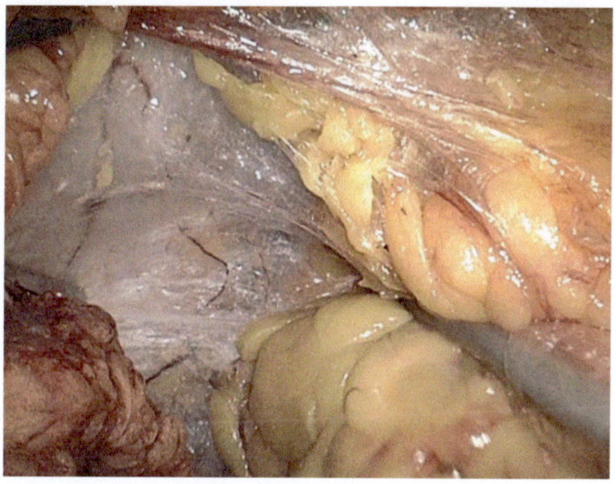

Fig. 7 Freeing the lower pole of the kidney

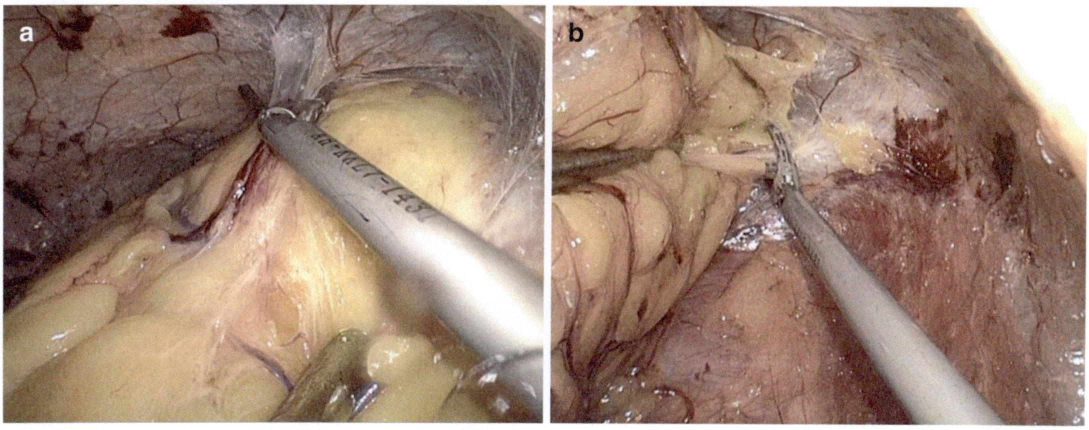

Fig. 8 Freeing the upper pole of the kidney (I and II)

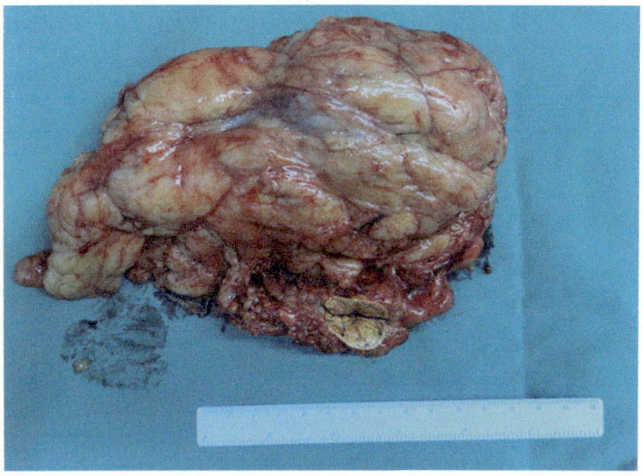

Fig. 9 Gross specimen of the left kidney and left adrenal gland

Expert Commentary

1. Cystic renal cell carcinoma generally has a lower degree of malignancy and develops slowly. This patient has a long disease course, so the maximum diameter of the tumor has increased to about 8 cm during surgery. Although most of the tumor is exophytic, considering that the tumor contains a large amount of fluid, partial nephrectomy can easily cause tumor rupture, thereby posing a risk of tumor implantation or spread. At the same time, preoperative renal blood flow imaging

suggested good renal function, so this patient chose radical nephrectomy.

2. For tumors at the upper pole of the kidney, if the tumor is not closely related to the adrenal gland, the ipsilateral adrenal gland can be considered for preservation. However, this patient's CT scan suggested a tumor of about 1.8 cm in the ipsilateral adrenal gland. Although PET/CT suggested that the adrenal tumor is likely benign, it cannot completely rule out the possibility of metastatic lesions. Therefore, this patient underwent ipsilateral adrenalectomy in one stage.
3. The biggest challenge in the surgery of cystic renal cell carcinoma is to avoid tumor rupture; therefore, it should be avoided to squeeze the tumor forcefully during the operation. If it is difficult to operate under laparoscopy, it should be timely changed to open surgery.

Kidney Surgery: Case 13 Laparoscopic Partial Nephrectomy via Retroperitoneal Approach

Guoyang Zheng

Chief Complaint

Right renal mass found on physical examination for over 4 months.

History

Male, 53 years old, visited a hospital due to upper abdominal discomfort 4 months ago. Abdominal and pelvic enhanced CT scan showed a small nodule of equal density in the lower pole of the right kidney, with mixed slightly low enhancement on enhanced scan, about 1 cm in diameter, considering the possibility of malignancy. The patient had no obvious back pain, gross hematuria, frequent urination, urgency, or pain. The hospital suggested continued follow-up observation. Two weeks ago, the patient had a follow-up abdominal and pelvic enhanced CT scan at the hospital, which showed a 1 cm equal density nodule in the lower pole of the right kidney, with mixed slightly low enhancement on enhanced scan, and no significant change compared to before (Fig. 1). The patient then visited our urology outpatient clinic and completed a urinary system ultrasound examination, which showed a mixed echo in the lower pole of the right kidney, 1.2 cm × 0.9 cm × 0.7 cm, regular shape, clear boundary, protruding outward, and no echo inside. CDFI: no clear blood flow signal, considered as cystic solid lesion in the lower pole of the right kidney. Presently, for further surgical treatment, the outpatient clinic admitted him with the diagnosis of "right renal tumor."

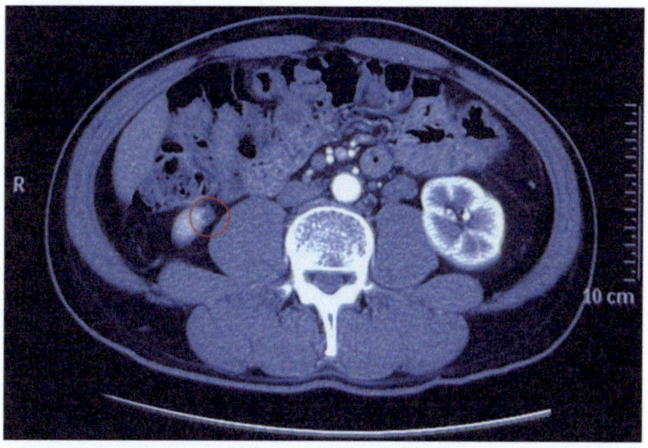

Fig. 1 Enhanced abdominal CT image

Past History

Generally healthy.

Supplementary Information The online version contains supplementary material available at https://doi.org/10.1007/978-981-96-8598-1_15.

G. Zheng (✉)
Beijing Union Medical College Hospital, Beijing, China

Y. Zhang, X. Zhao (eds.), *Laparoscopic Surgery in Urology*, https://doi.org/10.1007/978-981-96-8598-1_15

Physical Examination

Clear consciousness, good spirit, no special findings on heart, lung, and abdominal examination, no mass or percussion pain in both renal areas, no tenderness in the course of both ureters, and no palpable full bladder in the suprapubic area.

Imaging Data (Fig. 1)

Preoperative Assessment

Abdominal and pelvic enhanced CT scan showed a small nodule of equal density in the lower pole of the right kidney, about 1 cm in diameter, with mixed slightly low enhancement on enhanced scan, considering the possibility of malignancy. Urinary system ultrasound showed cystic solid lesion in the lower pole of the right kidney. Combined with the patient's clinical data, the diagnosis is right renal tumor, with a high possibility of renal cell carcinoma, clinical stage cTla-NOMO. The indication for surgery is clear.

Further assessment of heart and lung function showed no obvious abnormalities. Chest CT showed no distant metastasis. Renal blood flow imaging showed normal perfusion and function of both kidneys; GFR was 96.3 ml/(min·1.73 m^2), of which left kidney GFR was 46.8 ml/(min·1.73 m^2) and right kidney GFR was 49.5 ml/(min·1.73 m^2).

The surgical method is laparoscopic partial nephrectomy via retroperitoneal approach.

Surgical Procedure

1. The patient's position was the lateral position commonly used in retroperitoneal laparoscopic surgery, the surgical side was marked in the ward before the operation, general anesthesia was used, a urinary catheter was placed, and routine disinfection and draping were performed.
2. Establish the retroperitoneal space and insert the laparoscopic surgical sheath. This operation used four ports (two 5 mm sheaths, one 10 mm sheath, and one 12 mm sheath).
3. Clean the extraperitoneal fat (Fig. 2), identify the peritoneal reflection, and open the renal fascia longitudinally on the back side of the peritoneal reflection (Fig. 3), exposing the psoas major muscle and the perirenal fat capsule.
4. Use a suction device and an ultrasonic knife for blunt and sharp dissection, fully free the perirenal fat capsule along the surface of the psoas major muscle, and push it toward the abdominal side, fully exposing the surface of the psoas major muscle, exposing the inferior vena cava, and freeing the surface tissue along the surface of the inferior vena cava, looking for and freeing the right renal artery (Fig. 4).

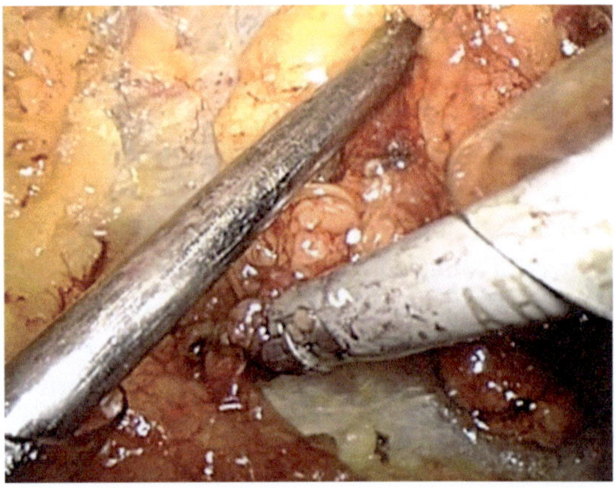

Fig. 2 Cleaning the extraperitoneal fat

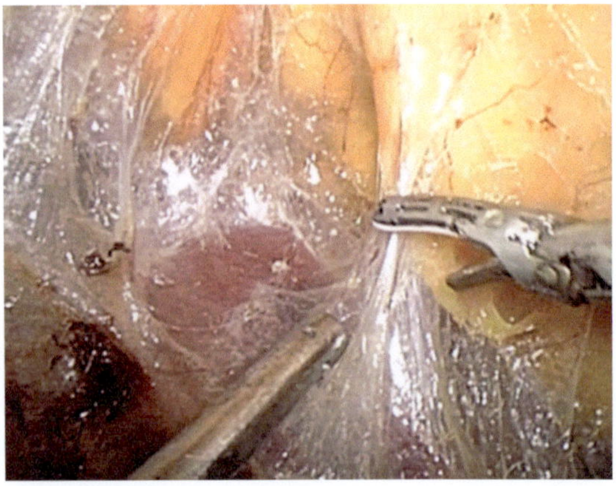

Fig. 3 Opening the renal fascia

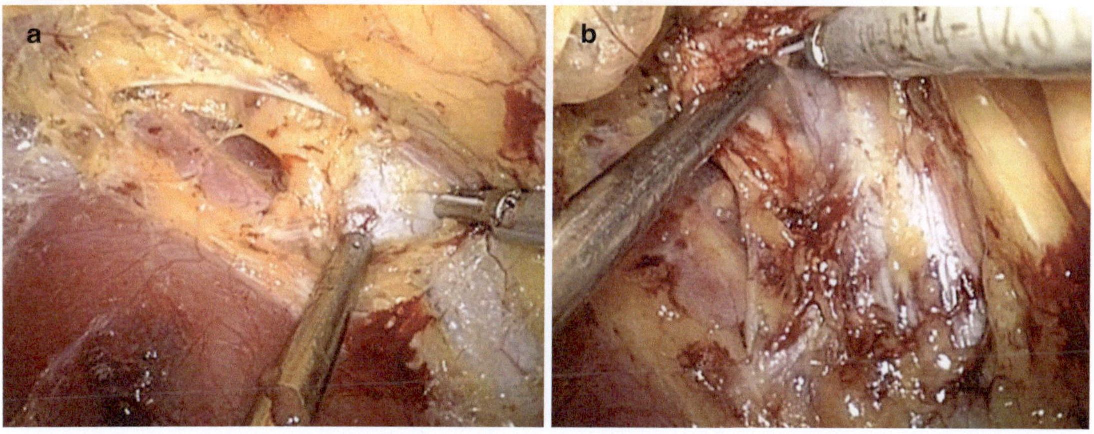

Fig. 4 Locating and exposing the renal artery (I and II)

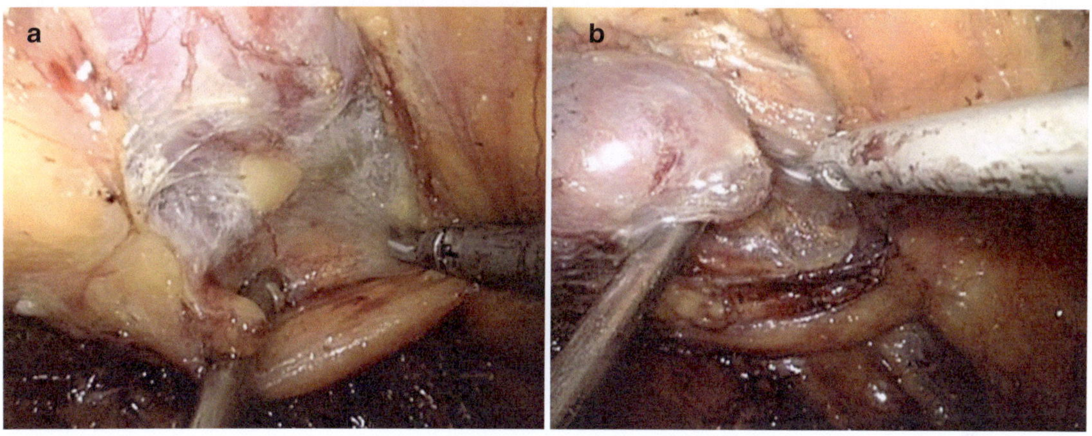

Fig. 5 Separating and exposing the kidney tumor (I and II)

5. At the position close to the peritoneum under the kidney, open the perirenal fat capsule, and combine blunt dissection and sharp cutting to free the middle and lower poles of the right kidney, fully exposing the solid tumor of the lower pole of the right kidney (Fig. 5).
6. Use a vascular occlusion clamp to block the right renal artery (Fig. 6). Cut the renal parenchyma 0.5 cm away from the tumor edge, use a combination of blunt and sharp methods to free the base of the tumor, completely remove the right kidney tumor, be careful to avoid rupture of the cystic tumor, and avoid excessive destruction of blood vessels and the collecting system (Fig. 7).

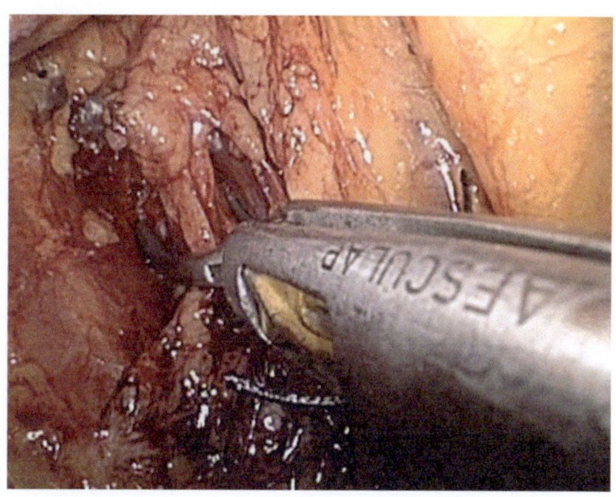

Fig. 6 Blocking the renal artery

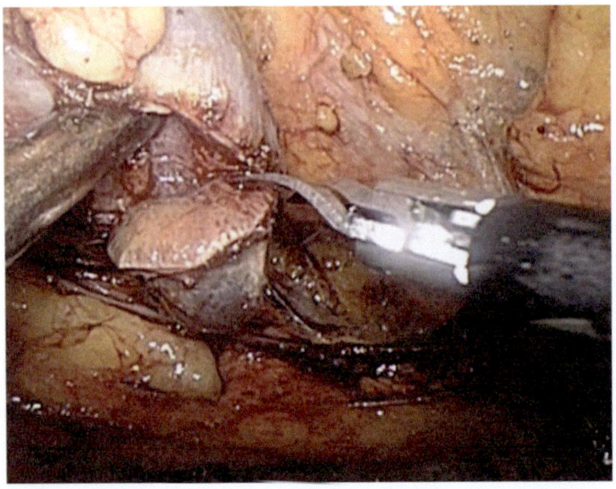

Fig. 7 Marking the removal of the kidney tumor

7. Use a layered suturing method, continuously suture the tumor base with 3-0 V-Loc thread, tighten it, and then use 1-0 V-Loc thread to continuously suture the wound. The thread end is fixed with Hem-o-lok (Fig. 8).
8. Remove the arterial occlusion clamp, and check for active bleeding in the renal hilum and renal wound (Fig. 9).
9. Insert a specimen bag through the auxiliary hole, put the right kidney tumor into the bag, remove the specimen, place a drainage tube, and close the incision (Fig. 10).

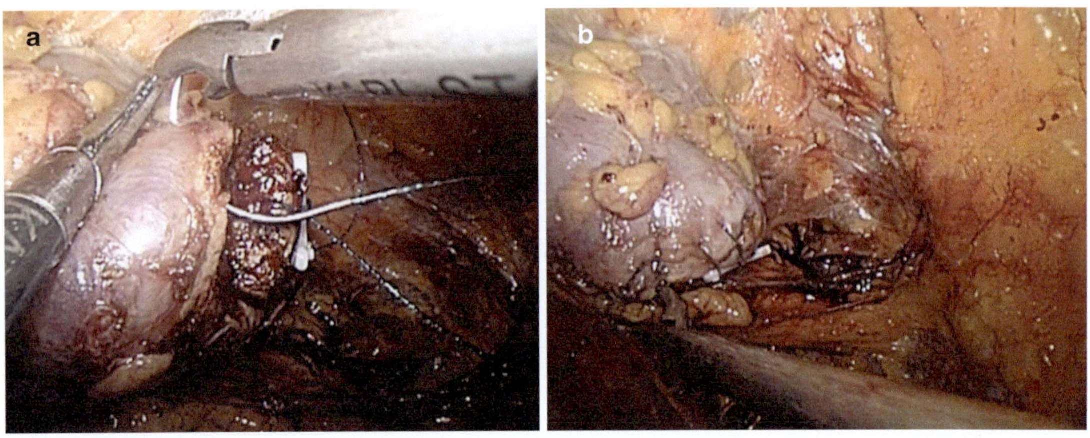

Fig. 8 Suturing the kidney wound (I and II)

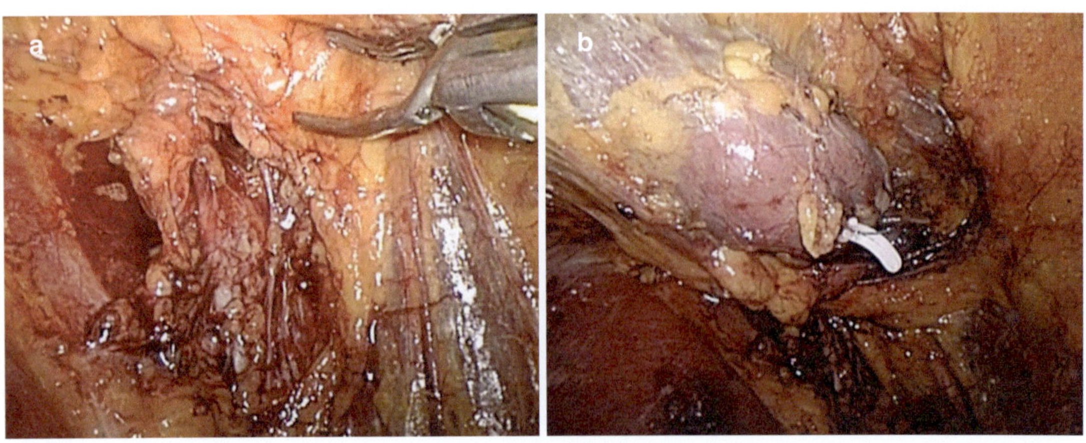

Fig. 9 Removing the occlusion clamp, checking for bleeding (I and II)

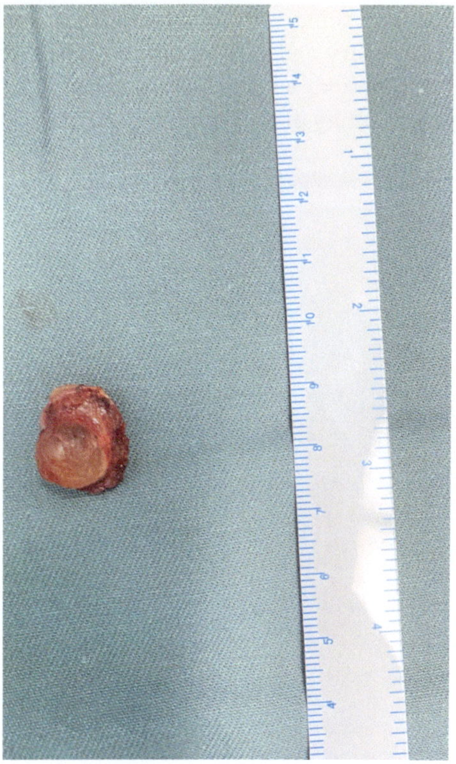

Fig. 10 Gross image of kidney tumor specimen

Expert Comments

1. The importance of preoperative diagnosis: If a renal cystic carcinoma ruptures during surgery, it may lead to tumor implantation in the surgical field, so preoperative differential diagnosis is very important. It should be fully combined with ultrasound, CT, or imaging examinations such as MRI, to distinguish whether the cystic mass is a simple cyst or a cystic tumor, to avoid blindly performing cyst decapitation surgery and causing tumor rupture.
2. Choice of surgical approach: The choice should be made in combination with the patient's own conditions and the surgeon's proficiency, considering either the intraperitoneal or retroperitoneal approach. Both paths can be considered. Because the retroperitoneal approach is more direct and has less impact on the intestinal tract in the abdominal cavity, patients recover faster after surgery, and our department more often uses the retroperitoneal approach for laparoscopic partial nephrectomy. However, for tumors on the upper or lower medial pole and anterior lip, there are certain visual and operational blind spots in the retroperitoneal approach, and the kidney should be fully mobilized during surgery.
3. Treatment of renal hilum vessels: In partial nephrectomy, whether the occlusion of the renal artery is complete determines the degree of bleeding in the surgical field during tumor resection. Therefore, before surgery, the images should be carefully reviewed to confirm whether there are accessory renal arteries or premature branches, and omission should be avoided when freeing the renal artery. To ensure the effect of arterial occlusion, multiple branches can be occluded separately. If the effect of renal artery occlusion is still not good under the premise of confirming that there are no other branch arteries, the possibility of incomplete closure of the renal artery should be considered, and two occlusion clamps can be tried side by side on the renal artery to achieve complete occlusion.
4. Treatment of cystic tumors: During surgery, rupture of cystic tumors should be avoided to prevent tumor implantation and spread. Therefore, the surgical operation should be careful and gentle, avoid violent contact with the tumor surface by surgical instruments, and ensure the integrity of tumor resection. For larger cystic tumors, excessive insistence on minimally invasive surgery should be avoided, and open surgery should be switched to in time if necessary, to avoid excessive squeezing of the tumor due to limited surgical field and narrow operating space. When removing the specimen, the surgical incision should be fully expanded to avoid violent pulling of the specimen.
5. Wound suturing: It is recommended to use layered suturing for renal wound suturing. The inner layer mainly uses 3-0 sutures to close the small openings in the blood vessels and collecting system formed during tumor resection, which also serves to reduce the

wound and reduce the tension of the outer layer suturing. Next, 1-0 sutures should be used for outer layer suturing of the wound, to accurately close the renal wound and achieve complete hemostasis and reconstruction. The needle entry and exit points should be at the renal capsule, with moderate force, to avoid suture cutting of the renal parenchyma.

Kidney Surgery: Case 14 Laparoscopic Retroperitoneal Partial Nephrectomy of the Right Kidney (Converted to Open Surgery During the Operation)

Yi Zhao

Chief Complaint

Right renal tumor found during physical examination 3 weeks ago.

Medical History

Male, 56 years old. Three weeks ago, during a local physical examination, an ultrasound suggested a slightly uneven, slightly high echo nodule of about 2.25 cm × 2.42 cm in the lower pole of the right kidney. Later, an abdominal enhanced CT scan at a local hospital suggested a quasi-circular equal density shadow in the lower pole of the right kidney, with plain CT values of 34 HU and enhanced scan three-phase CT values of 56 HU, 61 HU, and 68 HU (Figs. 1, 2, 3 and 4). The patient denied symptoms such as fever, hematuria, urgency, dysuria, back pain, and lumbar mass. He was admitted to our hospital for further treatment.

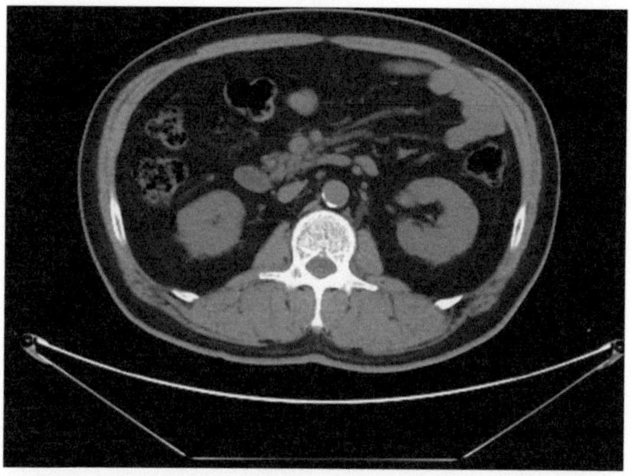

Fig. 1 Abdominal CT plain scan image

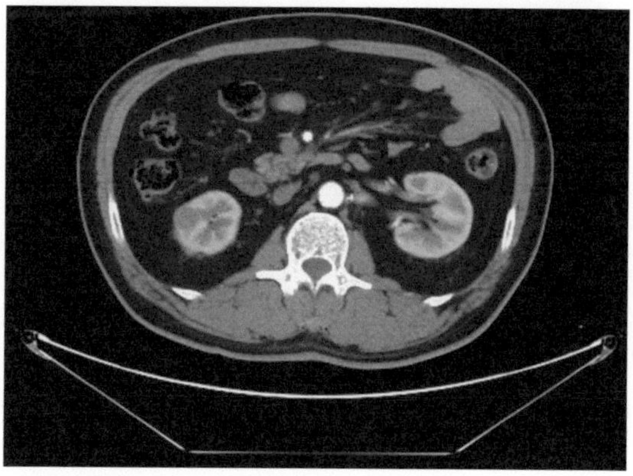

Fig. 2 Abdominal CT-enhanced image

Supplementary Information The online version contains supplementary material available at https://doi.org/10.1007/978-981-96-8598-1_16.

Y. Zhao (✉)
Beijing Union Medical College Hospital,
Beijing, China

Y. Zhang, X. Zhao (eds.), *Laparoscopic Surgery in Urology*,
https://doi.org/10.1007/978-981-96-8598-1_16

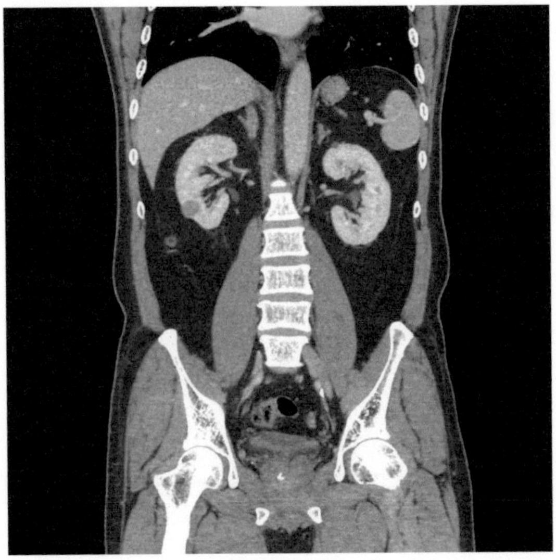

Fig. 3 Abdominal CT coronal image

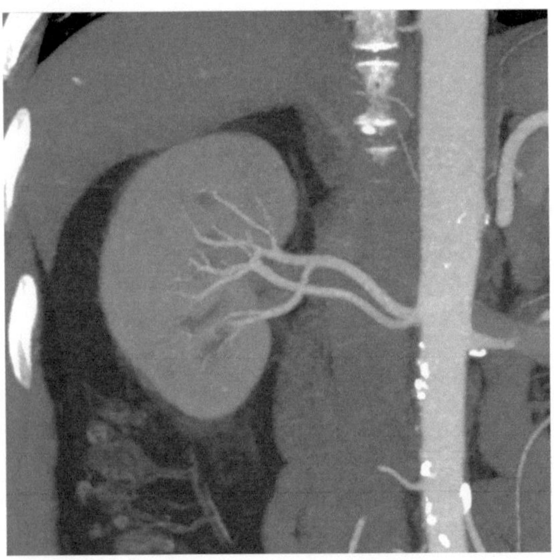

Fig. 4 Renal vascular imaging of abdominal CT

Past History

Nothing special.

Physical Examination

No percussion pain in both renal areas.

Imaging Data (Figs. 1, 2, 3 and 4)

Preoperative Assessment

The patient's imaging examination suggested a tumor in the lower pole of the right kidney, with a diameter of about 2 cm; considering the high possibility of malignancy, the surgical indications are clear.

In complete preoperative cardiopulmonary function assessment, no obvious abnormalities were seen. Lung CT showed no evidence of distant metastasis. The surgical method is laparoscopic partial nephrectomy of the right kidney converted to open surgery.

Surgical Process

1. The retroperitoneal approach was used, with the patient in the left lateral position. Preoperative CT assessment showed heavy adhesion around the kidney, and this operation used four holes (3 cm above the axillary midline, below the 12th rib of the axillary posterior line, below the 12th rib of the axillary anterior line, and between the first and third holes).
2. The surgical site was marked in the ward before the operation. General anesthesia with endotracheal intubation was used. A urinary catheter was placed. Routine disinfection and draping.
3. After establishing pneumoperitoneum, the upper urinary tract surgical channel was placed.
4. The extraperitoneal fat was cleaned, the peritoneal reflection was identified, and Gerota's fascia was longitudinally opened on the dorsal side of the peritoneal reflection, revealing the psoas major muscle and perirenal fat capsule (Fig. 5).
5. The perirenal fat capsule was fully freed along the surface of the psoas major muscle toward the head side, and the right renal artery was identified and dissected at the symmetrical

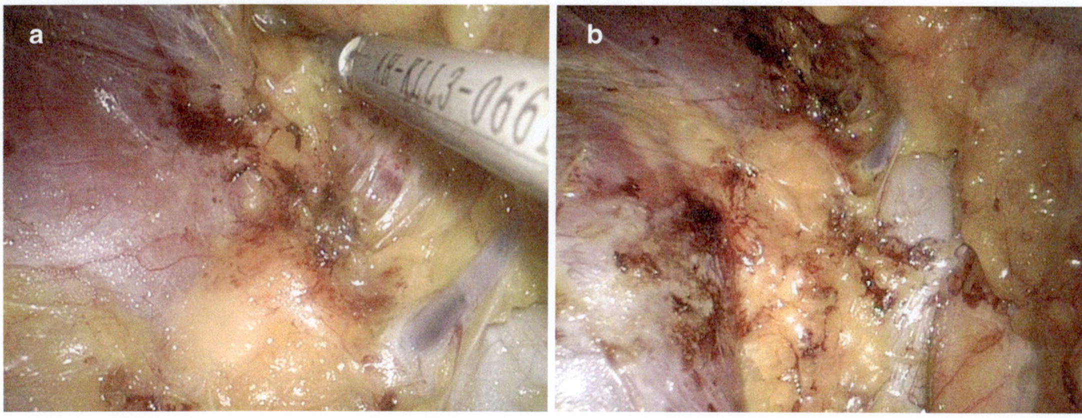

Fig. 5 (**a**, **b**) Cleaning the extraperitoneal fat, opening Gerota's fascia

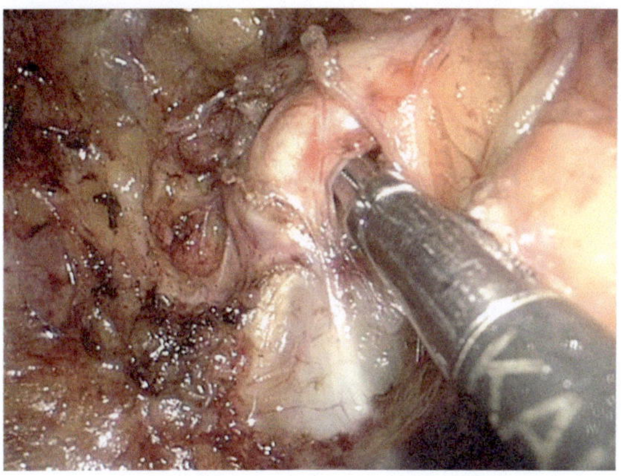

Fig. 6 Finding the renal artery

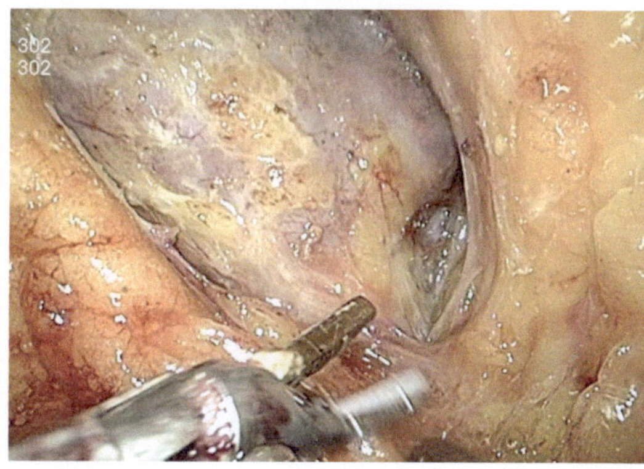

Fig. 7 Fully freeing the kidney

position of the arcuate ligament on the inner side of the surface of the psoas major muscle and the inner edge of the psoas major muscle (Fig. 6).

6. The kidney was fully freed along the surface of the kidney, revealing the lower pole tumor of the kidney. A slightly protruding tumor was visible in the lower pole of the kidney, with a diameter of 1–2 cm, and the surface was blue (Fig. 7).
7. The position of the renal tumor was marked with a monopolar hook (Fig. 8), the lower branch of the renal artery was selectively blocked (Fig. 9), and the tumor was completely removed along the tumor capsule with laparoscopic scissors (Fig. 10).
8. After the tumor is removed, the kidney wound is sutured with 3-0, 1-0 reverse barb sutures (Fig. 11). Because the tumor is located at the lower pole suturing was technically challenging. After suturing, the wound still bleeds a lot, so it was changed to open surgery (Fig. 12).

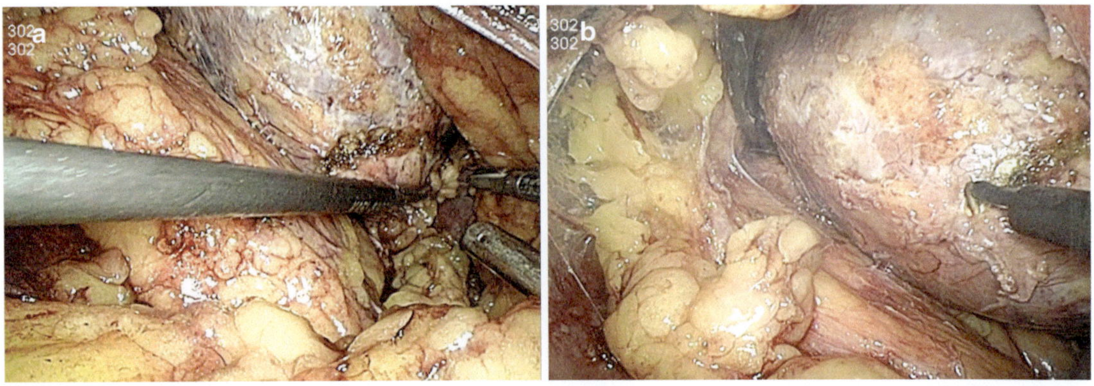

Fig. 8 (**a**, **b**) Locating the kidney tumor and marking

Fig. 9 Blocking the renal artery branch

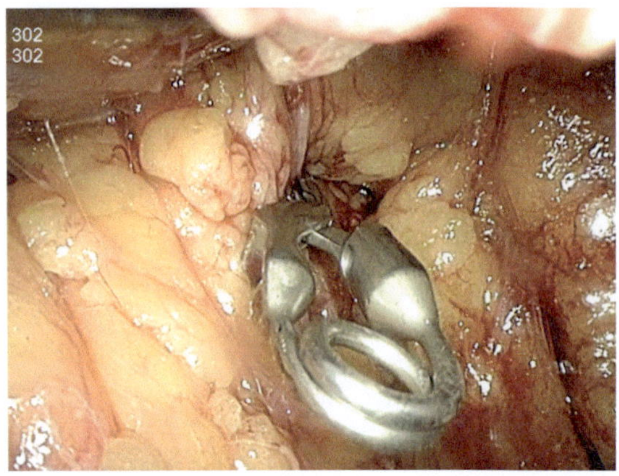

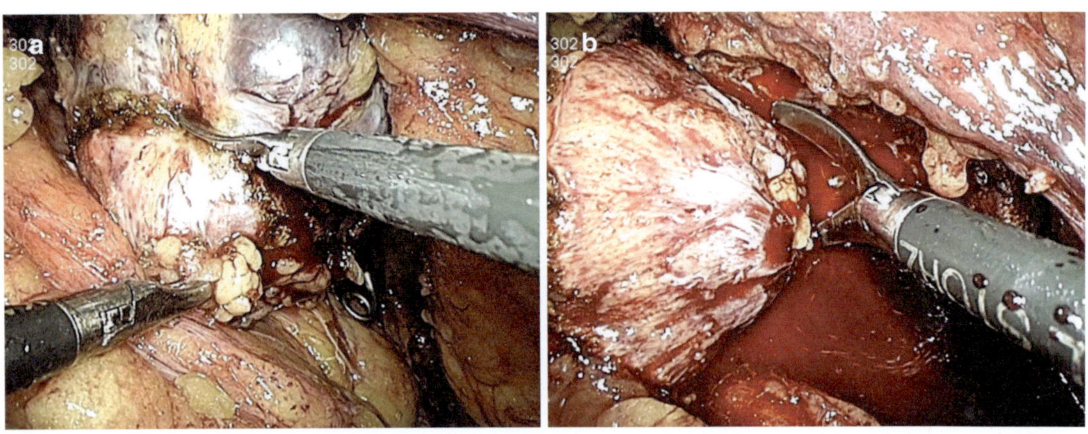

Fig. 10 (**a**, **b**) Removing the tumor along the marked line

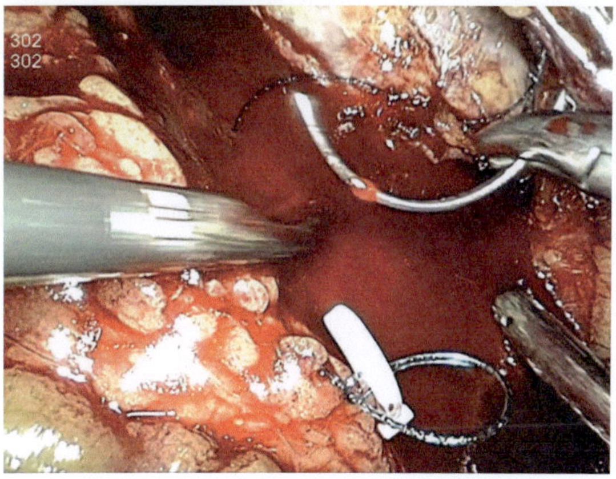

Fig. 11 Suturing the kidney wound

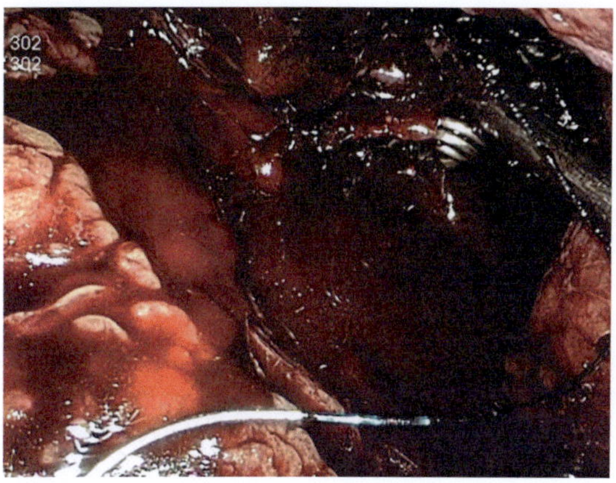

Fig. 12 Checking the wound after suturing

Expert Commentary

The main points of concern for laparoscopic partial nephrectomy are as follows: (1) the location of the tumor, (2) the size of the tumor, (3) the time of renal artery occlusion, and (4) suturing techniques. The location of the tumor growth determines the surgical method and also has a significant impact on suturing. The size of the tumor determines the range of resection. When removing the tumor, it should be cut as close to the tumor capsule as possible, which can both preserve normal kidney tissue and completely remove the tumor. It is important to note that the tumor capsule should not be cut to avoid tumor implantation. There is no specific time limit for renal occlusion, but it is generally best to control it within 30 min, which requires skilled suturing techniques.

The principle of renal artery treatment: Before the operation, the patient's preoperative renal artery angiogram should be carefully reviewed. In this case, the preoperative renal artery angiogram showed that there were multiple renal arteries supplying blood to the lower pole of the right kidney, and the preoperative plan should include blocking the main trunk of the renal artery. During the operation, management of the renal artery represents a relatively high-risk surgical maneuver. During the process of freeing and denuding the renal artery, the outer membrane around the renal artery should be appropriately opened, and the renal artery should not be overly exposed but should be fully freed. At the same time, the gap between the renal artery and the renal vein should be fully freed. The operation in between should be gentle to avoid damaging the renal vein. Finally, the renal artery should be blocked with a vascular occlusion clamp while maintaining a certain tension.

Kidney Surgery: Case 15 Laparoscopic Retroperitoneal Radical Nephrectomy for Right Renal Cancer (Radical Resection of Renal Collecting Duct Carcinoma After Neoadjuvant Immunotherapy)

Yi Zhao

Chief Complaint

Diagnosed with right renal collecting duct carcinoma, targeted combined immunotherapy for over 10 months.

Medical History

Male, 68 years old. The patient underwent an examination due to discomfort in the waist in May 2021, and a tumor was found in the right kidney (Fig. 1). A comprehensive PET-CT examination suggested the possibility of a malignant tumor in the right kidney, accompanied by liver capsule metastasis, right adrenal metastasis, bilateral lung metastasis, multiple lymph node metastasis, and bone metastasis that cannot be ruled out. On May 31, 2021, a CT-guided percutaneous biopsy of the right kidney tumor was performed under local anesthesia. The pathological result was poorly differentiated carcinoma of the right kidney tumor. Combined with morphology and immunohistochemistry, there was no evidence supporting urothelial carcinoma, and it was considered to be likely collecting duct carcinoma. Considering the patient was in the late stage of right kidney cancer, with multiple metastases throughout the body, and in poor performance status, surgery was not suitable at the time. The treatment plan was targeted therapy + immunotherapy. The specific plan was oral axitinib 5 mg bid and intravenous application of tislelizumab 200 mg, once every 3 weeks. After

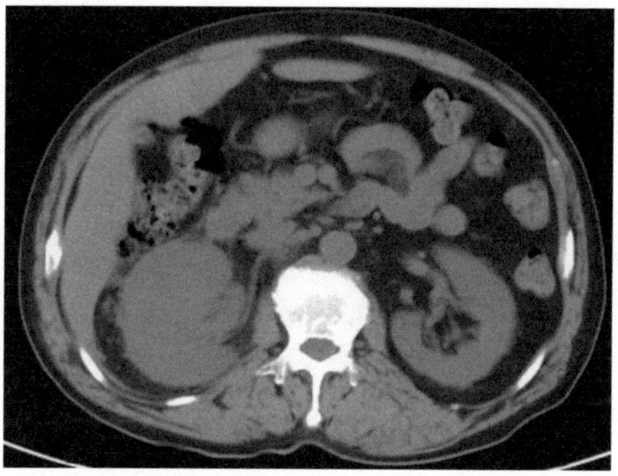

Fig. 1 CT before targeted + immunotherapy

Supplementary Information The online version contains supplementary material available at https://doi.org/10.1007/978-981-96-8598-1_17.

Y. Zhao (✉)
Beijing Union Medical College Hospital,
Beijing, China

Y. Zhang, X. Zhao (eds.), *Laparoscopic Surgery in Urology*,
https://doi.org/10.1007/978-981-96-8598-1_17

the patient completed three courses of immunotherapy, a follow-up abdominal and pelvic enhanced CT showed that the right kidney tumor had shrunk compared to before, the multiple enlarged lymph nodes in the retroperitoneal space had become smaller, and the lung metastases had shrunk. After completing six courses of immunotherapy, a follow-up PET-CT on October 8, 2021, showed the following: The volume of the right kidney had decreased, the metabolically active tumor in the original right kidney area was mostly not obvious this time, only the metabolism of the right kidney collecting system was increased, the original liver capsule metastasis and the uneven metabolism of the whole body bone marrow were not shown this time, the original right adrenal metastasis area was not obvious this time, the original multiple metastatic lymph nodes had decreased and become smaller compared to before, the metastatic nodules in the right upper lobe of the lung had decreased and the metabolism had decreased compared to before, and the original right lung micronodules were not shown. On October 8, 2021, no obvious bone metastasis was seen in the whole body bone scan. Considering the treatment was effective, targeted + immunotherapy was continued. After the fifth course of immunotherapy, the patient developed hypothyroidism and was given levothyroxine sodium 100 mg bid to supplement thyroid hormone. After the sixth course of immunotherapy, the patient developed liver and kidney function damage and was given polyene phosphatidylcholine 456 mg bid and glucuronolactone 100 mg bid for liver protection treatment. From October to November 2021, due to obvious chest tightness and shortness of breath, axitinib was reduced to 2.5 mg bid, and after the reduction, the chest tightness and shortness of breath did not significantly improve, so the dose was further reduced to 2.5 mg qd, and the chest tightness and shortness of breath improved compared to before. On November 24, 2021, a follow-up chest and abdominal pelvic plain CT scan showed a metastatic tumor in the right upper lobe of the lung, which was slightly smaller than before, and the primary lesion in the right kidney and the metastatic lymph nodes in the retroperitoneal space were roughly the same as before. A follow-up liver and kidney function and thyroid function test showed that the liver and kidney function had basically returned to normal levels, and the thyroid function had significantly improved compared to before. In December 2021, axitinib was restored to 2.5 mg bid, and then the patient experienced headaches and shortness of breath. In January 2022, axitinib was reduced to 2.5 mg qd. On February 8, 2022, the patient completed the 12th course of immunotherapy. During the hospitalization, an enhanced CT (Fig. 2) and PET-CT evaluation were performed. The patient's primary lesion was basically the same as before, the nodules in the right upper lobe of the lung were slightly smaller than before, some of the multiple lymph nodes throughout the body had shrunk compared to before, and the metabolism had decreased, but a new enhancing nodule was seen in the medial limb of the right adrenal gland, suggesting metastasis. Considering all factors, targeted + immunotherapy was continued, and at the same time, axitinib was adjusted to 2.5 mg bid and 2.5 mg qd to be taken every other day while continuing regular immunotherapy. The patient's diagnosis of right renal collecting duct carcinoma is basically clear, with multiple metastases throughout the body. After targeted combined immunotherapy, the right adrenal gland showed progression, while the remaining metastatic lesions and primary lesions decreased and shrank. It is planned to perform laparoscopic

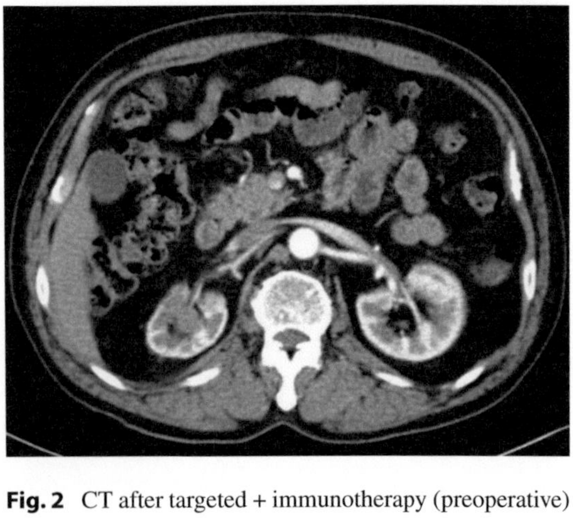

Fig. 2 CT after targeted + immunotherapy (preoperative)

right nephrectomy + right adrenal gland removal surgery (open surgery as a backup).

Past History

Postoperative hydrocele of the left testicle.

Physical Examination

No special findings in the heart, lungs, and abdomen, no percussion pain in both renal areas.

Imaging Data (Figs. 1 and 2)

Preoperative Assessment

The patient's imaging examination suggests that the right renal carcinoma has significantly shrunk compared to before, a new metastatic lesion is seen in the right adrenal gland, and the original lung metastatic lesions and multiple lymph node lesions have shrunk compared to before. Considering the patient's clinical data and general condition, it is considered that the best time to perform surgical treatment to remove the right kidney and right adrenal gland lesions is now. Renal blood flow imaging suggests that the perfusion function of the left kidney is normal and the perfusion function of the right kidney is slightly poor. The surgical method is laparoscopic radical right renal carcinoma + right adrenal gland removal surgery.

Surgical Process

1. The retroperitoneal approach was adopted, with the patient in the left lateral position. Preoperative CT assessment showed heavy adhesions around the kidney, and this surgery used four holes (3 cm above the xiphoid process on the midaxillary line, below the 12th rib on the posterior axillary line, below the 12th rib on the anterior axillary line, and between the first and third holes). The surgical side was marked in the ward before surgery. General anesthesia with endotracheal intubation was used. A urinary catheter was placed. Routine disinfection and draping.
2. After establishing pneumoperitoneum, the extraperitoneal fat was cleaned, the peritoneal reflection was identified, and Gerota's fascia was longitudinally opened on the back side of the peritoneal reflection, revealing the psoas major muscle and perirenal fat pad (Fig. 3).
3. Along the surface of the psoas major muscle, the perirenal fat pad was fully freed along the plane of the psoas major muscle toward the head side, and the right renal artery was found and fully freed at the symmetrical position of the arcuate ligament on the inner side of the surface of the psoas major muscle and

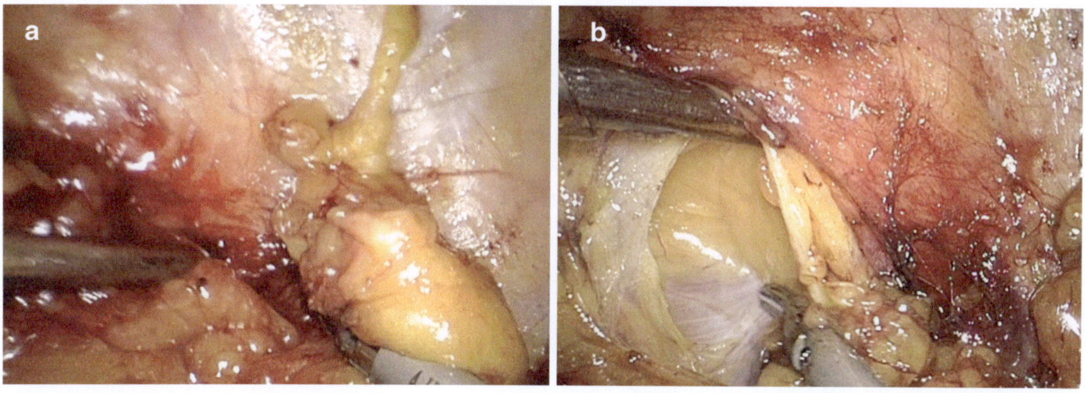

Fig. 3 (**a**, **b**) During the operation, Gerota's fascia was opened, revealing the psoas major muscle and perirenal fat pad

the inner edge of the psoas major muscle (Fig. 4). Two Hem-o-loks were applied at the proximal end of the right renal artery, and one Hem-o-lok was applied at the distal end to block it, and then the right renal artery was severed (Fig. 5).

4. Below and behind the right renal artery, using a combination of blunt and sharp methods, the right renal vein was found and freed. Hem-o-lok was used to clamp and sever it (Fig. 6).
5. Locate and sever the ureter at the lower pole of the kidney (Fig. 7), completely freeing the right kidney.
6. Continue to free the right renal perirenal fat pad along the psoas major muscle and peritoneum, freeing the upper pole and lateral and dorsal sides. The upper pole of the right renal perirenal fat pad is heavily adhered to the peritoneum (Fig. 8).
7. Carefully separate the renal perirenal fat pad from the peritoneum, locate the central vein of the right adrenal gland next to the inferior vena cava, fully free it, tie it with a Hem-o-Lok, and sever it (Fig. 9).
8. Use an ultrasonic dissector to sever the blood supply around the renal perirenal fat pad and adrenal fat pad until the right kidney and right adrenal gland are completely removed (Fig. 10).
9. After careful hemostasis, insert a specimen bag through the auxiliary hole, and place the right kidney and right adrenal gland in the bag. Place a drainage tube. Finally, after enlarging the auxiliary hole incision, the specimen is completely removed.

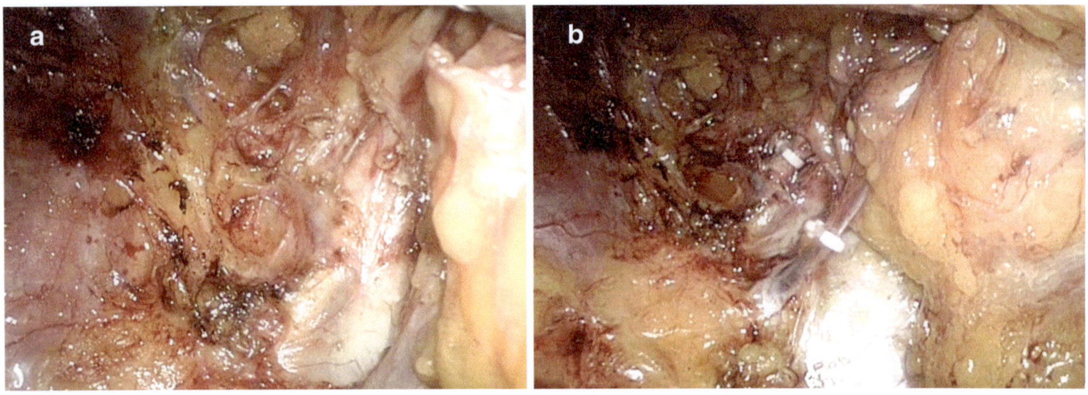

Fig. 4 (**a**, **b**) Finding the renal artery

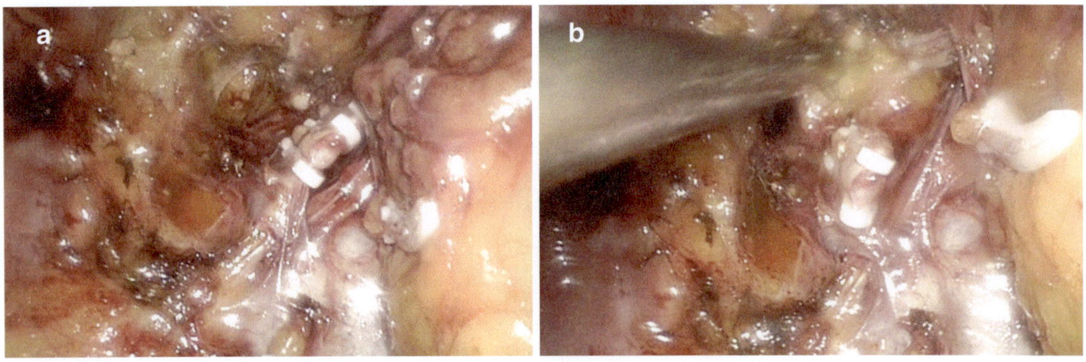

Fig. 5 (**a**, **b**) Hem-o-lok blocking the renal artery

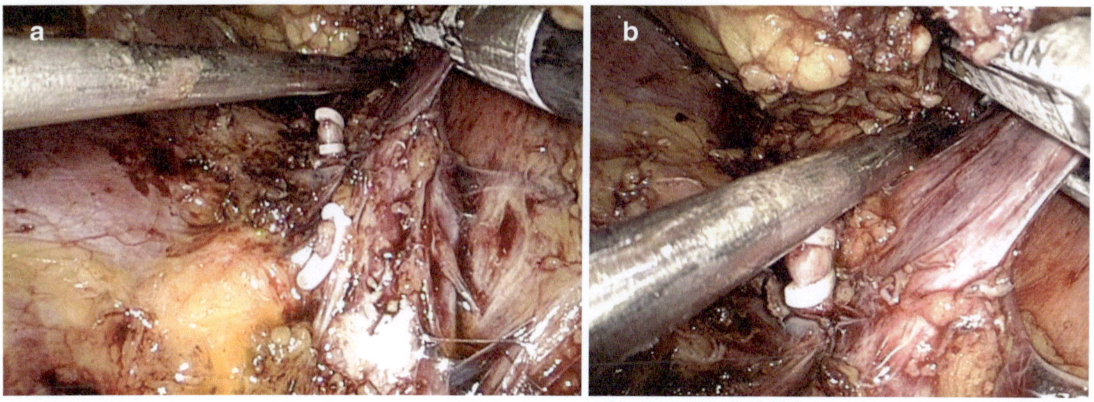

Fig. 6 (**a**, **b**) Locating and severing the renal vein

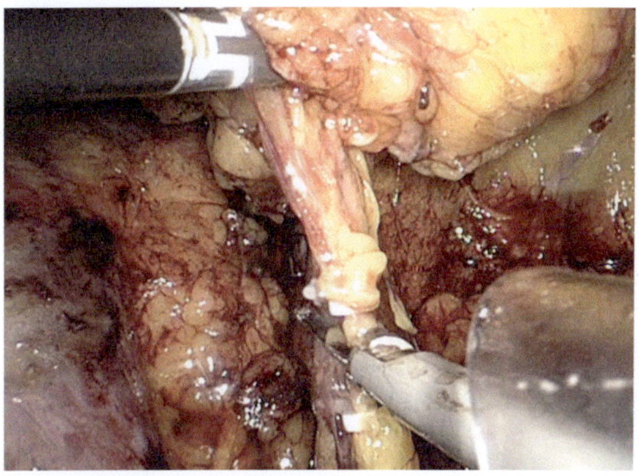

Fig. 7 Freeing and severing the ureter

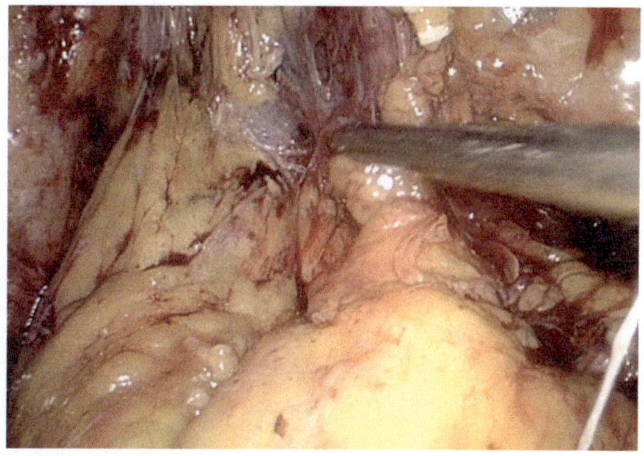

Fig. 8 Freeing the right renal perirenal fat pad (heavy adhesion at the upper pole)

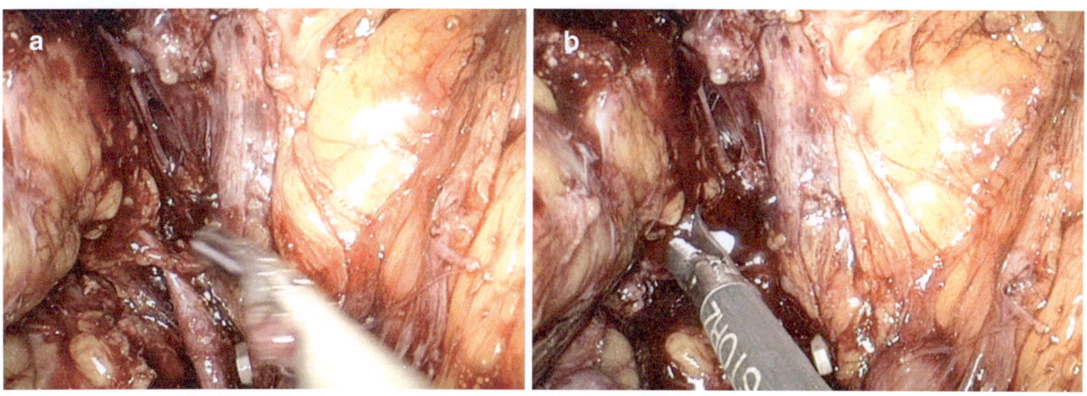

Fig. 9 (**a**, **b**) Freeing and severing the central vein of the adrenal gland

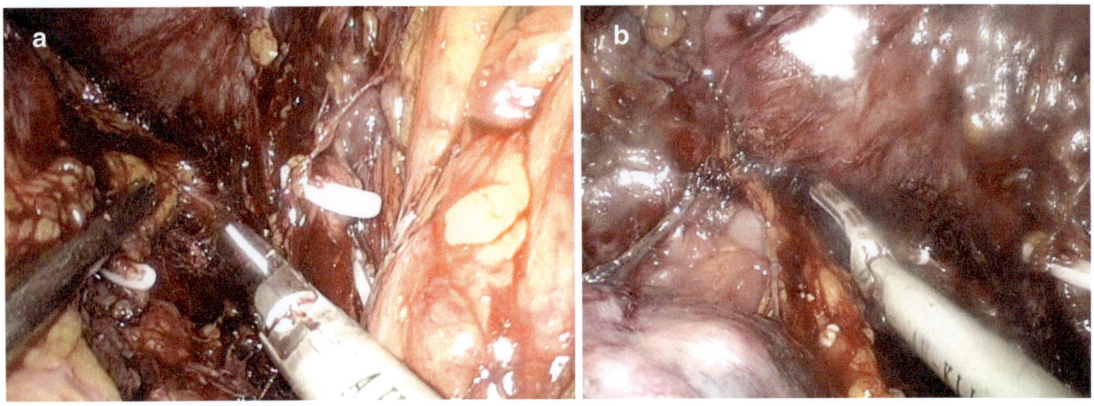

Fig. 10 (**a**, **b**) Complete removal of the right adrenal gland

Expert Commentary

Choice of surgical method and timing: For patients with advanced renal cancer, the traditional treatment method is targeted + surgical treatment, and presently targeted + immune + surgical treatment can usually be chosen. This patient had a good response to targeted + immune therapy; the tumor shrank significantly, creating favorable conditions for surgery. It should be noted that patients who have undergone targeted/targeted + immune therapy often face the problem of heavy adhesion of perirenal fat, which increases the difficulty of freeing the kidney during surgery. Care must be taken not to damage the renal capsule and renal parenchyma.

Handling of renal hilum vessels: In radical nephrectomy, the handling of renal hilum vessels is a relatively high-risk surgical step. During the process of freeing and exposing the vessels, it is necessary to maintain a certain degree of tension in the renal hilum vessels. Care must be taken to be gentle during operation to avoid tearing the vessels, especially the renal vein, which has a thin wall and requires extra caution when freeing. In addition, sometimes the patient may have multiple renal artery branches at the same time. Before surgery, it is necessary to carefully read the film, predict the number and course of the renal arteries through imaging examinations, and before ligating the renal vein during surgery, make sure to carefully check the renal hilum to ensure that all renal arteries have been severed.

Kidney Surgery: Case 16 Laparoscopic Retroperitoneal Partial Nephrectomy of the Right Kidney (Use of Intraoperative Ultrasound Localization)

Wenda Wang

Chief Complaint

Eight months after surgery for left renal clear cell carcinoma, a right kidney tumor was discovered one month ago.

Medical History

Female, 69 years old. The patient sought treatment at a local hospital for back pain following a fall 8 months ago. CT and MRI scans revealed a slightly low-density nodule on the dorsal side of the left kidney (report not available). Further consultation at our hospital and a complete urinary system ultrasound suggested a solid mass in the left kidney, with malignancy not excluded. One month later, a partial nephrectomy of the left kidney was performed under general anesthesia. Postoperative pathology reported: (left renal tumor) renal clear cell carcinoma, grade 2, no tumor identified on the cut surface; additionally, multiple foci of small lymphocyte infiltration were observed in the surrounding kidney tissue, suggesting involvement of small B-cell lymphoma/chronic lymphocytic leukemia. Immunohistochemistry results: PAX-8 (+), AE1/AE3 (+), CD10 (+), CK7 (−), MA (+), P504 (+), RCC (+), TFE3 (−), vimentin (+), CA9 (+), CD20 (diffuse positive in peripheral lymphocytes), CD3 (scattered positive in peripheral lymphocytes), Bcl-2 (+), Bcl-6 (−), and CD21 (focal positive in FDC). The patient recovered well after surgery and was discharged. One month prior, the patient had another fall and developed back pain, described as acid bilges feeling, with an NRS score reaching up to 8, worsening when turning over and standing, accompanied by bilateral hip pain. An MRI scan at another hospital showed abnormal signals in the right kidney. The patient then sought treatment at our hospital. A follow-up chest-abdomen-pelvis CT scan showed a slightly low-density round shadow on the posterior lip of the right kidney, about 1.5 cm in diameter. The lesion demonstrated significant enhancement in the arterial phase, with decreased enhancement in the venous and delayed phases, and RCC cannot be excluded (Figs. 1 and 2). The patient denied discomfort such as hematuria, and lumbar mass. She was admitted to the hospital for treatment of the right kidney tumor.

Supplementary Information The online version contains supplementary material available at https://doi.org/10.1007/978-981-96-8598-1_18.

W. Wang (✉)
Beijing Union Medical College Hospital, Beijing, China

Y. Zhang, X. Zhao (eds.), *Laparoscopic Surgery in Urology*, https://doi.org/10.1007/978-981-96-8598-1_18

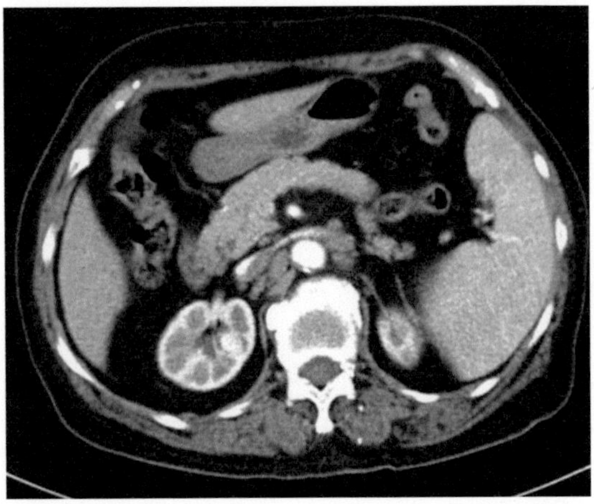

Fig. 1 Preoperative CT (arterial phase)

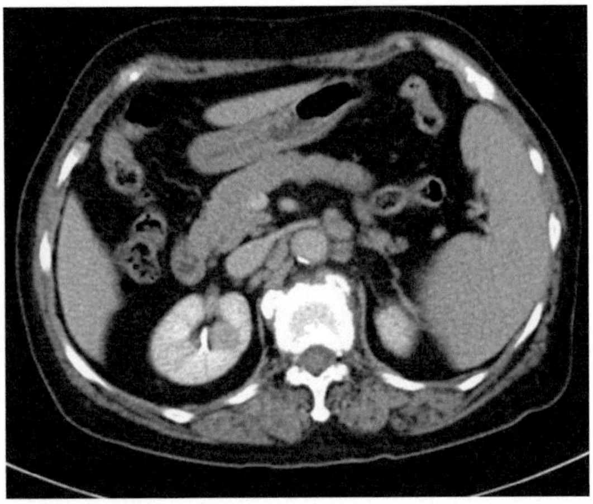

Fig. 2 Preoperative CT (venous phase)

Past History

Hypertension for more than 20 years, with BPmax 160/110 mmHg, usually taking one tablet of losartan potassium and hydrochlorothiazide once daily. History of chronic lymphocytic leukemia for 8 years. Eight months ago, she underwent percutaneous L1 vertebroplasty under local anesthesia due to a fall-induced fracture, along with L1 vertebral lesion puncture biopsy, and needle tract cement occlusion. On January 18, 2022, due to another fall-induced fracture, she underwent percutaneous T11 vertebroplasty under local anesthesia, as well as T11 vertebral lesion puncture biopsy, and needle tract cement occlusion.

Physical Examination

BP 148/83 mmHg. No anormal findings in the heart and lungs. An old surgical scar can be seen on the left abdomen. No bulging in both renal regions. Percussion of the right renal region elicits a dull aching and distending sensation, while no percussion pain in the left renal region. No tenderness is present along the course of both ureters, and the bladder is not distended.

Imaging Data (Figs. 1 and 2)

Preoperative Assessment

The patient's imaging examination suggests a 1.5 cm low-density shadow in the right kidney; enhanced scanning shows "fast in and fast out" enhancement characteristics, indicating a high probability of renal carcinoma. Combined with the patient's clinical data, the diagnosis of a right kidney tumor is basically clear, and renal carcinoma is suspected. The indications for surgery are clear. Further outpatient supplementary assessment of cardiopulmonary function showed no obvious abnormalities. Chest CT showed no evidence of distant metastasis. Renal blood flow imaging suggested that the GFR of both kidneys was 48.5 ml/(min·1.73 m^2), with the GFR of the right kidney being 28.5 ml/(min·1.73 m^2), and the GFR of the left kidney being 20.0 ml/(min·1.73 m^2). The surgical approach adopted was laparoscopic partial nephrectomy of the right kidney.

Surgical Process

1. The retroperitoneal upper urinary tract surgical approach was adopted. The surgical side was marked in the ward before surgery. General anesthesia with intubation was administered. A urinary catheter was placed. Routine disinfection and draping were performed.
2. After establishing pneumoperitoneum, the upper urinary tract surgical access was placed. Four ports were used in this surgery.

3. The extraperitoneal fat was dissected, the peritoneal reflection was identified, and the renal fascia was longitudinally opened on the dorsal side of the peritoneal reflection, exposing the psoas major muscle and the perirenal fat capsule (Fig. 3).
4. The perirenal fat capsule was fully freed along the surface of the psoas major muscle and pushed to the abdominal side. The arcuate ligament on the surface of the psoas major muscle was identified, and the right renal artery was found and freed at the symmetrical position of the ligament and the inner edge of the psoas major muscle (Fig. 4).
5. The perirenal fat capsule was fully freed along all surfaces of the kidney (Fig. 5).
6. The tumor location was identified by intraoperative ultrasound, and the tumor contour was outlined using a monopolar hook, and confirmation was re-obtained with ultrasound (Fig. 6).
7. The renal artery was occluded using a vascular occlusion clamp (Fig. 7). The renal parenchyma was incised along the outlined contour, and the tumor was located and resected (Fig. 8).
8. During the tumor resection, there was significant bleeding from the incision surface. The renal artery occlusion was checked, and another artery clamp was applied at the distal end (Fig. 9).
9. After the complete removal of the tumor, hemostasis of the wound surface was performed using a monopolar electrocautery (Fig. 10).
10. Using a layered suturing method, the tumor base was continuously sutured with 3-0 V-Loc (Fig. 11). After tightening, the wound surface was continuously sutured with 1-0 V-Loc (Fig. 12). The suture ends were secured with Hem-o-lok.
11. The arterial occlusion clamp was removed, and the renal hilum and renal wound surface were checked for active bleeding (Fig. 13).
12. Through the auxiliary hole, a specimen bag was placed, and the right kidney tumor was put into the bag (Fig. 14). A drainage tube was placed (Fig. 15). Finally, after enlarging the auxiliary hole incision, the specimen was completely removed.

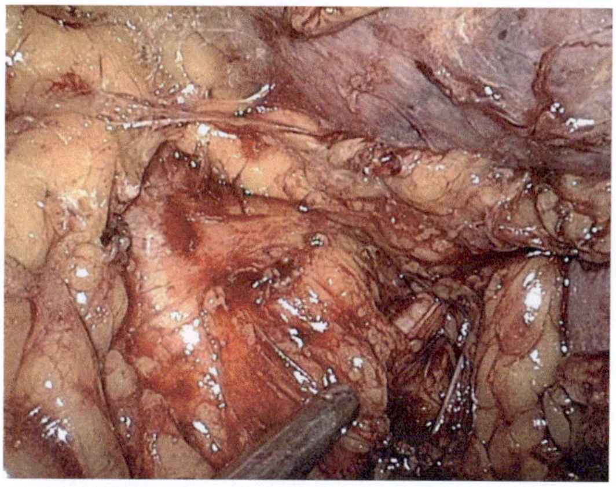

Fig. 4 Freeing the renal artery

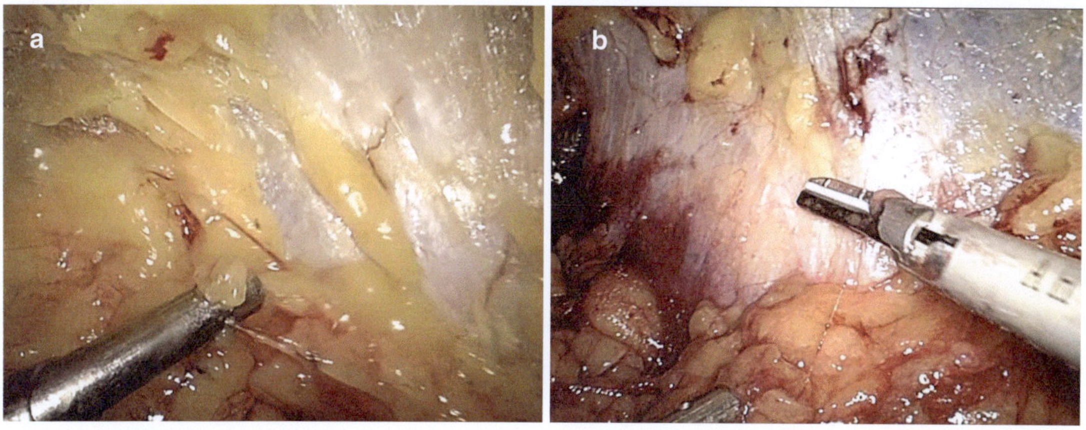

Fig. 3 (**a**, **b**) Opening the renal fascia

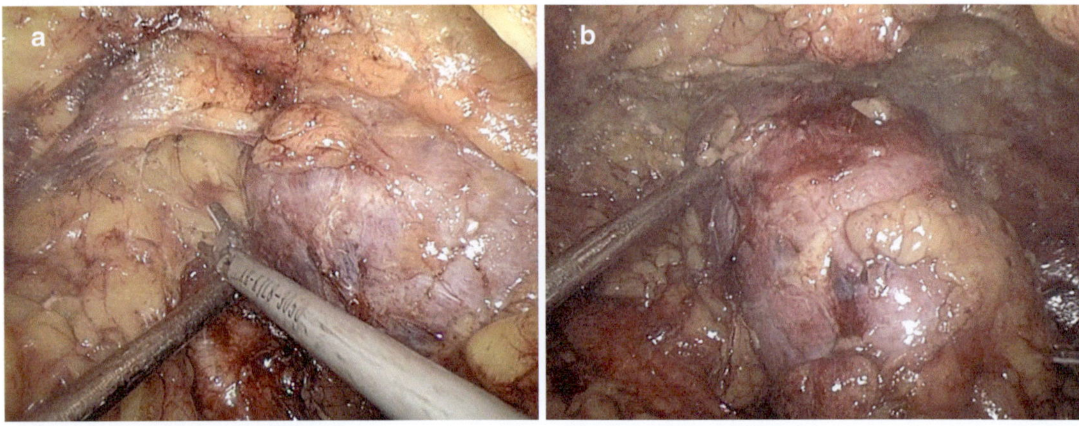

Fig. 5 (**a**, **b**) Fully freeing the perirenal fat

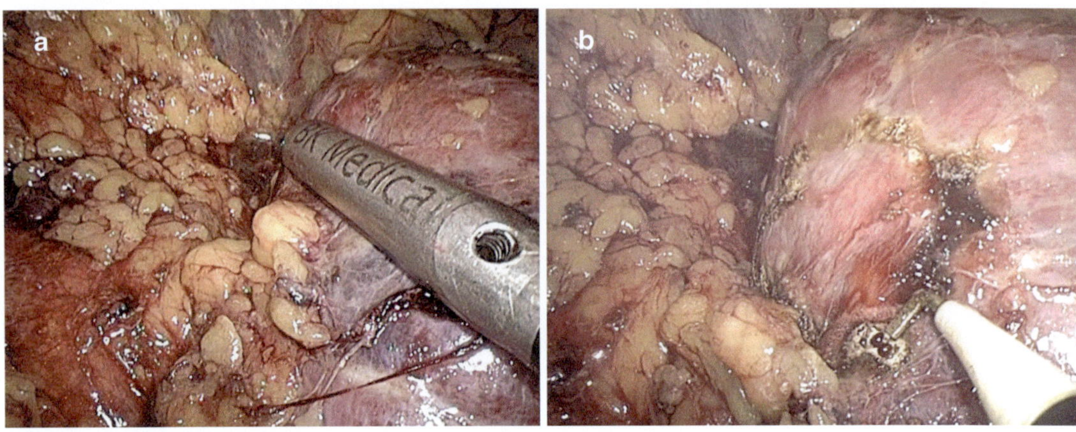

Fig. 6 (**a**, **b**) Intraoperative ultrasound location and outlining of the tumor contour

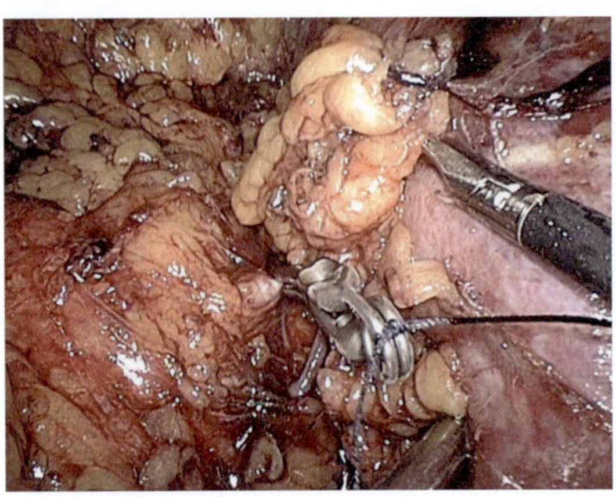

Fig. 7 Occluding the renal artery

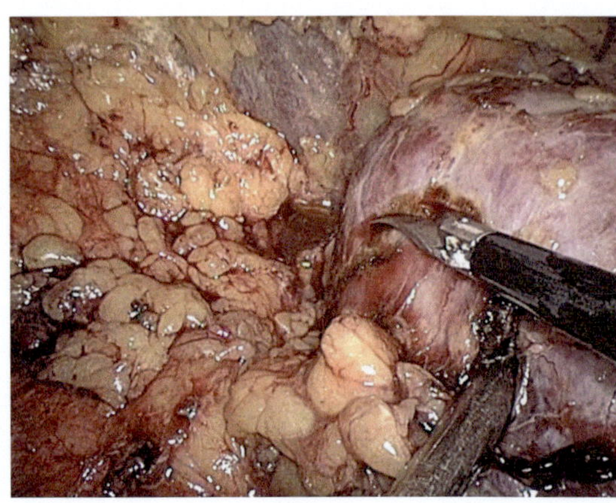

Fig. 8 Cutting the renal parenchyma and removing the tumor

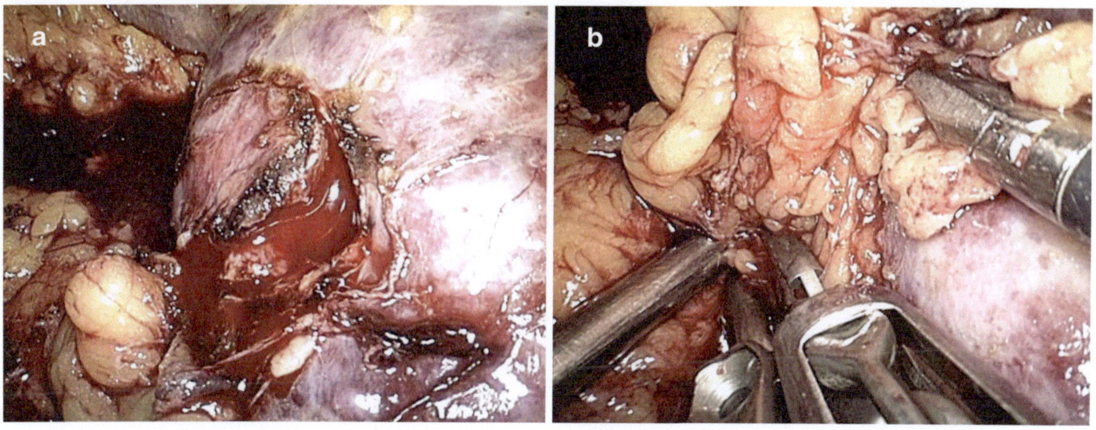

Fig. 9 (**a**, **b**) Significant bleeding from the wound, and the occlusion of the artery was enhanced

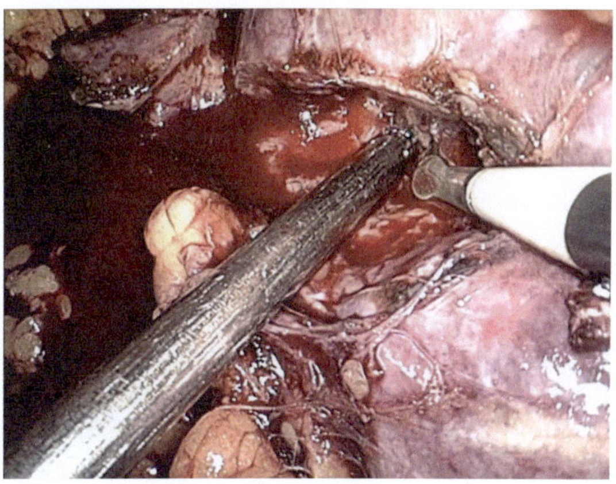

Fig. 10 Enhanced hemostasis of the wound surface

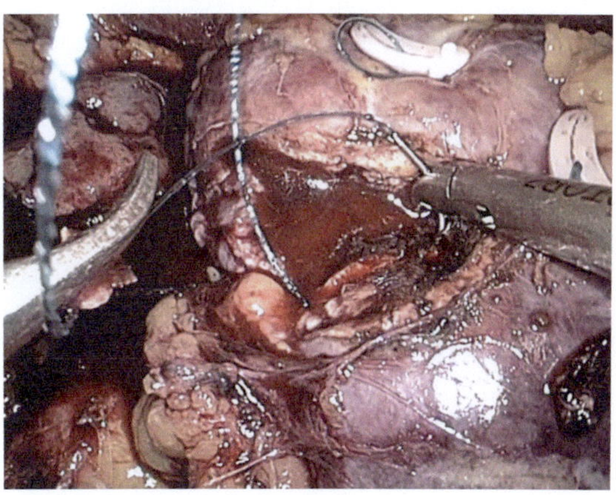

Fig. 11 Suturing the base with 3-0 V-Loc

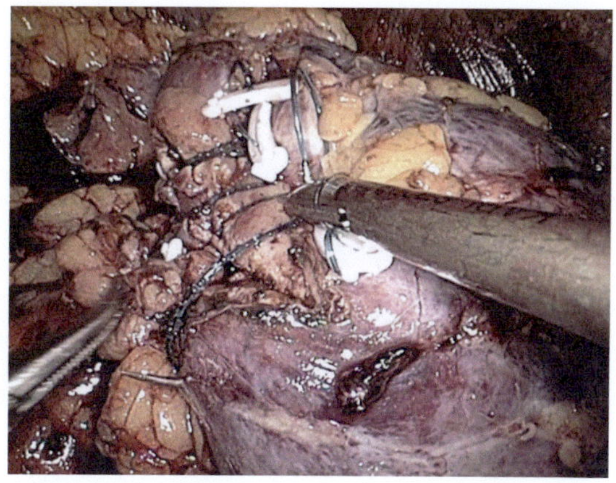

Fig. 12 Suturing the wound surface with 1-0 V-Loc

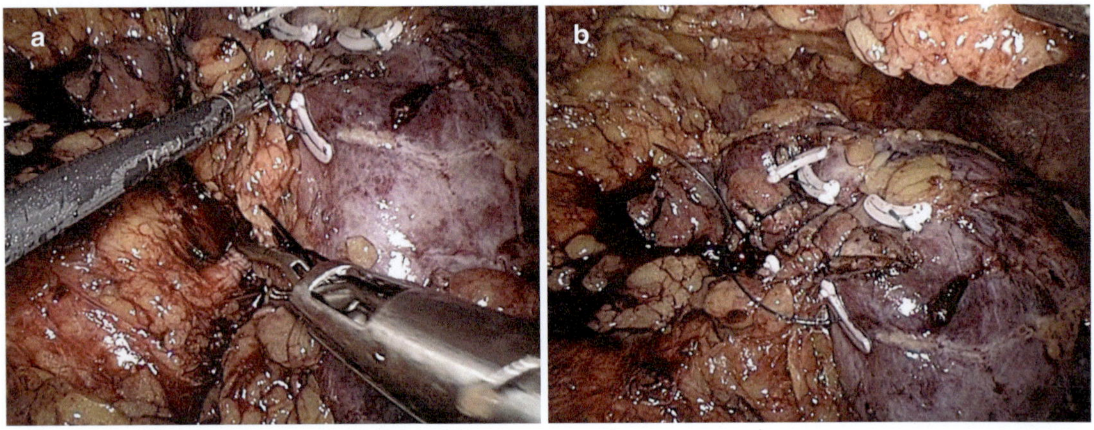

Fig. 13 (**a**, **b**) Removal of occlusion, observation of bleeding

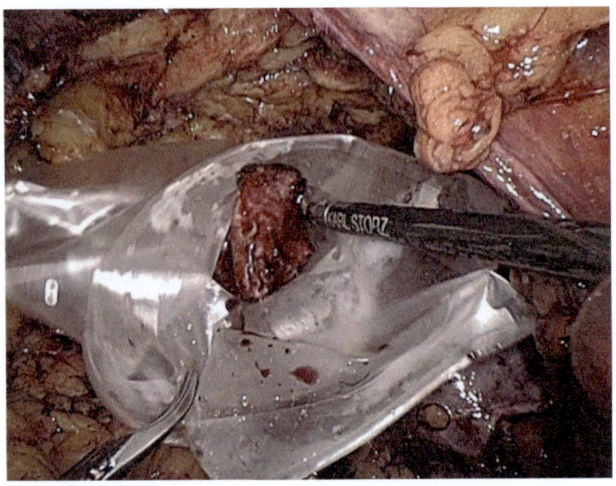

Fig. 14 Tumor placed in the specimen bag

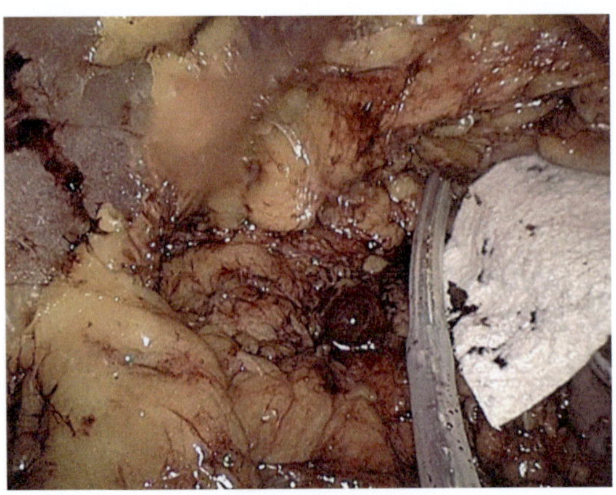

Fig. 15 Placement of the drainage tube

Expert Commentary

The patient had tumors in both kidneys and had undergone surgery on the left kidney. Considering the location and size of the tumor, partial nephrectomy was still the first choice for the right kidney tumor. The surgical approach chosen was laparoscopic retroperitoneal surgery because the tumor was located at the posterior lip of the right kidney. It was necessary to fully mobilize the right kidney to gain greater mobility, which would facilitate the operation of tumor removal. The tumor was endogenous, and its location could not be clearly identified from the surface of the kidney during surgery. Therefore, intraoperative ultrasound was very important for determining the location of the tumor.

Although renal artery occlusion was performed during surgery, some patients still had significant bleeding from the cut surface when the tumor was removed, indicating that the occlusion effect was not good. Therefore, it is necessary to fully understand the renal artery situation before surgery, pay attention to the number and location of renal arteries, and fully occlude before tumor removal; adjustments can be made to renal artery occlusion during the removal process to reduce bleeding from the cut surface and avoid affecting surgical operations. After the tumor is removed, the suturing of the wound surface should be accurate, and the suturing effect should be checked for satisfaction after the occlusion is released.

Kidney Surgery: Case 17 Laparoscopic Retroperitoneal Partial Nephrectomy (Treatment of Cystic Renal Carcinoma)

Wenda Wang

Chief Complaint

Renal cyst was found in the right kidney during physical examination 2 years ago.

Medical History

Female, 54 years old. The patient was found to have "bilateral renal cysts" (no report available) during a physical examination via ultrasound 2 years ago. She had no symptoms such as back pain, change in urine color, urinary urgency, frequent urination, or dysuria, and was advised to undergo regular follow-up examinations. In October 2020, a follow-up urinary ultrasound at our hospital showed a cyst in the upper pole of the right kidney, measuring 2.3 cm × 1.7 cm, with a medium-strong echo mass inside (approximately 0.8 cm in diameter), and a cyst in the upper pole of the left kidney, about 1.9 cm in diameter. Subsequent CTU showed a mixed low-density cyst in the upper pole of the right kidney, about 2.1 cm × 1.8 cm in size, with unclear boundaries, irregular adjacent renal cortex, heterogeneous density, and mild to moderate enhancement after enhancement, and an elliptical cyst in the upper pole of the left kidney, with clear boundaries and enhancement of the cyst septum after contrast administration. Malignancy of the cyst in the upper pole of the right kidney cannot be completely ruled out, and the cyst in the upper pole of the left kidney (was classified as Bosniak II type) (Figs. 1 and 2). Now for further diagnosis and treatment,

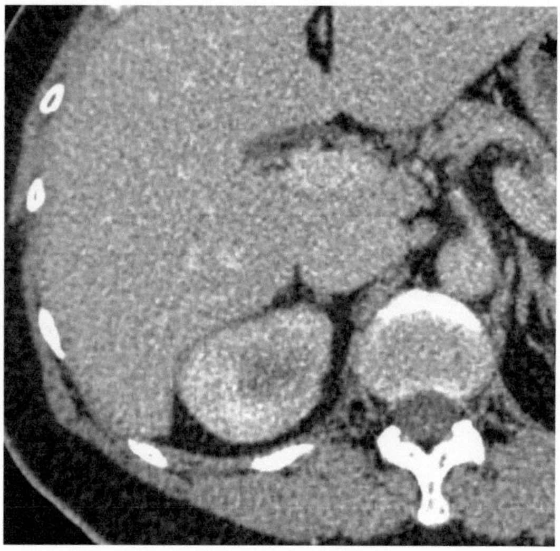

Fig. 1 Preoperative CT (cross section)

Supplementary Information The online version contains supplementary material available at https://doi.org/10.1007/978-981-96-8598-1_19.

W. Wang (✉)
Beijing Union Medical College Hospital,
Beijing, China

Y. Zhang, X. Zhao (eds.), *Laparoscopic Surgery in Urology*,
https://doi.org/10.1007/978-981-96-8598-1_19

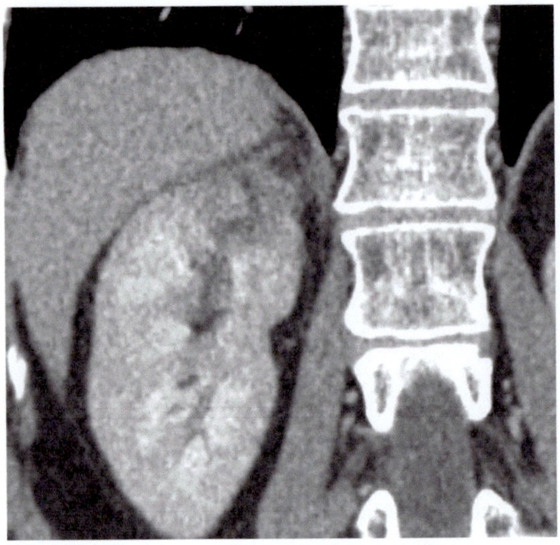

Fig. 2 Preoperative CT (coronal plane)

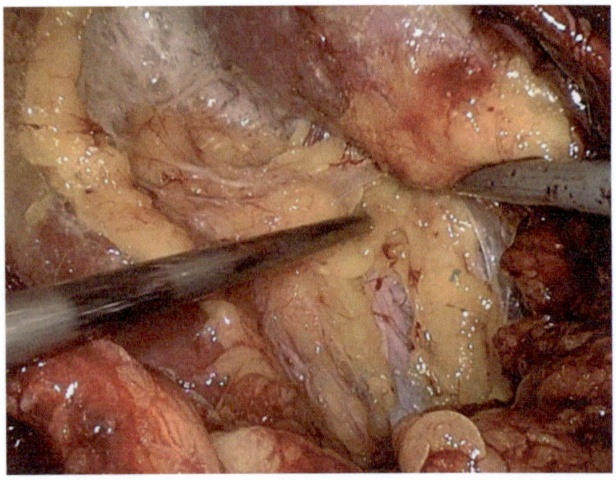

Fig. 3 Finding the renal artery along the course of the inferior vena cava

she was admitted to our department with the admission diagnosis of "bilateral renal cysts."

Past History

Denies a history of chronic disease history or surgical history.

Physical Examination

No abnormal findings were noted in the heart and lungs. There was no bulging in the upper abdomen or bilateral back regions, and no masses were palpable. There was no percussion tenderness in the bilateral renal regions, and no tenderness along the course of the bilateral ureters. The bladder area showed no distension and no tenderness.

Imaging Data (Figs. 1 and 2)

Preoperative Assessment

The patient's imaging examination suggests a 2.1 cm × 1.8 cm mixed low-density lesion in the upper pole of the right kidney, with unclear boundaries and mild to moderate enhancement, suggesting a high possibility of malignancy. Combined with the patient's clinical data, the diagnosis of right renal tumor is basically clear, and renal carcinoma is possible. The indication for surgery is clear.

During further outpatient evaluation of cardiac and pulmonary function, no obvious abnormalities were observed. Chest CT showed no evidence of distant metastasis. Renal blood flow imaging suggested that the GFR of both kidneys was 96.48 ml/(min·1.73 m^2), with the GFR of the right kidney was 47.25 ml/ (min·1.73 m^2), and the GFR of the left kidney was 49.23 ml/(min·1.73 m^2). The planned surgical approach is laparoscopic partial nephrectomy of the right kidney.

Surgical Procedure

1. The retroperitoneal approach for upper urinary tract surgery was adopted. The surgical side was marked in the ward before surgery. General anesthesia with intubation was administered. A urinary catheter was placed. Routine disinfection and draping were performed.
2. After establishing pneumoperitoneum, the upper urinary tract surgical access was placed. Four ports were used in this surgery.
3. After cleaning the extraperitoneal fat and identifying the peritoneal reflection, the renal fascia was incised longitudinally on the dorsal side of the peritoneal reflection, exposing the psoas major muscle and the perirenal fat cap-

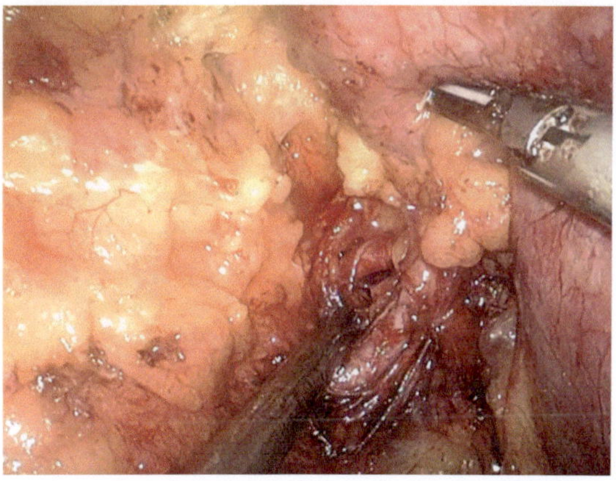

Fig. 4 Dissecting the two branches of the right renal artery

sule (Fig. 3). The right renal artery was located along the course of the inferior vena cava, and the two branches of the right renal artery were carefully dissected (Fig. 4).

4. Fully free the right kidney; the upper pole of the right kidney is severely adhered to the surrounding tissues. Carefully dissect the adhesion (Fig. 5).
5. Outline the tumor using a monopolar hook (Fig. 6).
6. Use a vascular occlusion clamp to occlude the dual renal arteries (Fig. 7). Incise the renal parenchyma along the outlined contour, and resect the tumor (Fig. 8).

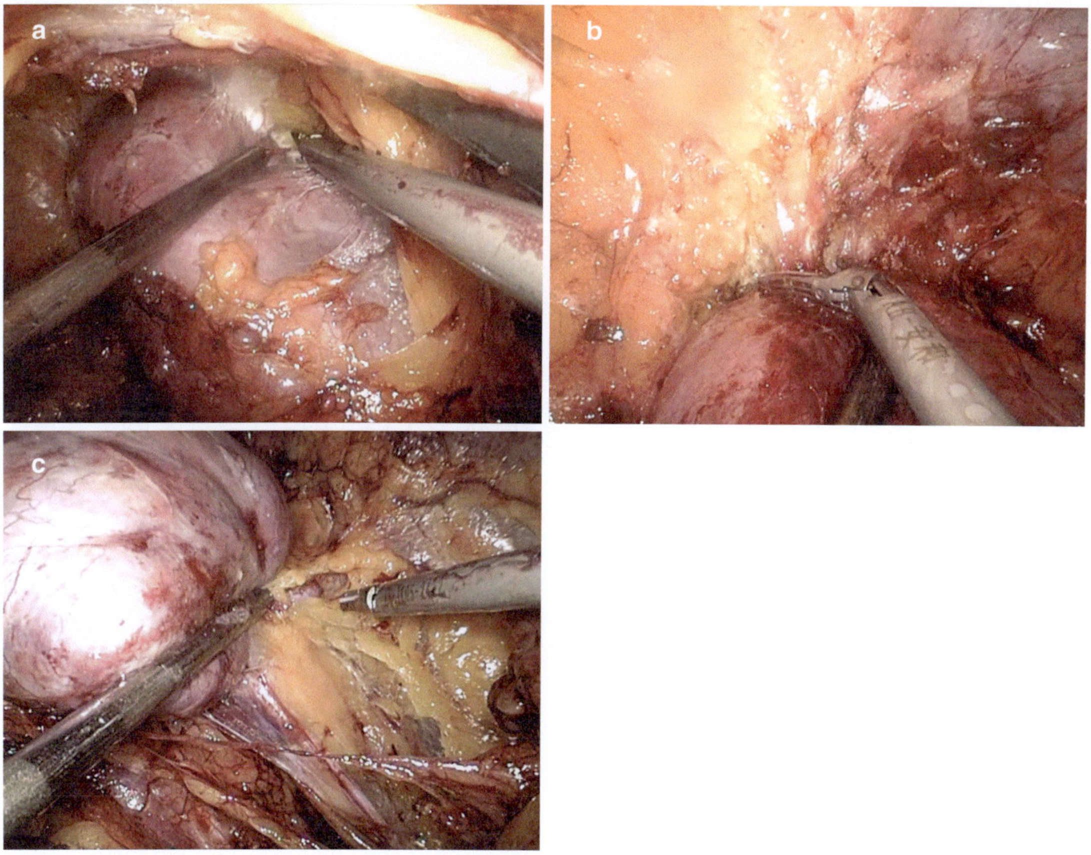

Fig. 5 (**a–c**) Free the right kidney, there is adhesion at the upper pole

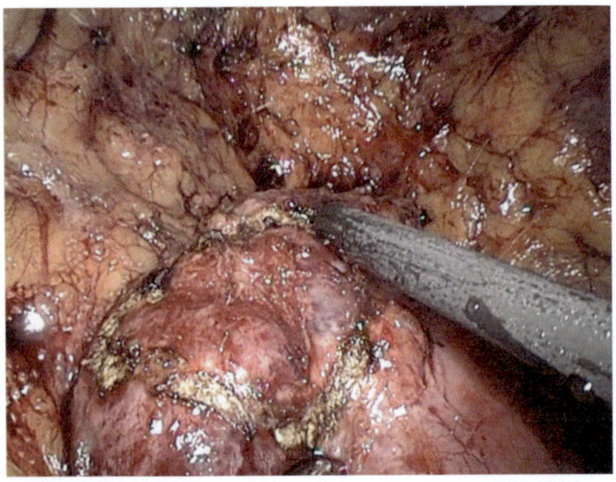

Fig. 6 Outline the tumor with an electric hook

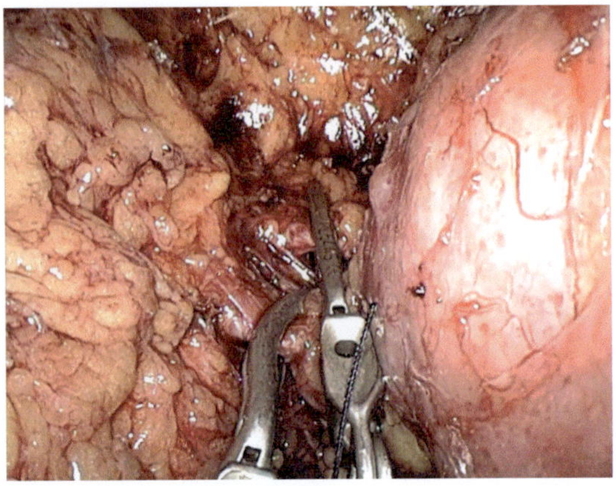

Fig. 7 Block the dual arteries

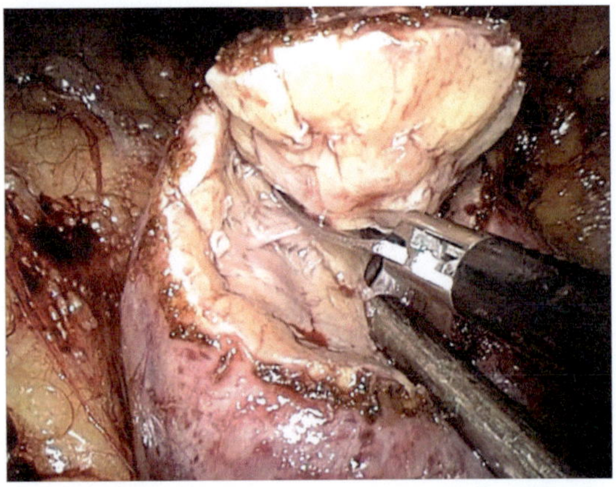

Fig. 8 Remove the tumor

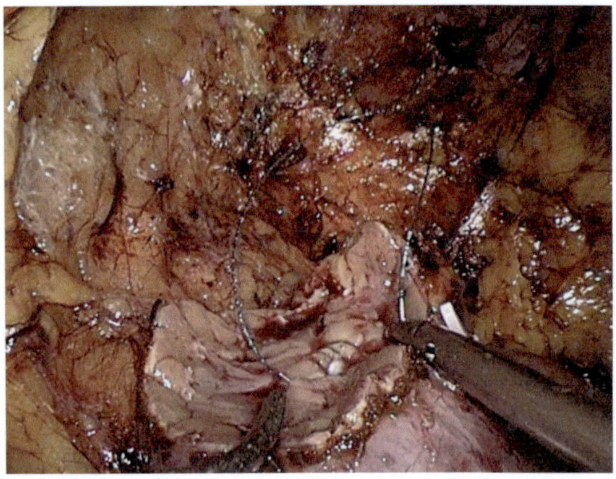

Fig. 9 3-0 V-Loc sutures suture the tumor base

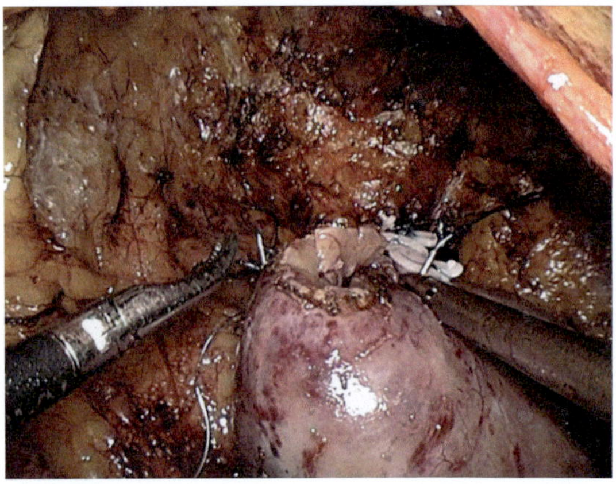

Fig. 10 1-0 V-Loc sutures suture the wound

7. After completely removing the tumor, use 3-0 V-Loc sutures to continuously suture the tumor base (Fig. 9); after tightening, use 1-0 V-Loc sutures to continuously suture the wound (Fig. 10). Secure the end of the suture with a Hem-o-lok clip.
8. Remove the arterial occlusion clamp, check for active bleeding in the renal hilum and renal wound (Fig. 11), and fix the kidney with sutures (Fig. 12).
9. Insert a specimen bag through the auxiliary port, and place the right kidney tumor in the bag (Fig. 13). Place a drainage tube (Fig. 14).

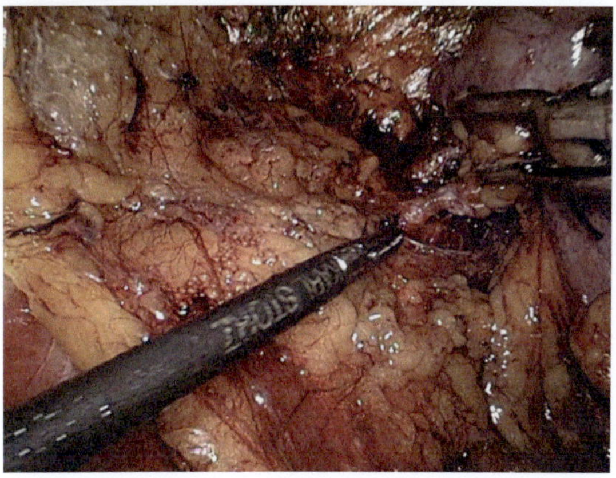

Fig. 11 Remove the occlusion clamp

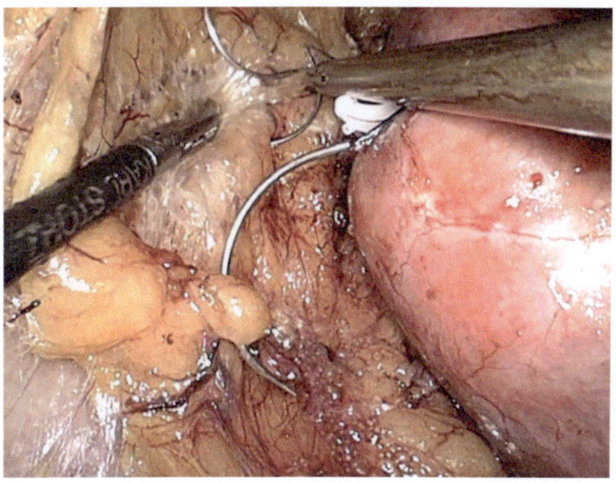

Fig. 12 Fix the kidney

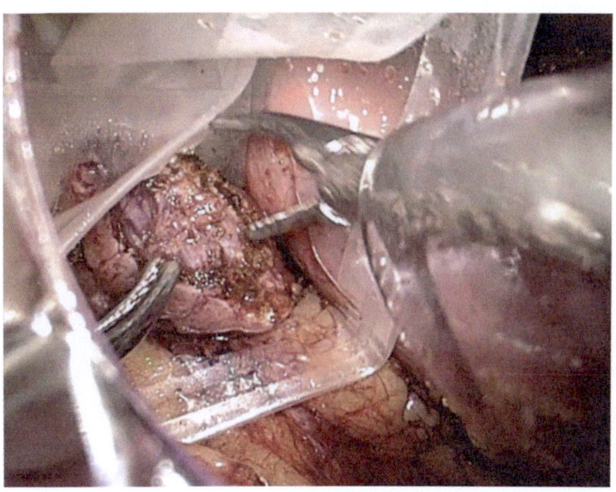

Fig. 13 Tumor placed in specimen bag

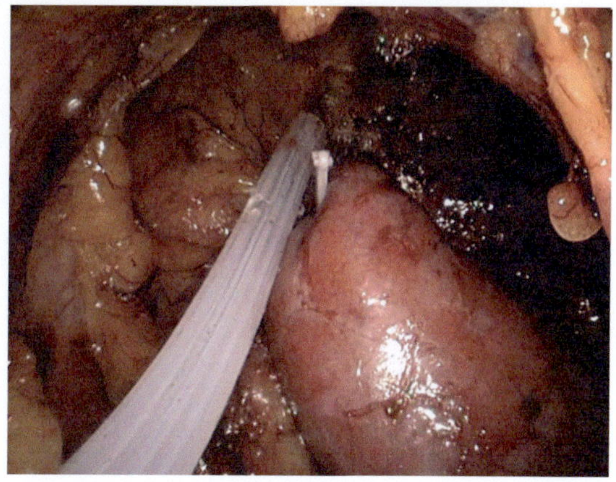

Fig. 14 Placement of drainage tube

Finally, after enlarging the incision of the auxiliary port, the specimen is completely removed.

Expert Commentary

The patient presents with a cystic mass at the upper pole of the right kidney, which is considered to be cystic renal cell carcinoma. Compared with solid masses, cystic masses require greater attention during surgery to avoid rupture. This patient's upper pole of the right kidney is significantly adhered to the surrounding tissues, and extreme care must be exercised during dissection to avoid damaging the kidney and adjacent cystic masses. When defining the range of tumor resection, it is also important to ensure the integrity of the tumor.

The preoperative CT reconstruction of this patient suggested dual renal arteries in the right kidney, guiding the thorough dissection and separation of the two renal arteries during surgery, with each artery clamped separately. There was no obvious bleeding on the surgical surface when the tumor was removed, and the clamping effect was satisfactory. The tumor is located at the upper pole of the right kidney, a relatively high anatomical position. This requires adequate mobilization of the kidney to achieve an optimal surgical field and operating angle. Postoperatively, the mobilized kidney can be fixed to the surrounding tissues.

Kidney Surgery: Case 18 Laparoscopic Retroperitoneal Radical Nephrectomy for Left Renal Carcinoma (Management of Large Renal Tumors)

Jingmin Zhou

Chief Complaint

Left renal tumor discovered 6 months ago. Medical history: Male, 67 years old. Six months ago, the patient was found to have a left renal tumor with a diameter of approximately 4 cm during a physical examination (no report available), and no special measures were taken. Three weeks ago, the patient had a re-examination at another hospital, and an ultrasound revealed a heterogeneous hypoechoic area in the lower pole of the left kidney, measuring approximately 86 mm × 68 mm × 65 mm. Further enhanced CT showed a mixed density mass in the lower pole of the left kidney with unclear boundaries. The enhanced scan showed obvious uneven enhancement, with the larger cross-sectional size about 97 mm × 66 mm. Multiple enlarged lymph nodes were seen in the retroperitoneal space, the larger one measuring about 13 mm × 11 mm. Both kidneys showed round low-density non-enhancing shadows (Fig. 1a, b). PET/CT showed increased FDG metabolism in the left renal mass, multiple nodular FDG metabolism in both lungs, and multiple nodular FDG metabolism in the liver. Considering the medical history, it is highly suspected of left renal carcinoma with multiple metastases. The patient occasionally has back pain but no hematuria, frequent urination, urgency, abdominal pain, or bloating.

Supplementary Information The online version contains supplementary material available at https://doi.org/10.1007/978-981-96-8598-1_20.

J. Zhou (✉)
Beijing Union Medical College Hospital,
Beijing, China
e-mail: zhoujm@pumch.cn

Y. Zhang, X. Zhao (eds.), *Laparoscopic Surgery in Urology*,
https://doi.org/10.1007/978-981-96-8598-1_20

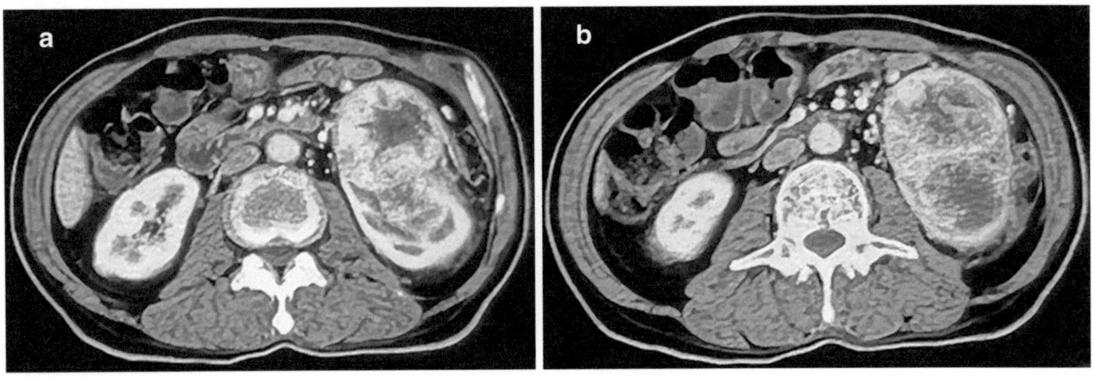

Fig. 1 (**a**, **b**) Preoperative CT

Past History

Diabetes for 2 years, presently controlled with insulin; blood sugar is stable.

Physical Examination

No special findings in the heart and lungs, no bulging in both renal areas, and no percussion pain.

Imaging Data (Fig. 1)

Preoperative Assessment

The patient's imaging examination suggests a tumor in the lower pole of the left kidney, measuring about 8.6 cm × 6.8 cm, with obvious enhancement, suggesting a high possibility of malignancy. Combined with the results of PET/CT, left renal carcinoma, multiple lung metastases, and liver metastases are considered. Considering the patient's clinical data, the diagnosis of left renal tumor is basically clear, with a high possibility of renal carcinoma and metastases in both lungs and liver. Presently, surgical removal of the left renal tumor is considered appropriate. Outpatient assessment of cardiac and pulmonary function showed no obvious abnormalities. Surgical method: laparoscopic radical nephrectomy for left renal carcinoma.

Surgical Procedure

1. Adopt the retroperitoneal upper urinary tract surgical position. The surgical side was marked in the ward before the operation. General anesthesia with endotracheal intubation was used. A urinary catheter was placed. Routine disinfection and draping.
2. After establishing pneumoperitoneum, the tract surgical channel was placed. This operation used four ports.
3. Clean the extraperitoneal fat, identify the peritoneal reflection, and open the Gerota's fascia longitudinally on the dorsal side of the peritoneal reflection to expose the psoas major muscle and the perirenal fat capsule (Fig. 2).
4. The perirenal fat capsule is fully freed along the surface of the psoas major muscle and pushed ventrally. Find the arcuate ligament on the surface of the psoas major muscle, and find the left renal artery at the symmetrical position of the ligament and the inner edge of the psoas major muscle. The artery is clamped and cut off with Hem-o-lok (Fig. 3).
5. Continue to free the left renal vein, which is usually located deep under the left renal artery. The left renal vein is a complex structure, with the central adrenal vein above and the gonadal vein merging below. Free it and disconnect at the distal end of the two merging veins (Fig. 4).

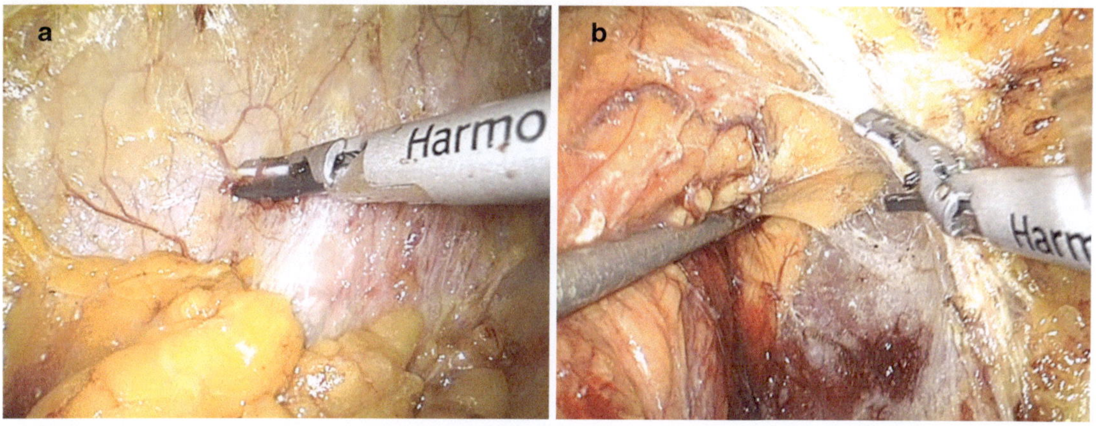

Fig. 2 (**a**, **b**) Clean the extraperitoneal fat, and open the Gerota's fascia

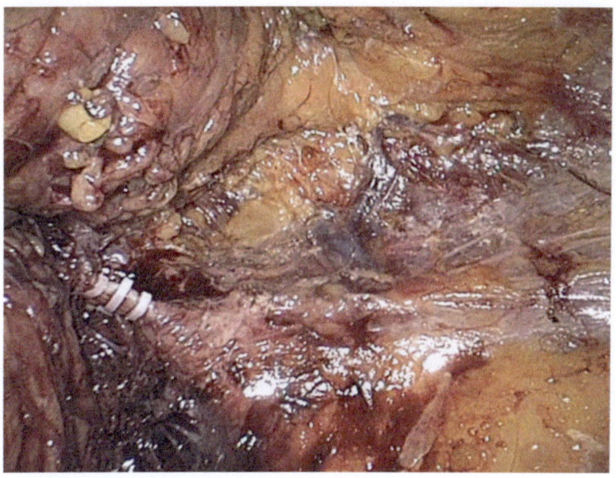

Fig. 3 Locate the renal artery, Hem-o-Lok occlusion and transection

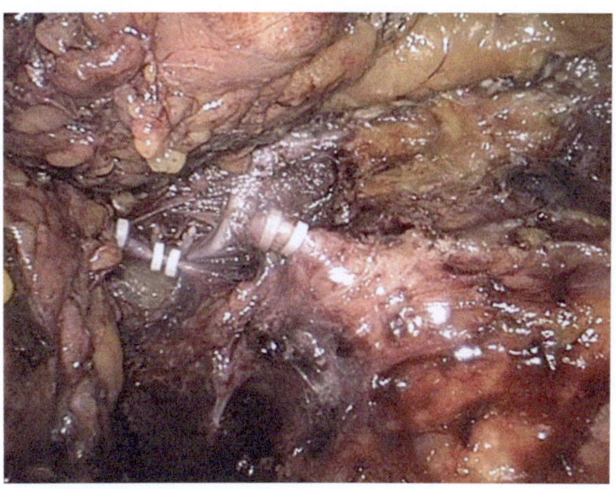

Fig. 4 Find the renal vein behind the renal artery and disconnect

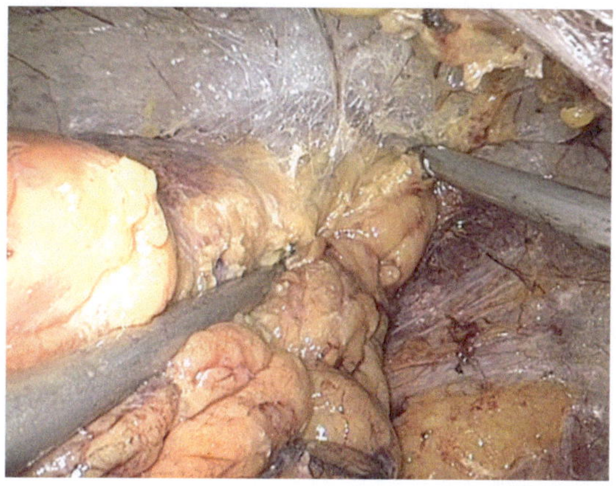

Fig. 5 Completely free the perirenal fat capsule

6. Free along the perirenal fat capsule, and completely remove the kidney, tumor, and perirenal fat capsule (Fig. 5).
7. Separate the upper pole of the kidney from the adrenal gland, preserving the adrenal tissue (Fig. 6).
8. Free the lower pole of the left kidney, locate and disconnect the left ureter, and completely free the left kidney (Fig. 7).
9. The ventral kidney tumor is heavily adhered to the peritoneum. After careful separation, the left kidney and tumor are completely removed (Fig. 8).
10. After careful hemostasis, place a drainage tube, put the left kidney and tumor into a specimen bag, enlarge the incision, and completely remove the specimen (Fig. 9).

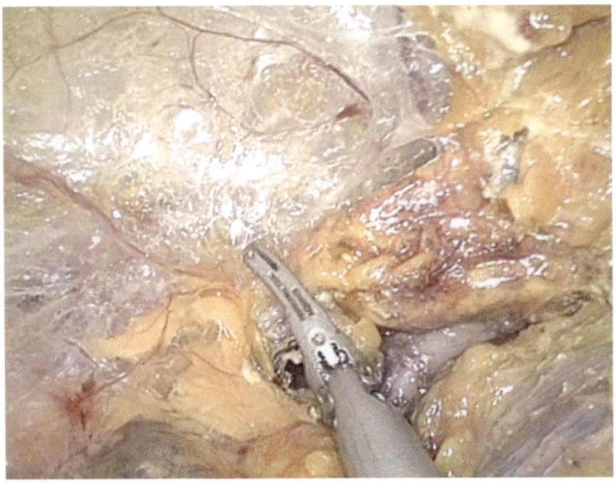

Fig. 6 Separate the kidney from the adrenal gland

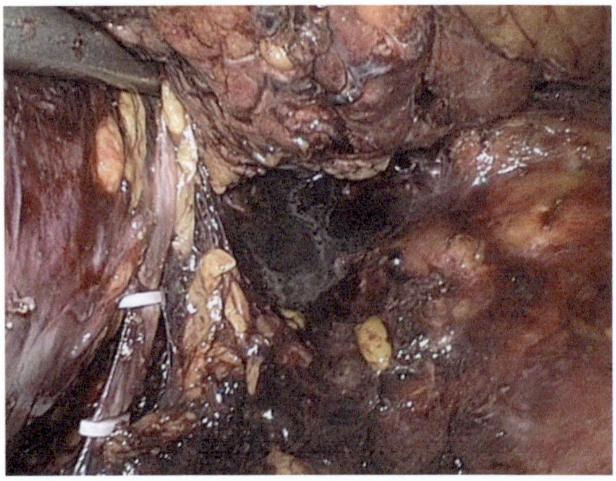

Fig. 7 Disconnect the ureter

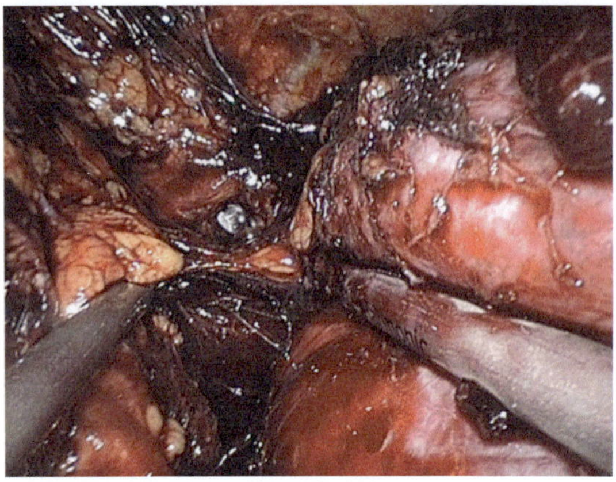

Fig. 8 Completely separate the kidney tumor from the peritoneum

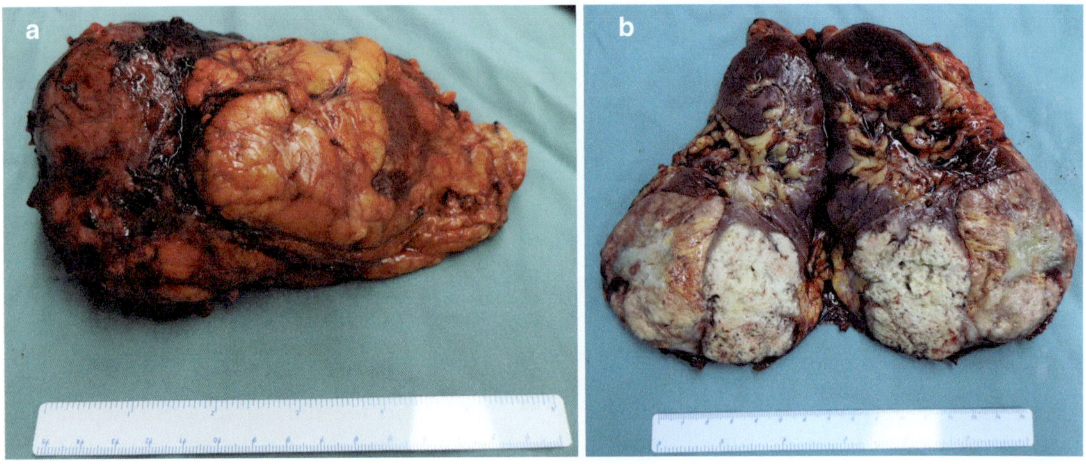

Fig. 9 (a, b) Tissue specimen

Expert Comments

Treatment of Renal Hilum Vessels: During the radical nephrectomy, the treatment of renal vessels is a key step in the surgery. Preoperatively, the number of arteries should be determined based on imaging. If there are multiple arteries or early branches, they should be carefully freed and cut separately. After confirming the artery to be disconnected, the renal vein should be attempt to clamp. If there is still significant reflux, continue to look for other branch arteries. The left renal vein is a complex structure and should be carefully freed and cut. The left renal vein is located behind and below the left renal artery. During radical tumor removal, there are occasional difficulties in freeing the vein. The kidney can be fully freed first, and the renal vein can be cut last.

The ventral kidney tumor is usually heavily adhered to the peritoneum and intestines and should be carefully separated. For the left kidney, pay attention to whether it affects the tail of the pancreas. For the right kidney, pay attention to whether it affects the duodenum. These are all easily damaged parts and organs. If the right-sided tumor is located at the upper pole, there are occasional situations where the boundary with the liver is unclear. After separation, there may be bleeding from the liver wound that is difficult to stop. All of these should be paid special attention to, and adequate preparation should be made before surgery.

Adrenal Preservation: For tumors at the upper pole of the kidney, the adrenal gland is generally not preserved; if the tumor is located at the middle or lower pole, the adrenal gland can be preserved, and the upper pole of the kidney and the adrenal gland are separated during surgery. If there are special circumstances before surgery, such as the removal of the adrenal gland on the opposite side or reduced adrenal cortical function, the adrenal gland can be preserved.

Scope of Radical Nephrectomy for Renal Cancer: The scope of radical nephrectomy for renal cancer should include the perirenal fat capsule and, when necessary, the adrenal tissue on the same side. The specimen should be completely removed, and if conditions permit, a specimen bag should be used to prevent tumor rupture due to compression, leading to local implantation or wound implantation.

Kidney Surgery: Case 19 Laparoscopic Retroperitoneal Partial Nephrectomy (Treatment of Renal Tumor)

Jingmin Zhou

Chief Complaint

Right renal mass found on examination for 12 days. Male, 65 years old. Twelve days ago, he underwent an enhanced abdominal CT scan in our hospital, which revealed a right upper pole renal mass measuring approximately 4.1 cm × 3.7 cm (he had a chest CT scan due to coughing, which incidentally found multiple slightly low-density shadows in both kidneys; further enhanced abdominal CT scan was performed to clarify the condition) marked heterogeneous enhancement in the corticomedullary phase, with hypoenhancement in the nephrographic and excretory phases (Figs. 1a, b and 2a, b), suggesting the possibility of right renal cancer, and

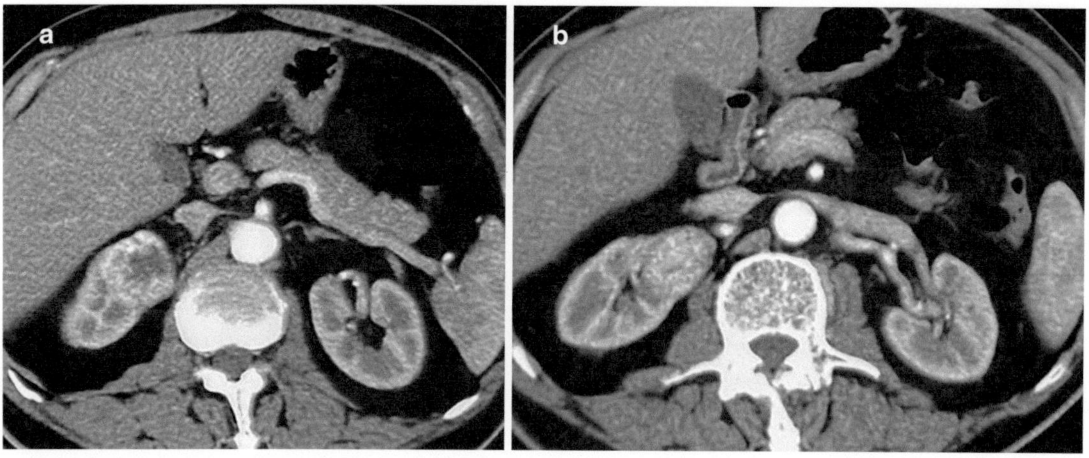

Fig. 1 (**a**, **b**) Abdominal enhanced CT (arterial phase)

Supplementary Information The online version contains supplementary material available at https://doi.org/10.1007/978-981-96-8598-1_21.

J. Zhou (✉)
Beijing Union Medical College Hospital, Beijing, China
e-mail: zhoujm@pumch.cn

Y. Zhang, X. Zhao (eds.), *Laparoscopic Surgery in Urology*,
https://doi.org/10.1007/978-981-96-8598-1_21

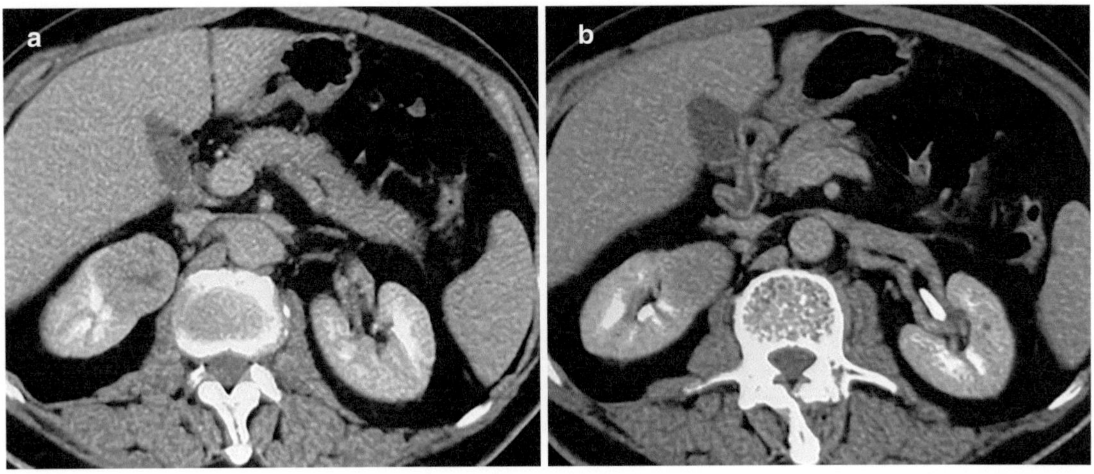

Fig. 2 (**a**, **b**) Abdominal enhanced CT (excretory phase)

surgical treatment was recommended. The patient had no discomfort such as abdominal pain, gross hematuria, frequent urination, urgency, dysuria, chills, or fever.

Past History

He had a right femoral fracture due to a car accident, which healed after conservative treatment.

Physical Examination

No special findings in the heart and lungs, no bulging in both renal areas, and no percussion pain.

Imaging Data (Figs. 1 and 2)

Preoperative Assessment

The patient's imaging examination suggested a right renal tumor, about 4.1 cm × 3.7 cm in size, with significant enhancement, suggesting a high possibility of malignancy. Combined with the patient's clinical data, the diagnosis of right renal tumor is basically clear, and renal cancer is possible. The indication for surgery is clear. Outpatient assessment of heart and lung function, no obvious abnormalities, and no evidence of metastasis to other parts. Surgical method: laparoscopic partial nephrectomy of the right kidney.

Surgical Procedure

1. The retroperitoneal upper urinary tract surgical position is adopted. The surgical side is marked in the ward before surgery. General anesthesia with endotracheal intubation is used. A urinary catheter is placed. Routine disinfection and draping.
2. After establishing the retroperitoneal space, the tract surgical channel is placed. This operation uses four ports.
3. After cleaning the extraperitoneal fat and identifying the peritoneal reflection, the Gerota's fascia is longitudinally opened on the dorsal side of the peritoneal reflection, revealing the psoas major muscle and the perirenal fat capsule (Figs. 3 and 4).
4. Along the surface of the psoas major muscle, the perirenal fat capsule is fully freed and pushed toward the abdominal side. Look for the medial arcuate ligament on the surface of the psoas major muscle, and find and free the right renal artery at the symmetrical position

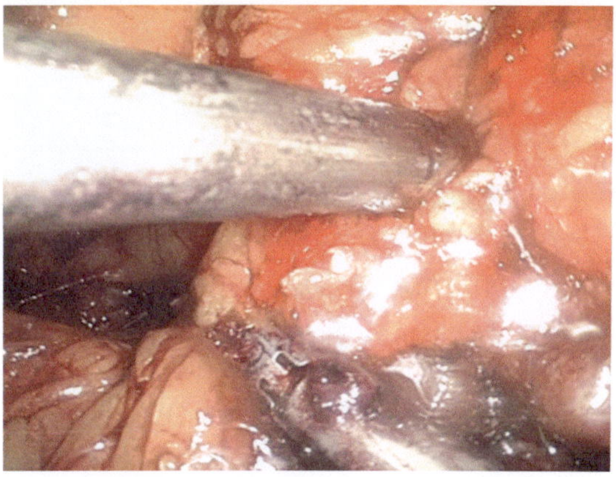

Fig. 3 Opening the renal fascia

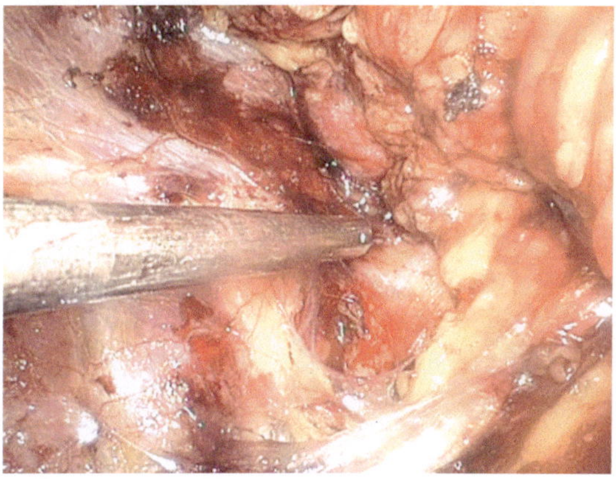

Fig. 4 Exposing the psoas major muscle and perirenal fat

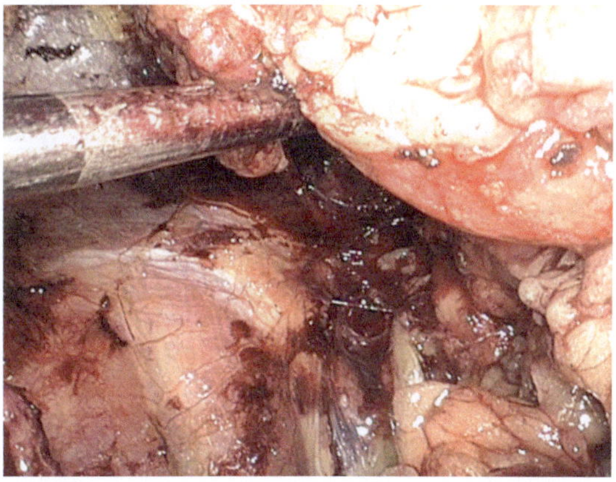

Fig. 5 Locating the medial arcuate ligament of the psoas major muscle

of this ligament and the inner edge of the psoas major muscle (Figs. 5 and 6).

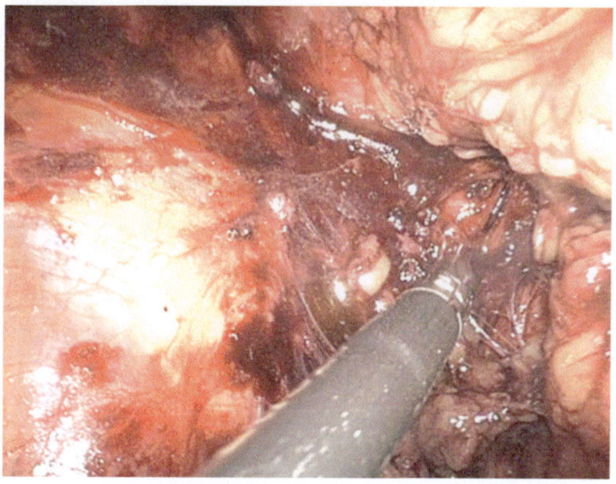

Fig. 6 Locating the renal artery

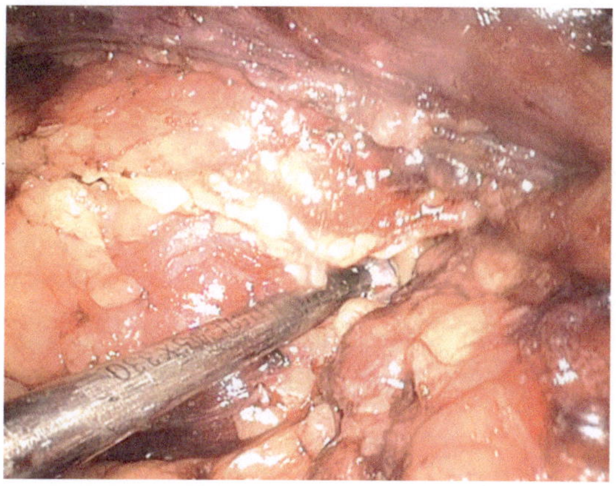

Fig. 7 Freeing the surface of the kidney

5. At a position close to the peritoneum, longitudinally split the renal fat capsule, free the right kidney, and expose the tumor (Figs. 7 and 8).
6. Use a monopolar hook to mark the edge of the tumor, which is beneficial for determining the boundary of the tumor during the tumor removal process (Fig. 9).
7. Use a vascular occlusion clamp to block the renal artery (Fig. 10). Cut the renal parenchyma 0.5 cm away from the edge of the tumor, and use a combination of blunt and sharp methods to free the base of the tumor while avoiding damaging the blood vessels and collecting system as much as possible (Fig. 11).
8. Using a layered suturing method, continuously suture the base of the kidney with

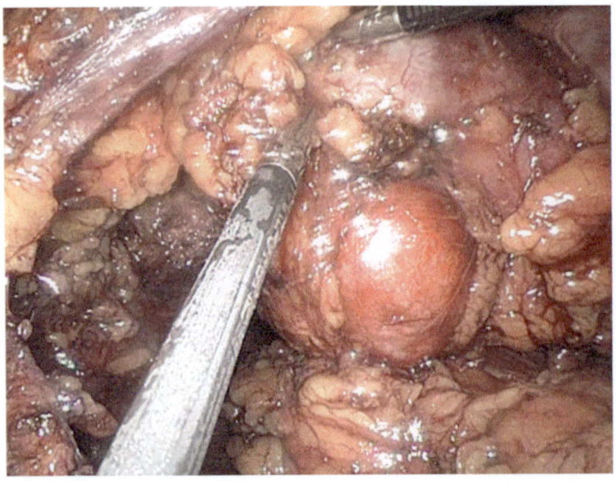

Fig. 8 Exposing the tumor

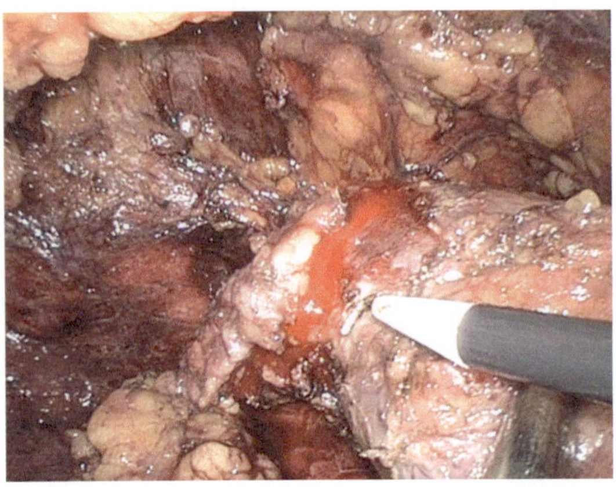

Fig. 9 Outlining the tumor with an monopolar hook

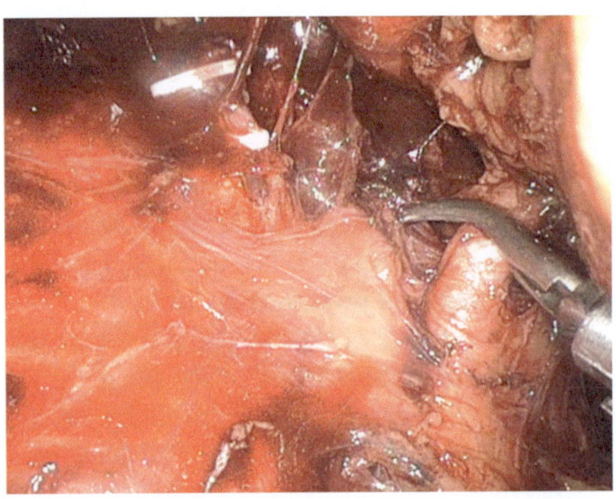

Fig. 10 Blocking the renal artery

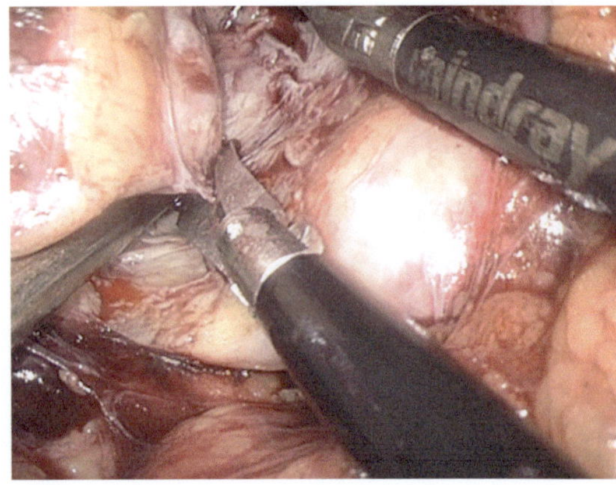

Fig. 11 Removing the tumor

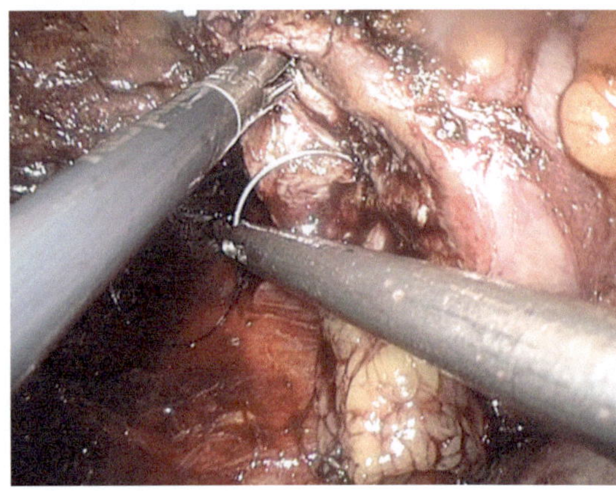

Fig. 12 Suturing the base with 3-0 V-Loc thread

3-0 V-Loc suture, and then continuously suture the wound with 1-0 V-Loc suture, making sure that the 1-0 suture enters and exits the needle on the renal capsule. The suture tail is fixed with Hem-o-lok (Figs. 12 and 13).

9. Remove the arterial occlusion clamp and check for active bleeding at the renal hilum and the wound on the kidney (Fig. 14).
10. Place a drainage tube. Finally, after enlarging the auxiliary hole incision, the specimen is bagged and completely removed (Figs. 15 and 16).

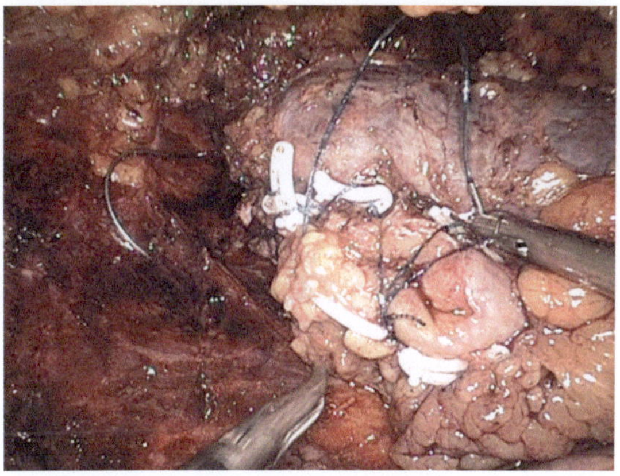

Fig. 13 Suturing the wound with 1-0 V-Loc thread

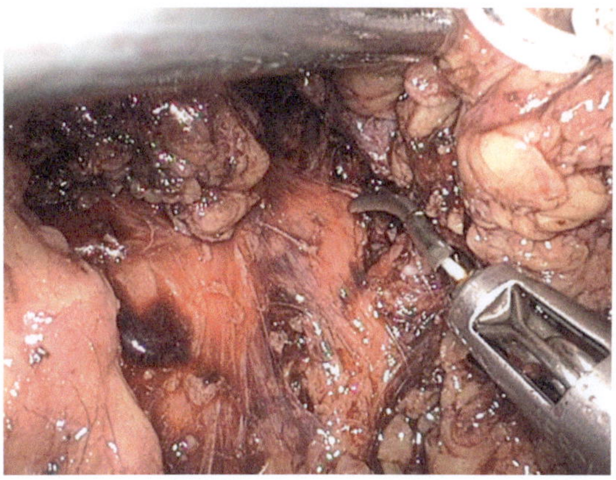

Fig. 14 Removing the arterial occlusion clamp

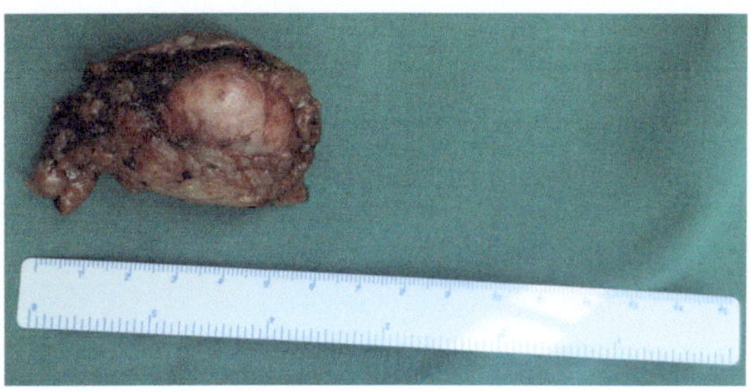

Fig. 15 Gross specimen (complete)

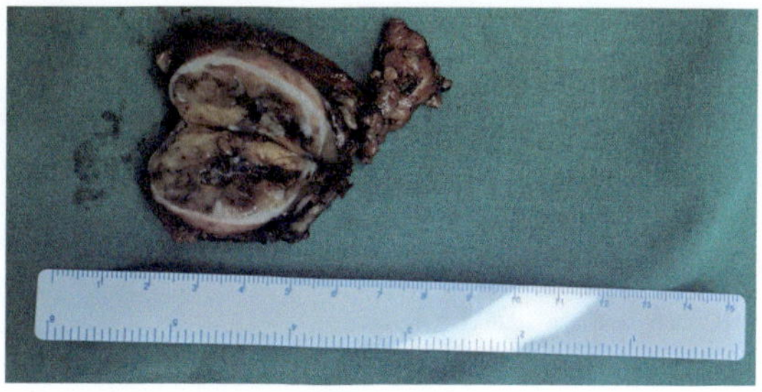

Fig. 16 Gross specimen (cut open)

Expert Comments

Choice of surgical approach: Laparoscopic partial nephrectomy can be performed through the abdominal cavity or retroperitoneal approach. The choice should be based on the surgeon's habits, tumor location, tumor size, relationship with renal vessels, and other factors. Generally, tumors on the dorsal side of the kidney are more suitable for the retroperitoneal approach. The advantage of the retroperitoneal approach is that it can avoid intestinal interference and is less affected by surrounding organs, but the disadvantage is that the operating space is small, so for beginners or those who are not proficient in the operation, the abdominal approach may be a better choice. The abdominal approach can provide a relatively spacious operating space, and this approach can be chosen for tumors on the ventral side of the kidney. Both approaches can be used by surgeons who are proficient in the operation.

Handling of renal hilum vessels: During partial nephrectomy, for patients with multiple arteries or early branches, preoperative imaging should be used for early judgment, and occlusion should be performed separately to achieve a better occlusion effect. The occlusion time is crucial for the recovery of renal function after surgery, so all preparations for resection and suturing should be done before occlusion. After the suturing is completed, the occlusion should be loosened before cutting the suture and removing the needle, paying attention to details and trying to shorten the occlusion time.

Full mobilization of the kidney: Full mobilization of the kidney is particularly critical for partial nephrectomy via the retroperitoneal approach, especially for renal tumors in some locations, where resection and suturing are difficult. Full mobilization of the kidney can even allow the kidney to be rotated to some degree along the renal hilum, reducing the difficulty of resection and suturing. Suturing of the renal wound: For the suturing of the wound after partial nephrectomy, especially when the renal wound is deep, a layered suturing method is recommended. The deep layer mainly closes the blood vessels and collecting system opened during tumor resection. It also reduces tension on the wound by approximating the deep renal medulla. The outer layer suturing can achieve complete hemostasis and reconstruction, but the suturing entry and exit points must be on the renal capsule; otherwise, the suturing thread may cut the renal parenchyma, leading to local bleeding after surgery.

Kidney Surgery: Case 20 Laparoscopic Retroperitoneal Right Renal Hamartoma Excision (Treatment of Multiple Renal Hamartomas)

Jiaquan Zhou

Chief Complaint

Bilateral renal tumors found during physical examination for over 7 years.

Present Illness History

Female, 52 years old. The patient was found to have multiple bilateral renal tumors during an ultrasound examination 7 years ago, with the largest one on the right side measuring about 1 cm in diameter, suggesting the possibility of hamartomas. She usually has a feeling of distension in the right waist, without back pain, hematuria, or other discomforts, and has regular follow-ups. Two months ago, a reexamination at another hospital showed a strong echo mass measuring about 7.9 cm × 3.5 cm between the liver and kidney, closely related to the kidney, and multiple strong echo masses could be detected in both kidneys. One month ago, a CTU examination at our hospital showed multiple fat density lesions in both kidneys, some of which exceeded the contour, with the largest one located in the upper part of the right kidney, measuring about 5.5 cm × 3.0 cm × 3.5 cm. After enhancement, flaky slightly high-density shadows could be seen inside, and the lipid component did not enhance, suggesting a high possibility of bilateral renal hamartomas (Figs. 1, 2, and 3).

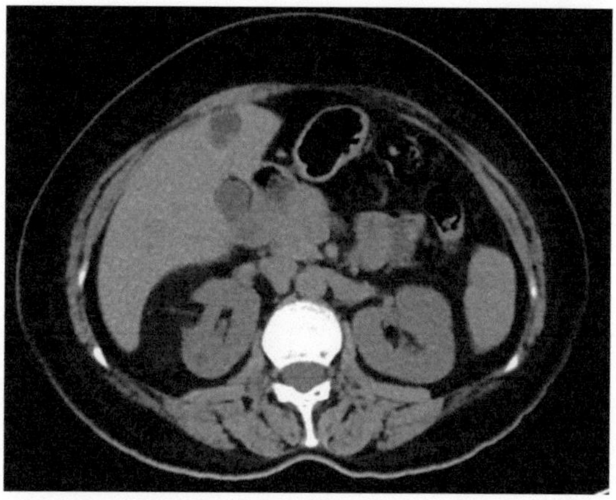

Fig. 1 CT plain scan image of the largest tumor of the right renal hamartoma

Supplementary Information The online version contains supplementary material available at https://doi.org/10.1007/978-981-96-8598-1_22.

J. Zhou (✉)
Hainan Affiliated Hospital of Hainan Medical University, Haikou, Hainan, China

Y. Zhang, X. Zhao (eds.), *Laparoscopic Surgery in Urology*,
https://doi.org/10.1007/978-981-96-8598-1_22

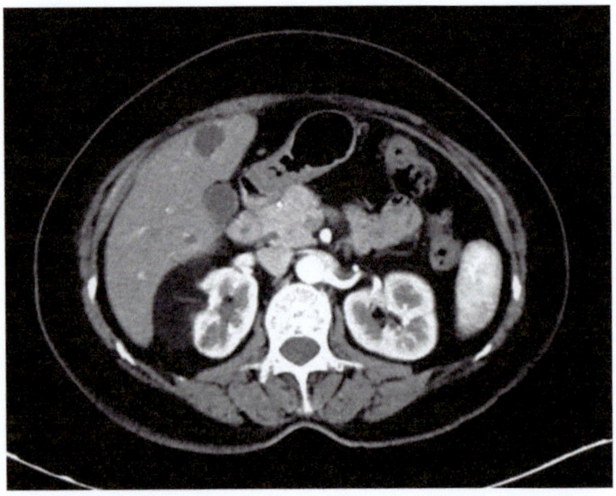

Fig. 2 CT-enhanced image of the largest tumor of the right renal hamartoma

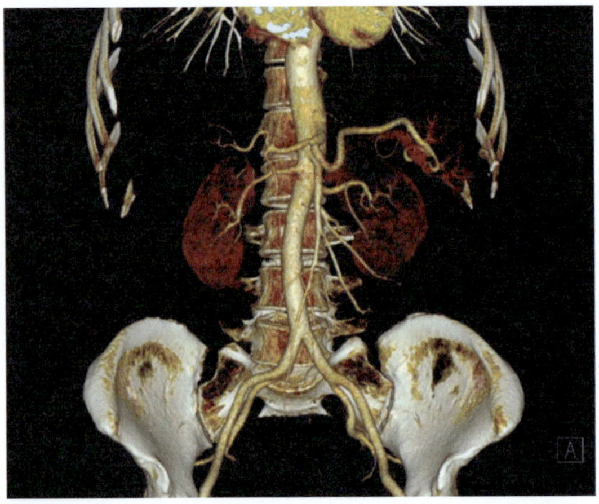

Fig. 3 CT three-dimensional arterial reconstruction

Past History

In 2014, she underwent laparoscopic liver cyst fenestration for liver cysts, and in May 2022, she underwent laparoscopic bilateral adnexectomy + myomectomy for right ovarian mucinous adenocarcinoma and uterine fibroids.

Physical Examination: No special vital signs were stable, no special heart and lung auscultation, no bulging in both renal areas, no percussion pain, no tenderness along both ureteral routes, no bladder filling, and no tenderness.

Auxiliary Examination

1. Urinary system color ultrasound: A relatively strong echo of about 7.9 cm × 3.5 cm can be seen between the liver and kidney, closely related to the kidney. Multiple relatively strong echoes can be detected in both kidneys, the larger one in the right kidney is about 1.9 cm × 1.7 cm, and the larger one in the left kidney is about 2.3 cm × 1.5 cm.
2. CTU: No obvious abnormalities in the size and shape of both kidneys. Multiple lipid density lesions can be seen in both kidneys, some of which exceed the outline. The larger one is located in the upper part of the right kidney, about 5.5 cm × 3.0 cm, considering the possibility of multiple angiomyolipomas (AML) in both kidneys.
3. Renal blood flow imaging: The total glomerular filtration rate (GFR) is 63.7 ml/(min•1.73 m^2), right kidney GFR is 27.7 ml/(min•1.73 m^2), and left kidney GFR is 36.0 ml/(min•1.73 m^2). The blood flow perfusion and function of the left kidney are slightly poor, the blood flow perfusion and function of the right kidney are relatively poor, and the renal pelvis drainage is not smooth.

Preoperative Assessment

The patient only had a feeling of soreness in the right waist during the course of the disease. The bilateral renal tumors were found by physical examination ultrasound. Combined with ultrasound and CTU examination, it is considered that the bilateral renal tumors contain fat components, and the possibility of bilateral renal hamartomas is high. The right kidney hamartoma is larger, and there is a risk of spontaneous bleeding, which can be considered for surgical removal; the left kidney hamartoma is smaller and does not need surgical intervention for the time being. The patient's creatinine was normal before surgery, but renal blood flow imaging suggested mild impairment of renal function in both kidneys, and prolonged renal artery occlusion should be avoided during surgery to further damage renal function. Preoperative assessment of cardiopulmonary function: no obvious abnormalities were found.

Surgical Procedure

1. General anesthesia with endotracheal intubation, placement of a urinary catheter, left lateral position, routine disinfection, and draping.
2. The first incision is made 2 cm above the axillary midline crest, longer than 2 cm, successively cutting the skin, subcutaneous tissue, and fat, expanding the muscle layer with a curved clamp, and entering the retroperitoneal space.
3. With the index or middle finger closely attached to the inner wall of the muscle layer, bluntly separate the retroperitoneal fat to establish a retroperitoneal space. Under the guidance of the finger, make the second incision below the rib edge of the posterior axillary line, and place a 5 cm trocar. Parallel to the second incision, make the third incision on the anterior axillary line, and place a 12 cm trocar; parallel to the first incision, make the fourth incision 2 cm to the outside of the anterior axillary line, and place a 5 cm trocar.
4. A 10 cm trocar is placed in the first incision as an observation hole to establish pneumoperitoneum.
5. Free the retroperitoneal fat to expose the posterior peritoneum, taking care to avoid damaging the peritoneum during the freeing process. If there is a hole in the peritoneum, it is recommended to close it before proceeding to the next step of the operation (Fig. 4).
6. Identify the peritoneal reflection, open Gerota's fascia, and expose the perirenal fat (Fig. 5).
7. Free the perirenal fat along the psoas major muscle (Fig. 6). First, expose the vena cava (Fig. 7), and then expose the renal artery along the vena cava (Fig. 8).
8. Free the kidney closely to the ventral side of the kidney, fully expose the renal hamartoma, and only free the root of the largest diameter hamartoma when freeing it, to form a natural suspension state, which is conducive to spatial exposure (Figs. 9 and 10).

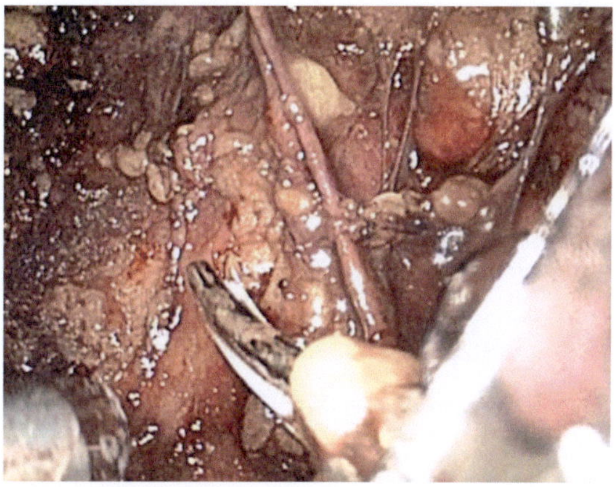

Fig. 4 Freeing the retroperitoneal fat

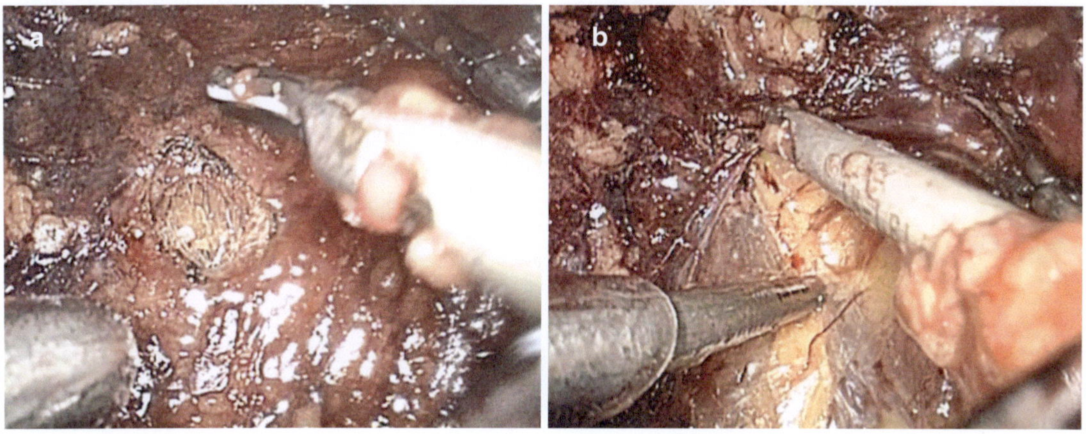

Fig. 5 (**a**, **b**) Opening Gerota's fascia

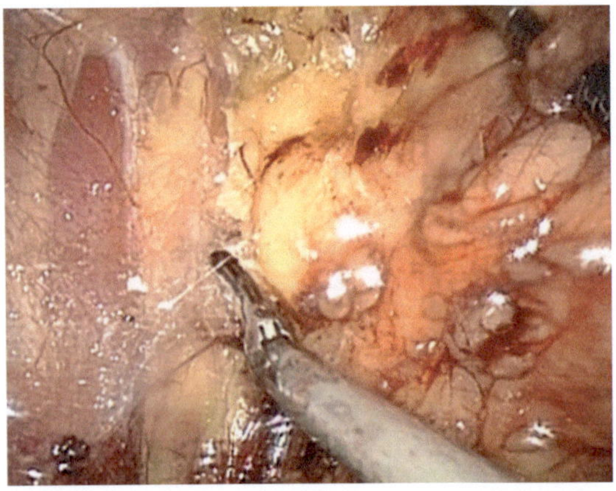

Fig. 6 Free the surface of the lumbar muscle around the kidney

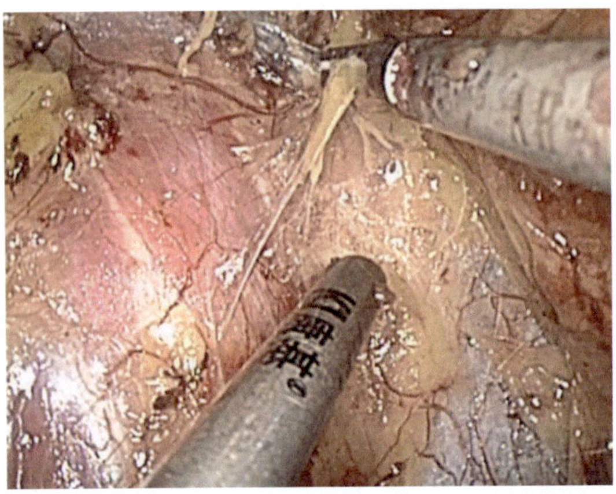

Fig. 7 Expose the vena cava

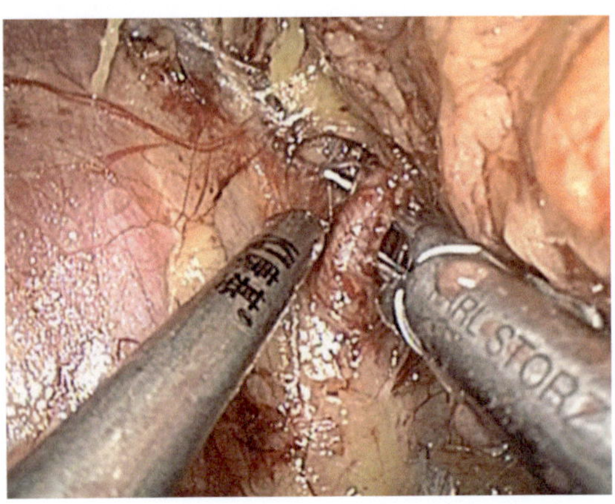

Fig. 8 Expose the renal artery

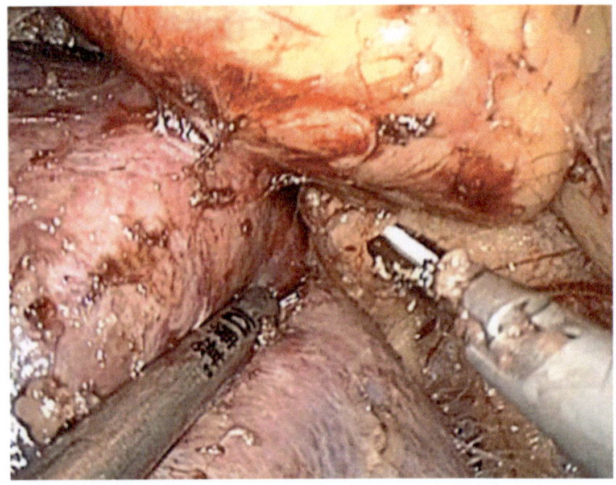

Fig. 9 Fully free the upper tumor

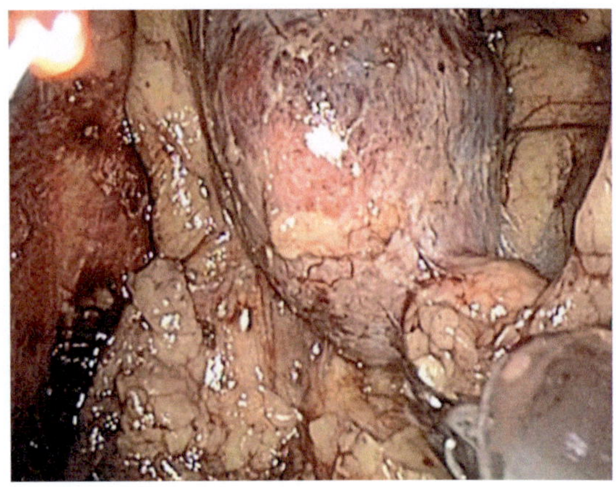

Fig. 10 Fully free the lower tumor

9. Temporarily block the renal artery with a bulldog clamp (Fig. 11), cut along the root of the tumor with scissors (Fig. 12), and remove some of the base hamartoma tumor tissue with a suction device (Fig. 13).
10. Suture the tumor cavity tightly with a continuous 1-0 V-Loc thread (Fig. 14), release the bulldog clamp (Fig. 15), and evaluate for any wound bleeding.
11. Free the largest diameter hamartoma from the peritoneal side (Fig. 16), place the tumor tissue in a specimen bag, and remove it (Fig. 17).
12. Leave a drainage tube and suture the incision.

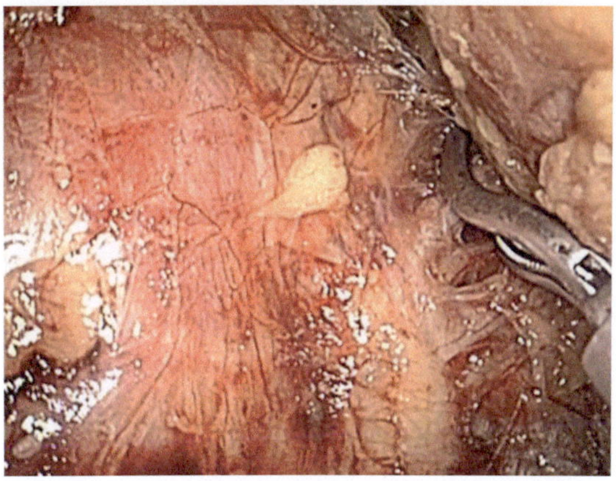

Fig. 11 Block the renal artery

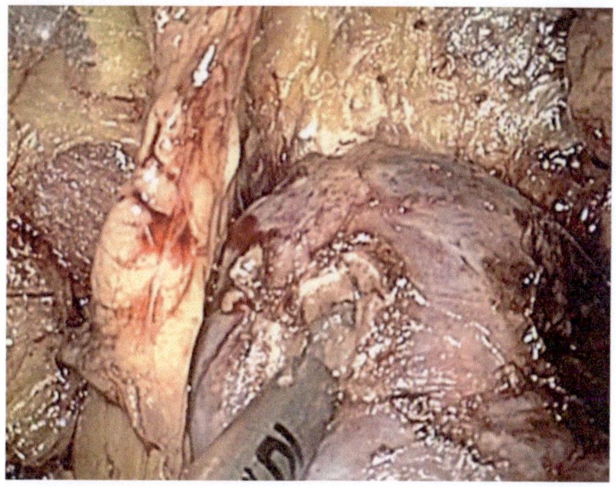

Fig. 13 Suction the residual hamartoma tissue at the base

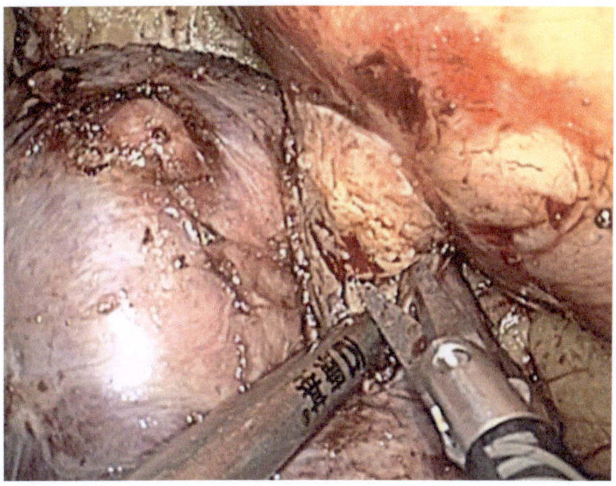

Fig. 12 Cut the tumor along the root

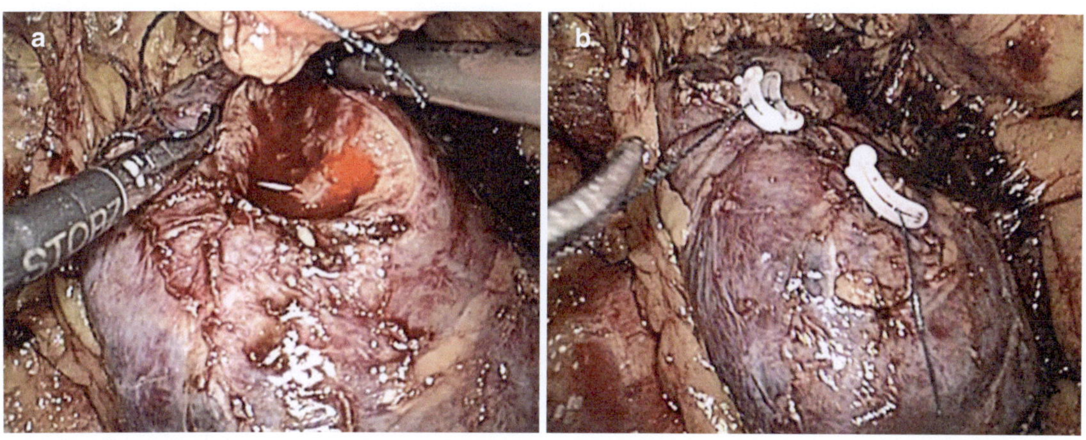

Fig. 14 (**a**, **b**) Suturing the tumor cavity with V-Loc suture

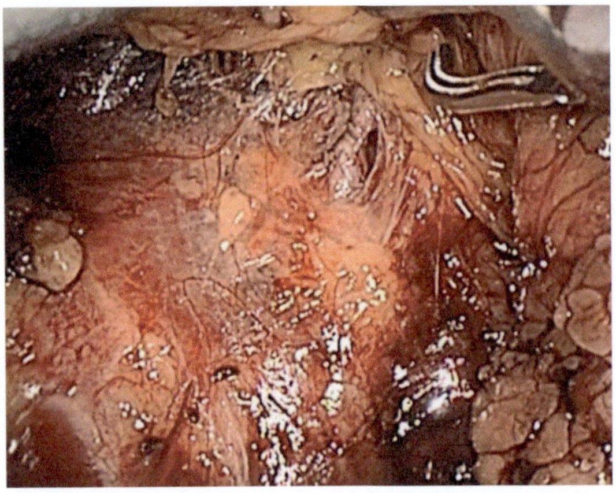

Fig. 15 Remove the renal artery blockage

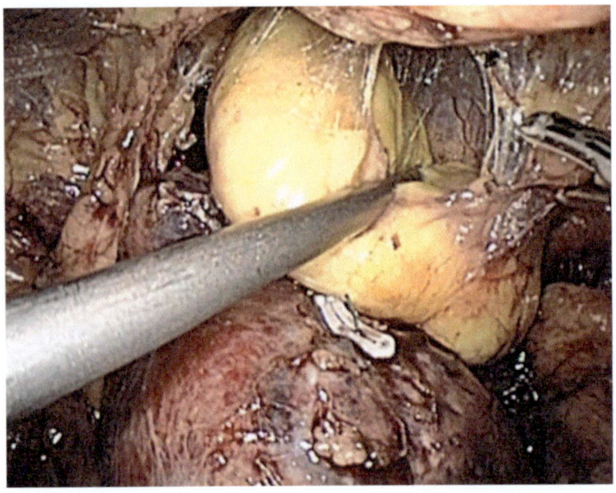

Fig. 16 Free the tumor from the peritoneal side

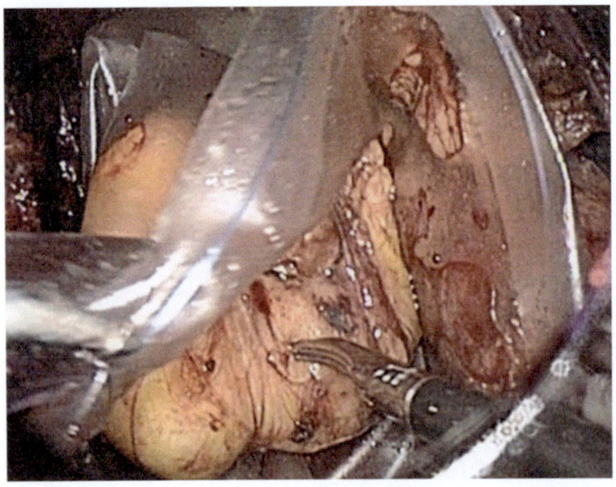

Fig. 17 Place the tumor in a specimen bag

Expert Comments

1. Hamartoma is the most common benign tumor of the kidney, generally unilateral, but also bilateral and multiple. For such multiple renal hamartomas, it is necessary to rule out tuberous sclerosis-related renal hamartoma. This patient only has bilateral renal hamartoma and does not have other signs and lesions related to tuberous sclerosis, so it is not considered for now.
2. Considering that hamartoma is a benign lesion, smaller renal hamartomas do not require surgical treatment, but this patient's right renal hamartoma is larger, and there is a risk of spontaneous bleeding, so active surgical treatment is required, while the left renal hamartoma is smaller and the risk of bleeding is not high, so there is no need for surgical intervention for now.
3. The surgery for renal hamartoma is similar to that for renal cancer, where only the tumor needs to be excised. Depending on the composition of the hamartoma, different surgical strategies can be adopted. For instance, if the hamartoma contains less fat and is relatively hard, it is recommended to adopt the same partial nephrectomy method as for renal cancer, and a small amount of normal renal parenchyma around the tumor should be excised together; if the hamartoma contains a large amount of fat or is mainly composed of fat, suction can be used to avoid loss of normal renal unit tissue and protect renal function as much as possible. Especially for this patient, the renal blood flow imaging suggests mild impairment of bilateral renal function, so renal function should be protected as much as possible.
4. Preoperative enhanced CT suggests that there is a branch artery supplying blood to the largest diameter of the tumor. After excision, attention should be paid to closing this branch artery, or the suturing should be more rigorous to avoid postoperative bleeding.

Kidney Surgery: Case 21 Laparoscopic Retroperitoneal Partial Nephrectomy (Locating the Renal Artery During Bleeding in Partial Nephrectomy)

Xin Zhao

Chief Complaint

A right renal tumor was found during a physical examination 9 years ago, and it has grown in the past month.

Medical History

Female, 49 years old. The patient was found to have a right renal hamartoma during an ultrasound examination 9 years ago. The initial tumor diameter was considered to be 0.6–0.7 cm. The patient had no discomfort, back pain, hematuria, dysuria, frequent urination, urgency, abdominal pain, bloating, etc., and was regularly reviewed. In 2021, the ultrasound showed a tumor diameter of about 0.7 cm. In October 2022, the ultrasound showed a high echo at the upper pole of the right kidney, about 2.5 cm × 2.0 cm, with blood flow signals inside. MRI suggested a high echo at the upper pole of the right kidney, about 2.1 cm × 1.9 cm, slightly long T2, slightly long T1 signal, considering the possibility of right renal hamartoma (Figs. 1 and 2). The outpatient clinic admitted her

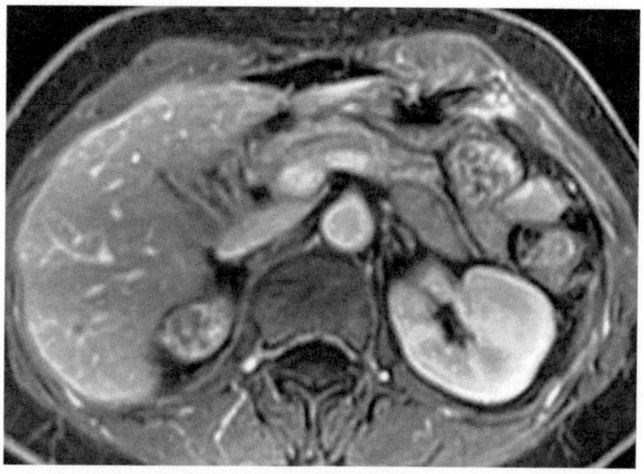

Fig. 1 MRI transverse section

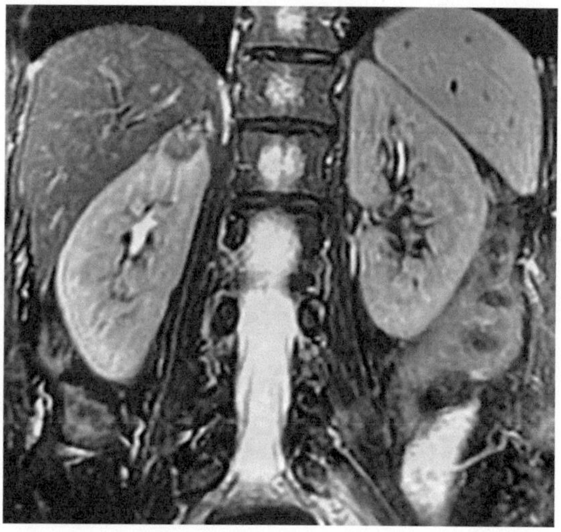

Fig. 2 MRI coronal section

Supplementary Information The online version contains supplementary material available at https://doi.org/10.1007/978-981-96-8598-1_23.

X. Zhao (✉)
Beijing Union Medical College Hospital,
Beijing, China

Y. Zhang, X. Zhao (eds.), *Laparoscopic Surgery in Urology*,
https://doi.org/10.1007/978-981-96-8598-1_23

with the diagnosis of "right renal tumor, high possibility of right renal hamartoma."

Past History

She underwent a cesarean section in 1997, with no other special conditions.

Physical Examination

No special abnormalities were observed.

Imaging Data (Figs. 1 and 2)

Preoperative Assessment

After admission, the preoperative assessment was completed. Coagulation, infection screening (eight items), liver full + kidney full + lipid full, whole blood cell analysis, and ECG showed no obvious abnormalities. The reexamined urinary system ultrasound showed a medium-high echo in the upper part of the right kidney, 2.4 cm × 1.7 cm, suggesting the possibility of a vascular smooth muscle lipoma. Abdominal CT scan showed a mixed density lesion in the upper pole of the right kidney, containing fat, about 2.4 cm × 2.2 cm, suggesting the possibility of a right renal vascular smooth muscle lipoma. Renal blood flow imaging showed normal perfusion and function of both kidneys.

Based on the patient's condition, a retroperitoneal partial nephrectomy of the right kidney is planned.

Surgical Procedure

1. The retroperitoneal upper urinary tract surgical position is adopted. The surgical side is marked in the ward before surgery. General endotracheal anesthesia is used. A urinary catheter is placed. Routine disinfection and draping are performed.
2. Establish a retroperitoneal approach for upper urinary tract surgery. This operation uses four ports.
3. Clean the retroperitoneal fat. The patient was relatively thin, so care should be taken not to damage the peritoneum when cleaning the extraperitoneal fat (Fig. 3).
4. Open the renal fascia (Fig. 4).
5. Separate the renal artery. This operation initially found one renal artery (Fig. 5).
6. Free the perirenal fat along the surface of the kidney to find the tumor. Preoperative MRI imaging suggested that the tumor was located at the upper pole of the right kidney.
7. Fully expose the right kidney tumor (Fig. 6).
8. Use a monopolar electrocautery marker to mark the periphery of the tumor. Considering the tumor's rapid growth and the potential malignancy of the epithelioid angiomyolipoma, a partial nephrectomy was performed instead of a tumor excision (Fig. 7).
9. Block the renal artery. After blocking, touch the kidney and find that the texture of the kidney has not softened, and the color of the kidney has not turned pale, suspecting that there may be multiple arteries (Figs. 8 and 9).
10. Remove the tumor, find that there is more bleeding on the kidney wound surface, consider the existence of multiple renal arteries, immediately flip the kidney to the abdominal side and look for the branch renal artery around the original renal artery,

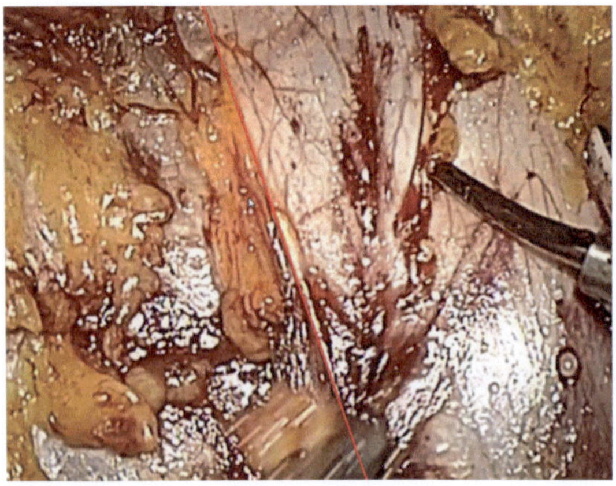

Fig. 3 Cleaning the extraperitoneal fat

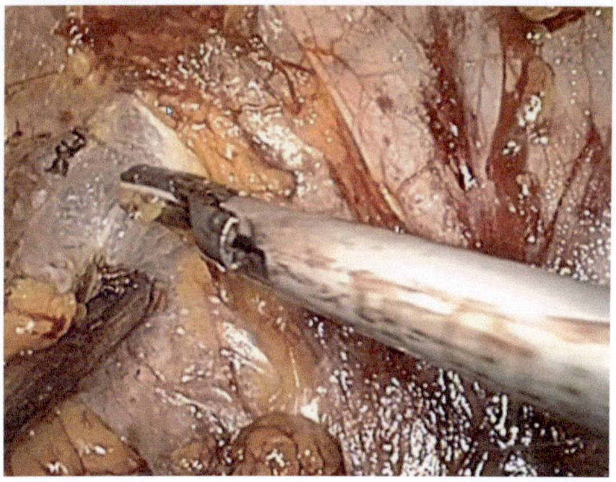

Fig. 4 Opening the renal fascia

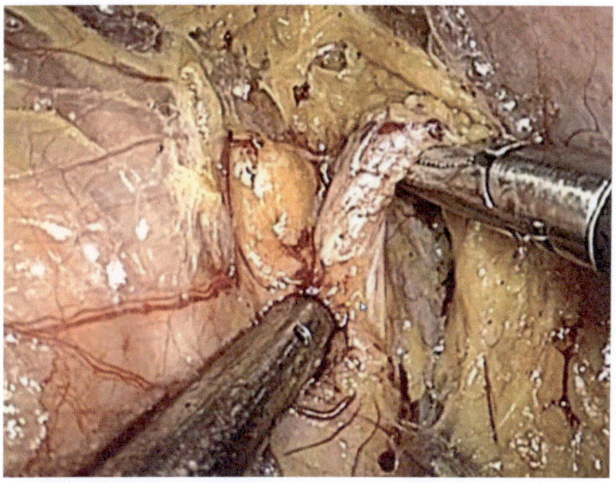

Fig. 5 Finding the renal artery

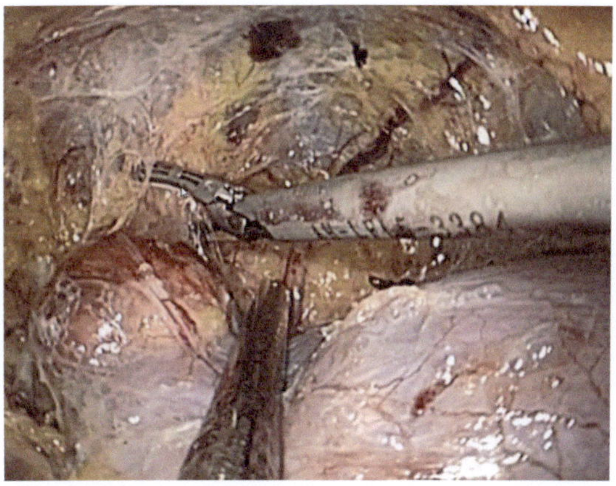

Fig. 6 Freeing the kidney surface to reveal the tumor

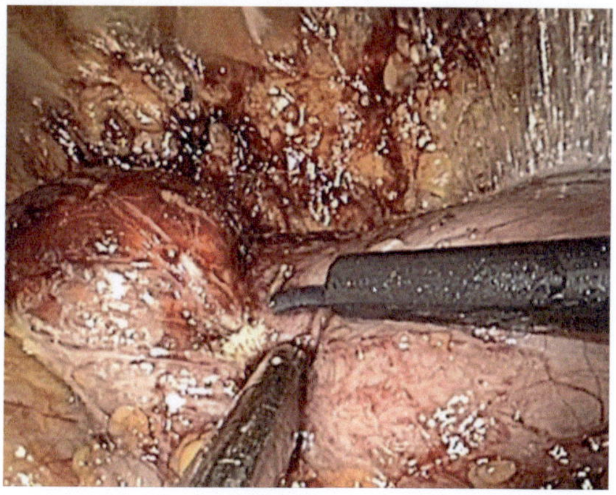

Fig. 7 Using an electrocautery hook to outline the tumor

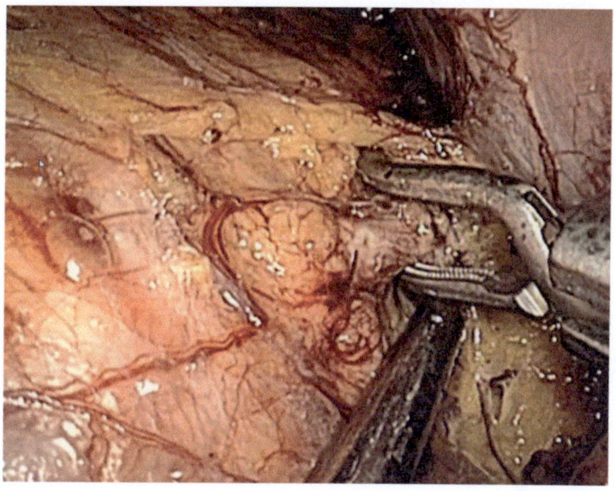

Fig. 8 Blocking the renal artery

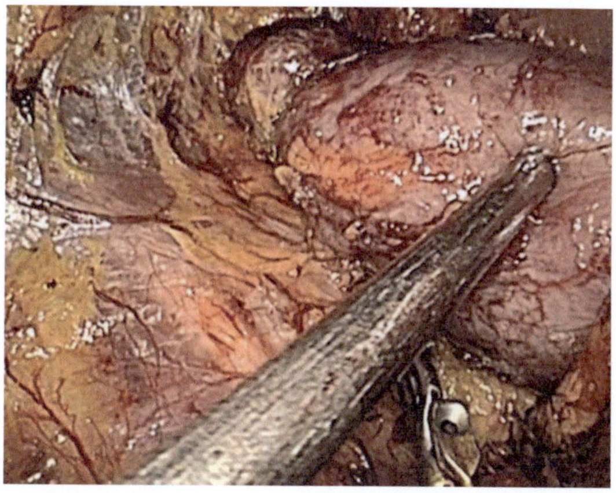

Fig. 9 No significant color change in the kidney after blocking the renal artery

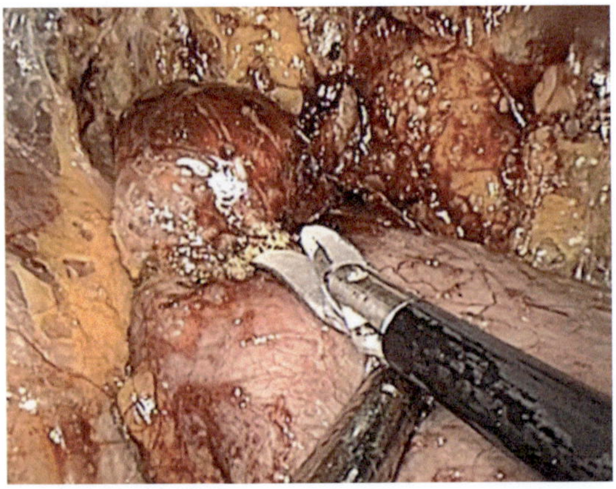

Fig. 10 Removing the tumor

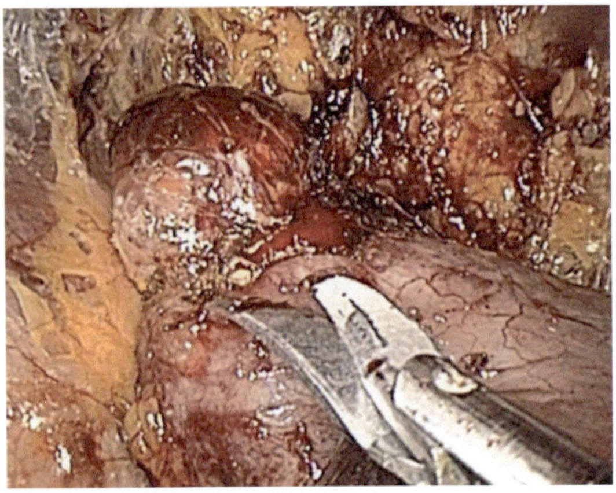

Fig. 11 More bleeding from the wound surface

then find another renal artery on the side of the blocked renal artery, and block the newly found renal artery again. After blocking, the bleeding from the kidney wound surface significantly reduced (Figs. 10, 11, 12, 13, 14, and 15).

11. Completely remove the tumor (Fig. 16).
12. Use 3-0 V-Loc sutures to sew the base. Use 1-0 V-Loc sutures to sew the renal parenchyma (Figs. 17 and 18).
13. Release the blockage and observe if there is active bleeding at the suture site.
14. Remove the tumor.
15. Place local hemostatic materials and leave a drainage tube. The operation is over, and the gross specimens are shown in Figs. 19 and 20.

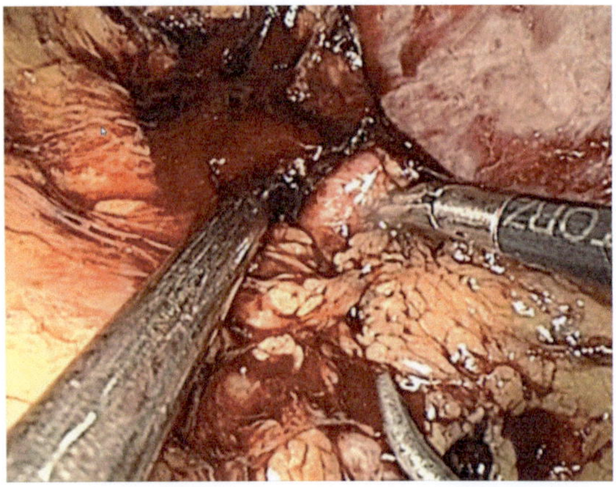

Fig. 12 Looking for the renal artery again, another renal artery can be seen

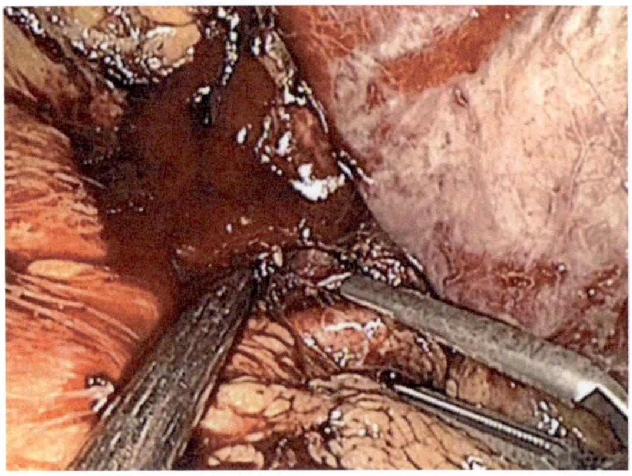

Fig. 13 Re-blocking the renal artery

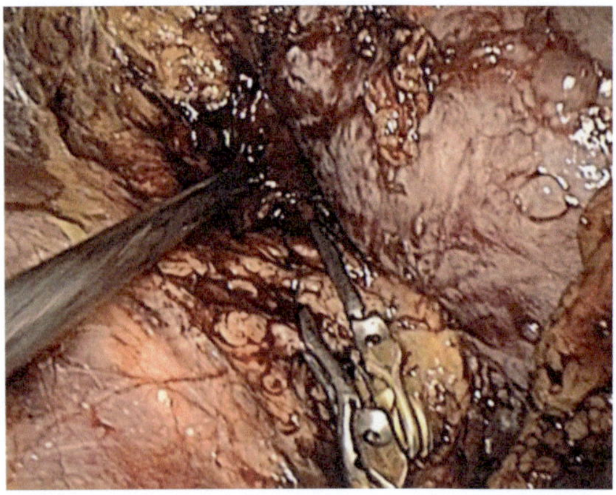

Fig. 14 Both renal arteries are blocked

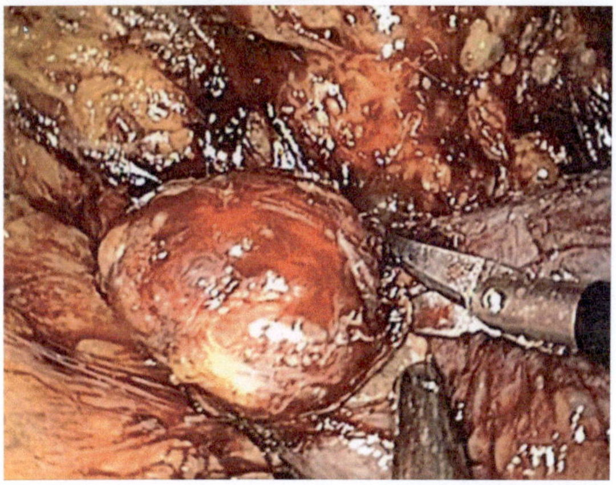

Fig. 15 Continue to remove the tumor, bleeding reduced

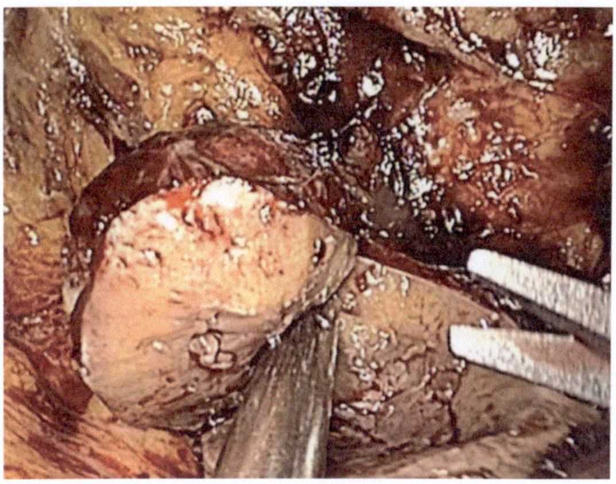

Fig. 16 Completely removing the tumor

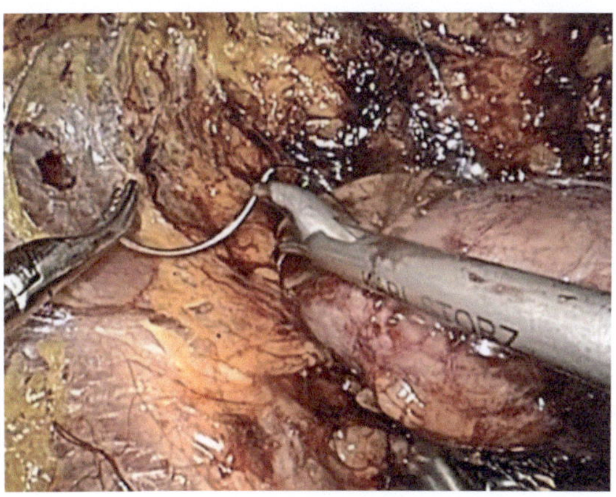

Fig. 17 3-0 V-Loc sutures sewing the base

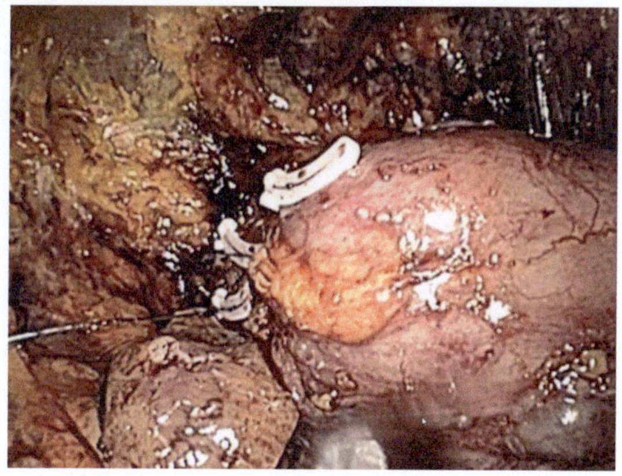

Fig. 18 1-0 V-Loc sutured wound

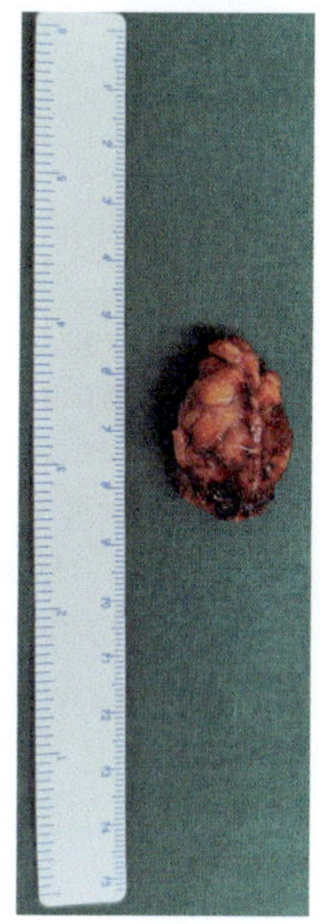

Fig. 19 Gross specimen (intact)

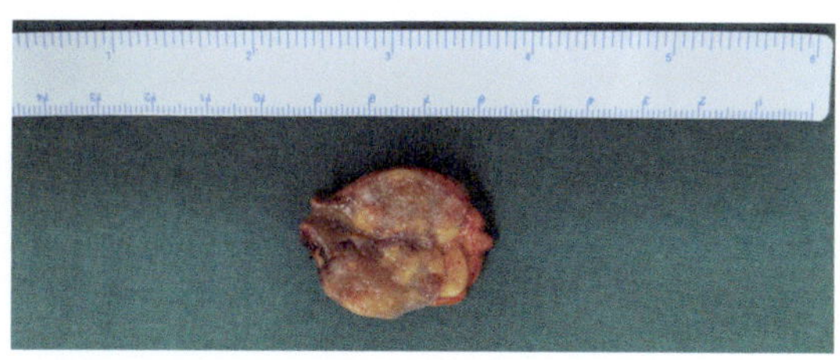

Fig. 20 Gross specimen (cut open)

Expert Comments

1. Choice of surgical indications: Hamartoma is a benign disease, and the right kidney tumor in this case is relatively small and can continue to be observed. However, the patient found that the tumor volume had significantly increased during a physical examination in the past month, and the possibility of epithelioid angiomyolipoma with malignant potential in renal hamartoma should be considered. The patient strongly desired treatment, so it was decided to admit her for surgical treatment. Considering the rapid growth of the tumor and the possibility of malignancy, a laparoscopic partial nephrectomy was chosen instead of a typical excision for hamartoma.
2. Clarify the renal blood supply: The preoperative review did not clearly identify the number of renal arteries, and it was believed that there was only a single renal artery. The renal blood flow supply was not completely blocked, leading to more bleeding during the operation. Therefore, the patient's renal blood supply should be clarified before surgery. The main method is to clarify the course and branches of the renal vessels through preoperative enhanced CT. Hospitals with the necessary facilities can perform a CTA of the renal vessels before partial nephrectomy. In this case, the preoperative review did not find a branch of the renal artery, so only one renal artery was isolated during the operation. How to judge whether the renal artery is completely blocked during the operation: ① After blocking the renal artery, you can press the kidney with an instrument to feel whether the texture of the kidney has softened and whether the color of the kidney has turned pale. ② After cutting open the renal capsule and part of the renal parenchyma with scissors, check if there is clear active arterial bleeding, mainly characterized by abundant bleeding, rapid flow, and bright red color. If the above situation occurs, stop removing the tumor immediately and lift the kidney to find if there is a branch of the renal artery. This is the method used in this case. ③ Some patients have early branches of the renal artery. When isolating the renal artery, it should be as close to the root as possible to avoid just blocking the branch of the renal artery.

Kidney Surgery: Case 22 Laparoscopic Transperitoneal Treatment of Multiple Large Volume Hamartomas in the Right Kidney

Wenda Wang

Chief Complaint

Facial rash for 27 years, bilateral renal masses detected during physical examination for 10 years.

History

Female, 37 years old. Twenty-seven years ago, the patient first developed scattered multiple hard, waxy papules on the facial skin, ranging in size from pinhead to rice grain, which were distributed in a butterfly shape on both sides of the nose. The color of the papules fades slightly when pressed, with no symptoms of itching or pain. She received laser treatment at a dermatology clinic, and currently the papules have decreased. Ten years ago, during a physical examination, multiple small nodules were found in both kidneys by abdominal ultrasound, with a diameter of no more than 1 cm (report not available). Multiple hamartomas are considered. In addition, the patient has a single periungual fibroma on the little toe of the right foot, with a diameter of approximately 2 mm. The patient has no specific discomfort and has not sought further to diagnosis and treatment for these conditions. One year ago, the periungual fibroma on the little toe of the right foot increased in size, and periungual fibromas subsequently appeared on the other four toes of the right foot and all toes of the left foot. The patient sought treatment at a local hospital, and a complete urinary system ultrasound suggested multiple renal hamartomas, leading to a consideration of tuberous sclerosis complex (TSC). The patient had no symptoms such as hematuria, frequent urination, urgent urination, dysuria, back pain, headache, etc., and thus came to our hospital for treatment. Chest and abdominal contrast-enhanced CT showed multiple round mixed-density lesions of varying sizes (composed of fat and soft tissue) in both kidneys, with clear boundaries. The larger one was in the left kidney, about 77 mm × 96 mm in size, and the surrounding tissues were compressed and displaced. No obvious enhancement was observed in the enhanced scan, and blood vessels were visible in some lesions (Fig. 1a, b). Diffuse distribution of ground-glass density small nodules and tiny nodules in the lungs and diffuse distribution of thin-walled lucencies in both lungs,

Supplementary Information The online version contains supplementary material available at https://doi.org/10.1007/978-981-96-8598-1_24.

W. Wang (✉)
Beijing Union Medical College Hospital,
Beijing, China

Y. Zhang, X. Zhao (eds.), *Laparoscopic Surgery in Urology*,
https://doi.org/10.1007/978-981-96-8598-1_24

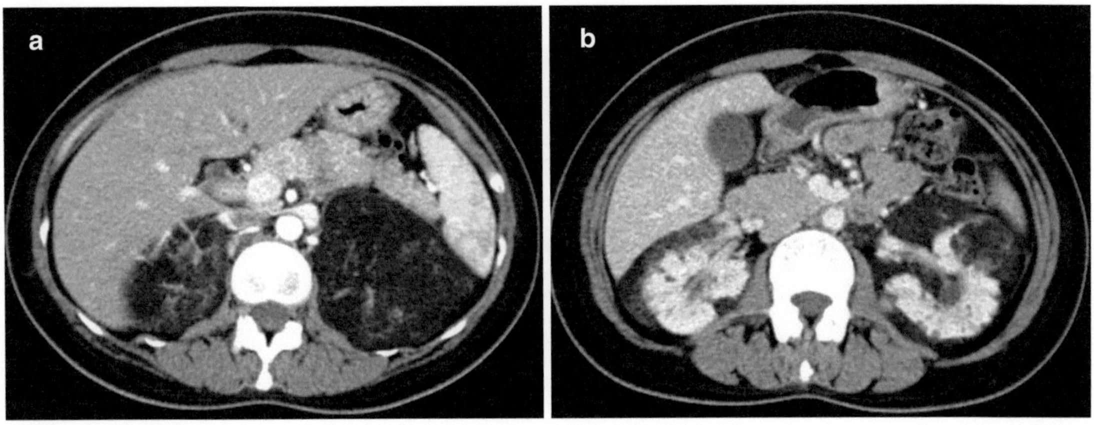

Fig. 1 (**a**, **b**) Abdominal enhanced CT

consistent with TSC-related lung changes. Further genetic testing revealed a mutation in the TSC2 gene. The patient's diagnosis of tuberous sclerosis complex was confirmed, and he was presently admitted to the hospital for surgical removal of renal angiomyolipoma.

Past History

Thyroid nodule surgery and cervical conization surgery have been performed.

Physical Examination

No special findings in the heart, lungs, and abdomen; and no percussion tenderness in both renal regions.

Imaging Data (Fig. 1)

Preoperative Assessment

The imaging examination of the patient suggests multiple renal angiomyolipomas. Combined with the patient's clinical manifestations in other systems 删除逗号 and the results of genetic testing, the diagnosis of TSC is confirmed. The largest angiomyolipoma in the patient's left kidney is about 77 mm × 96 mm, which is large in volume and has a high risk of bleeding, indicating the need for surgery.

Further assessment of cardiac and pulmonary function after admission revealed no obvious abnormalities. Renal blood flow imaging suggests that the perfusion and function of both kidneys are normal. GFR is 73.1 ml/(min 1.73 m^2), with the left kidney GFR being 36.0 ml/(min·1.73 m^2) and the right kidney GFR being 37.1 ml/(min·1.73 m^2). The surgical approach is laparoscopic partial nephrectomy of the left kidney.

Surgical Process

1. The retroperitoneal approach for partial nephrectomy position is adopted. The surgical side is marked in the ward before the operation. Endotracheal intubation general anesthesia is administered. A urinary catheter is retained. Routine disinfection and draping are performed.
2. After establishing the retroperitoneal cavity, a renal surgical access is placed. Four ports are used in this operation.
3. Clean the extraperitoneal fat (Fig. 2), identify the peritoneal reflection, and make a longitudinal incision on the renal fascia at the posterior aspect of the peritoneal reflection to expose the psoas major and renal fat capsule.

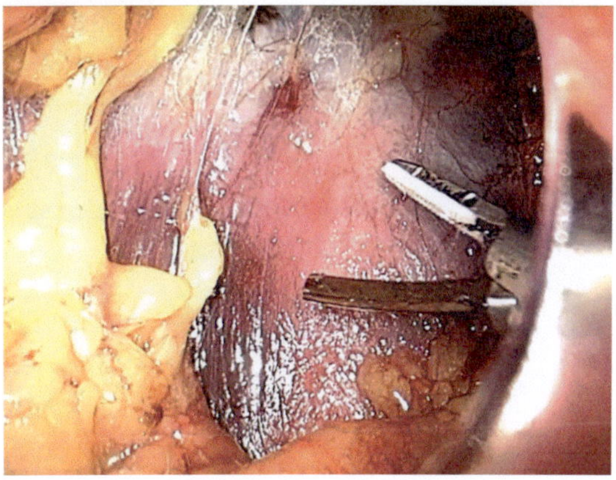

Fig. 2 Cleaning the extraperitoneal fat

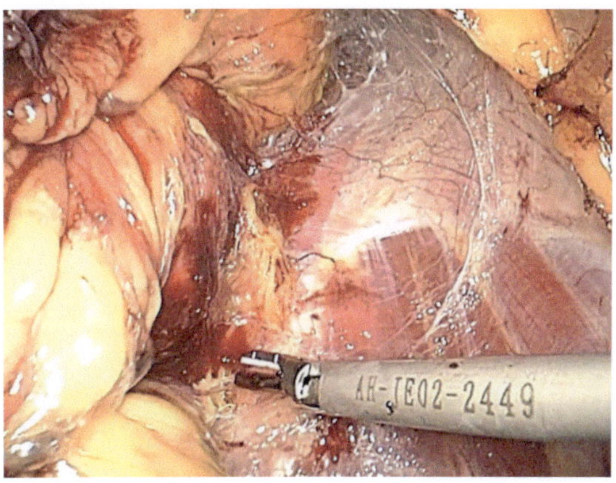

Fig. 3 Freeing the perirenal fat along the psoas major muscle

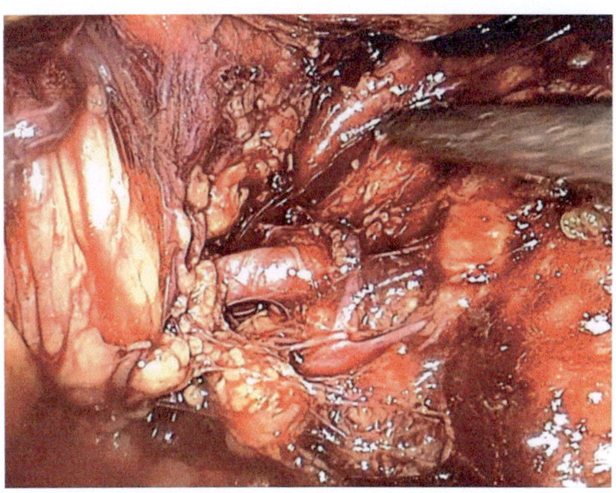

Fig. 4 Exposing the renal artery

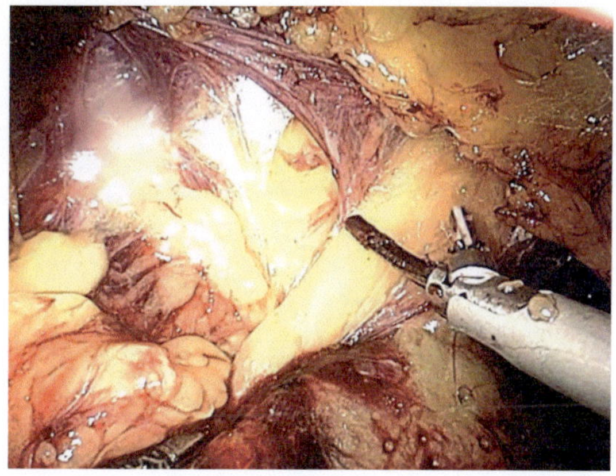

Fig. 5 Freeing the left renal tumor

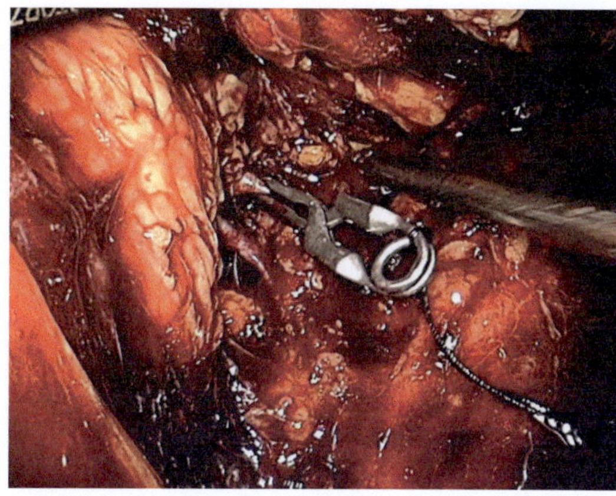

Fig. 6 Blocking the renal artery

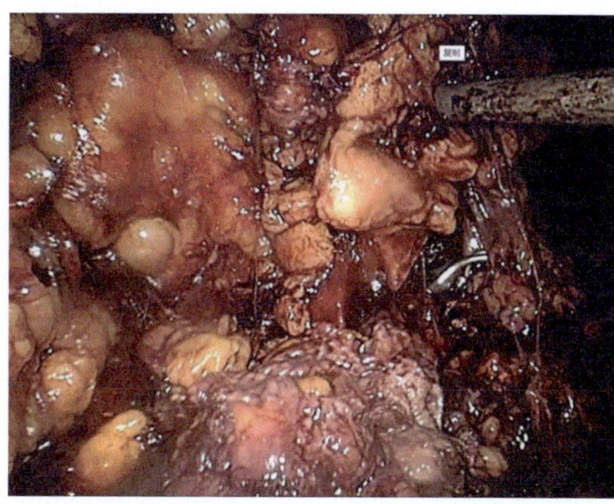

Fig. 7 Removing the renal tumor

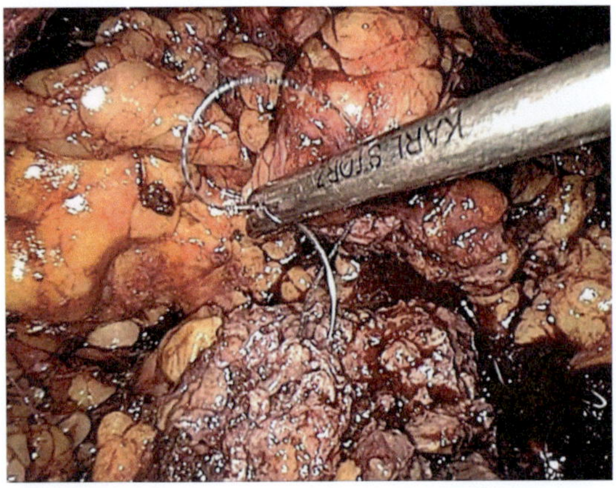

Fig. 8 1-0 V-Loc thread suturing the cut surface of the kidney

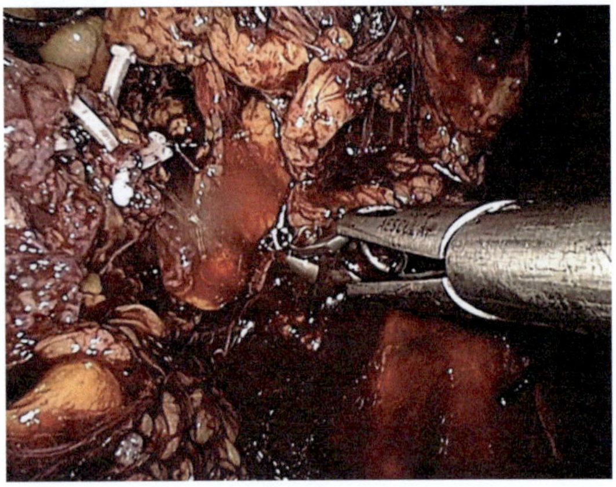

Fig. 9 Removing the arterial clamp

4. The perirenal fat pad is fully freed along the surface of the psoas major muscle and pushed toward the abdominal side (Fig. 3). Locate the medial arcuate ligament on the surface of the psoas major muscle, then find and free the left renal artery at the symmetrical position between this ligament and the medial edge of the psoas major muscle (Fig. 4).
5. Free the left renal tumor (Fig. 5).
6. Use a vascular clamp to occlude the renal artery (Fig. 6), and resect the left renal tumor from the kidney (Fig. 7).

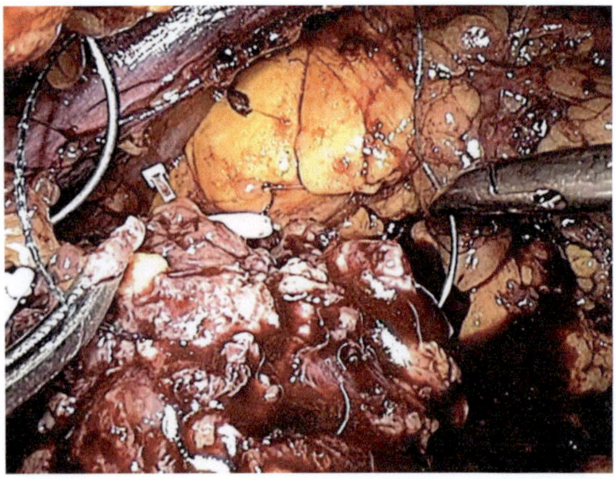

Fig. 10 Reinforcing the sutured wound

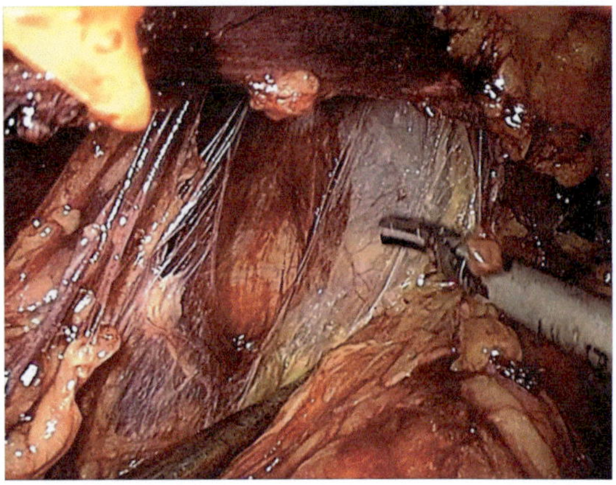

Fig. 11 Freeing the tumor on the peritoneal side

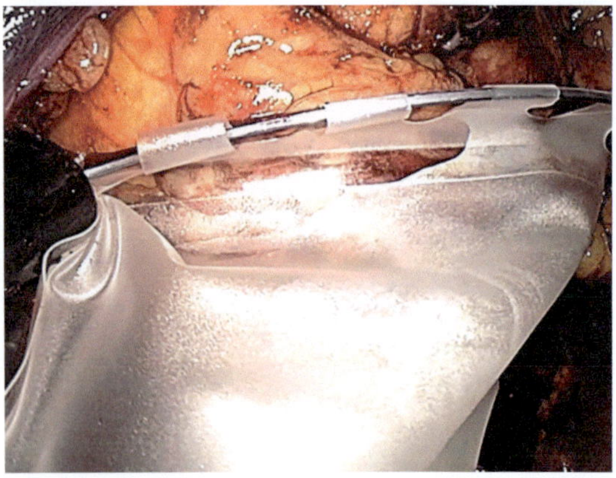

Fig. 12 Placing the tumor in the specimen bag

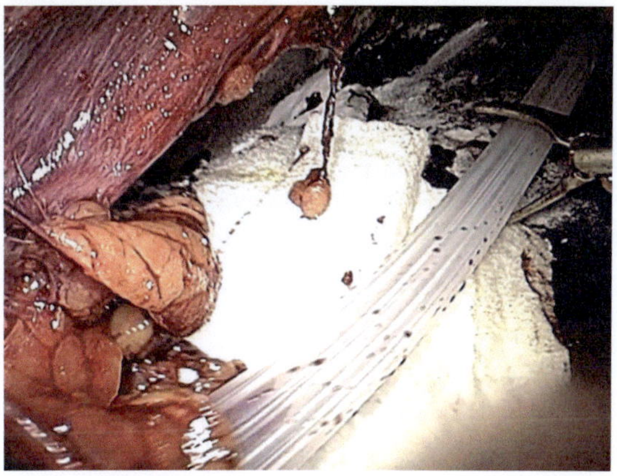

Fig. 13 Placing the drainage tube

7. Suture the cut surface of the kidney continuously with 1-0 V-Loc thread (Fig. 8). Remove the arterial clamp (Fig. 9), check for residual bleeding at the kidney wound, and continue suturing for reinforcement (Fig. 10).
8. Continue to free the resected tumor and surrounding tissue (Fig. 11).
9. Insert a specimen bag through the auxiliary port, and place the left renal tumor in the bag (Fig. 12). Check the renal hilum and wound again, achieve hemostasis, and place a drainage tube (Fig. 13). Finally, after enlarging the auxiliary port incision, the specimen is completely removed.

Expert Commentary

Tuberous sclerosis is a relatively rare autosomal dominant genetic disease, with the causative genes including TSC1 and TSC2. In terms of renal lesions, the main manifestation is renal angiomyolipoma (AML). The treatment of AML includes monitoring, mTOR inhibitors, interventional embolization, and surgery. For renal angiomy olipomas with a diameter of ≥4 cm, due to their significantly increased risk of bleeding, it is recommended to intervene with medication or surgery. Since renal angiomyolipomas often occur in multiple locations, for eligible surgical patients, nephron-sparing surgery, i.e., partial nephrectomy, is preferred to protect the patient's renal function. If surgery is required on both kidneys, staged surgery may be considered, and the order of surgery is determined based on a comprehensive assessment of the patient's tumor size and renal function.

The surgery was performed via a retroperitoneal approach for laparoscopic partial nephrectomy of the left kidney. After blocking the renal artery, the tumor was excised along its boundary from the surface of the kidney. Although the patient's left-side tumor was large, considering the tumor's shallow location, a single-layer suture was applied. Due to the large wound surface after excision, bleeding was still visible after releasing the blockage, requiring additional suturing to ensure hemostasis.

Kidney Surgery: Case 23 Robot-Assisted Laparoscopic Radical Nephrectomy of Right Kidney Cancer

Jie Dong

Chief Complaint

Right kidney tumor found during physical examination 5 days ago. Female, 51 years old. The patient accidentally discovered a right kidney tumor during a urinary system ultrasound examination 5 days ago at a local clinic. Further enhanced CT showed a round mass in the right kidney, with equal or low density, and obvious uneven enhancement in the arterial phase, about 49 mm × 45 mm, suggesting a right kidney tumor, with a high possibility of kidney cancer (Fig. 1). PET/CT suggested a round soft tissue mass about 4.8 cm × 4.3 cm in the right kidney, with clear boundaries, uneven density, and slightly increased metabolism, SUV about 1.36; the lesion protrudes into the right renal pelvis. It is considered a right kidney soft tissue mass, high possibility of kidney. The patient had no symptoms such as hematuria, back pain, or fever.

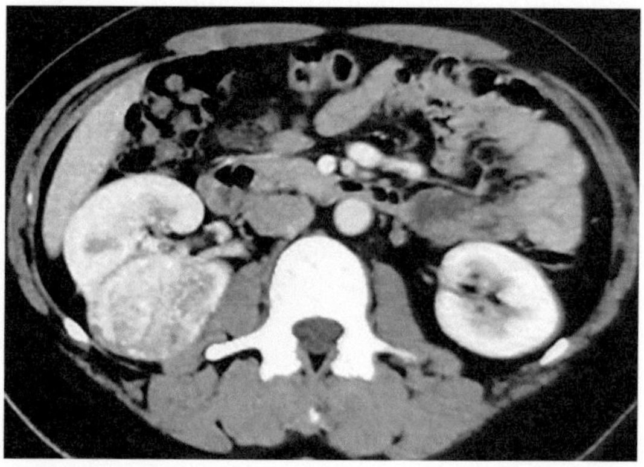

Fig. 1 Abdominal enhanced CT

Past History

History of cesarean section.

Physical Examination

No special findings in the heart and lungs, an old cesarean section scar can be seen in the lower abdomen, and there is no percussion pain in both kidney areas.

Supplementary Information The online version contains supplementary material available at https://doi.org/10.1007/978-981-96-8598-1_25.

J. Dong (✉)
Beijing Union Medical College Hospital,
Beijing, China

Y. Zhang, X. Zhao (eds.), *Laparoscopic Surgery in Urology*,
https://doi.org/10.1007/978-981-96-8598-1_25

Imaging Data (Fig. 1)

Preoperative Assessment

The patient's imaging examination suggested a right kidney tumor, with a diameter of about 5 cm, and a high possibility of malignancy, and there is a possibility of renal pelvis invasion. Combined with the patient's clinical data, the diagnosis of right kidney tumor is basically clear, and kidney cancer is possible. The indication for surgery is clear.

The outpatient clinic further supplemented the assessment of cardiopulmonary function, and no obvious abnormalities were found. Lung CT did not show evidence of distant metastasis. Renal blood flow imaging suggested that the GFR of both kidneys was 103.47 ml/(min·1.73 m^2), the GFR of the right kidney was 54.28 ml/(min·1.73 m^2), and the GFR of the left kidney was 49.19 ml/(min·1.73 m^2). The surgical method is robot-assisted laparoscopic radical nephrectomy of the right kidney.

Surgical Procedure

1. The transabdominal upper urinary tract surgical position was adopted. The surgical side was marked in the ward before surgery. Intubation general anesthesia was used. A urinary catheter was placed. Routine disinfection and draping.
2. After establishing pneumoperitoneum, the upper urinary tract surgical pathway was placed. This surgery used six holes (including the trocar below the xiphoid process and the auxiliary holes on both sides of the lens hole).
3. It was observed that the liver significantly obstructed the right kidney, so the hepatocolic ligament and the right triangular ligament of the liver were first cut off. A needle holder was placed through the trocar below the xiphoid process to lift the liver (Fig. 2).
4. Open the lateral peritoneum along the ascending colon, up to the hepatic colonic ligament, down to the sacral promontory. Push the colon inward along the outer layer of Gerota's fascia until the duodenum is exposed (Fig. 3). Then, push the duodenum inward along the outer side of the descending part of the duodenum to expose the inferior vena cava (Fig. 4).
5. At the level of the lower pole of the kidney, separate laterally to the inferior vena cava toward the dorsal side, entering the loose avascular area on the surface of the psoas major muscle. Lift the kidney and extend this plane toward the head side, to the renal hilum vessels (Fig. 5).
6. At the renal hilum, the right renal vein can be seen originating from the inferior vena cava.

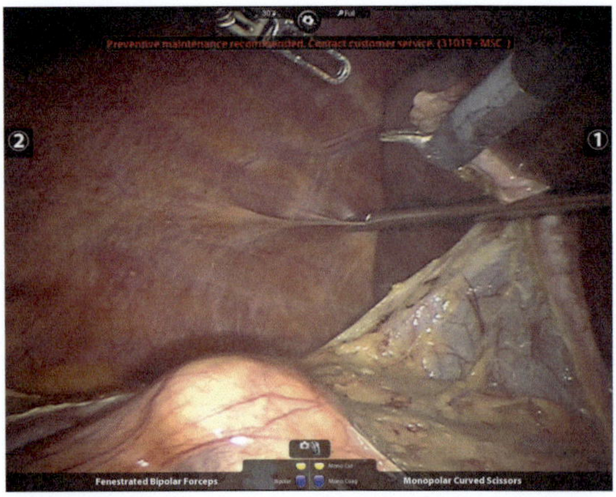

Fig. 2 Lifting the liver to assist in exposure

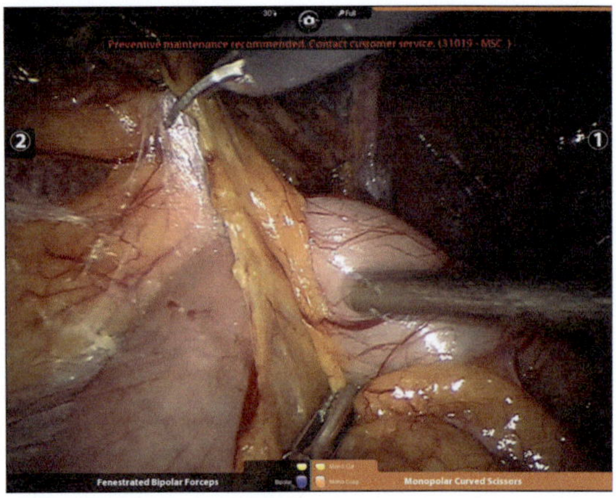

Fig. 3 Exposing the duodenum

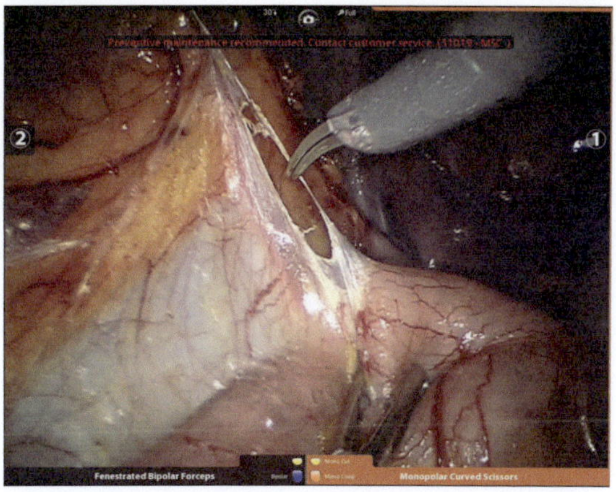

Fig. 4 Exposing the inferior vena cava

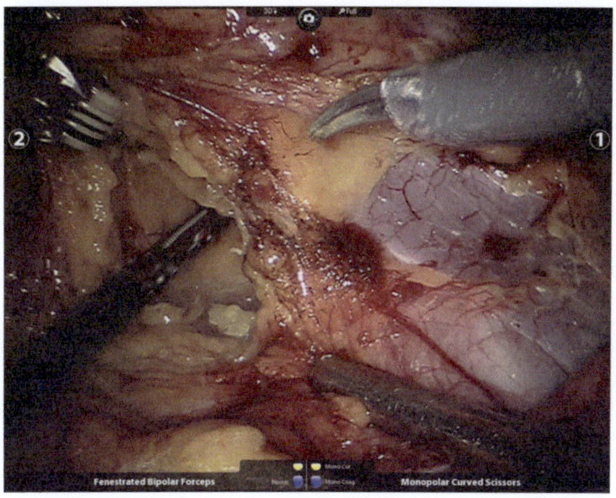

Fig. 5 Freeing along the surface of the psoas major muscle toward the renal hilum

Usually, using a combination of blunt and sharp methods, locate and free the right renal artery below and behind the renal vein (Fig. 6). Hem-o-lok is used to clamp and cut off (Fig. 7).

7. After confirming that the renal artery is properly handled, free and cut off the right renal vein in the same way (Figs. 8 and 9).
8. Continue upward along the inferior vena cava, and free the upper pole of the right kidney and the lateral and dorsal side of the right kidney outside the right adrenal gland (Figs. 10 and 11).
9. Find and cut off the ureter at the lower pole of the kidney (Figs. 12 and 13), completely freeing the right kidney.

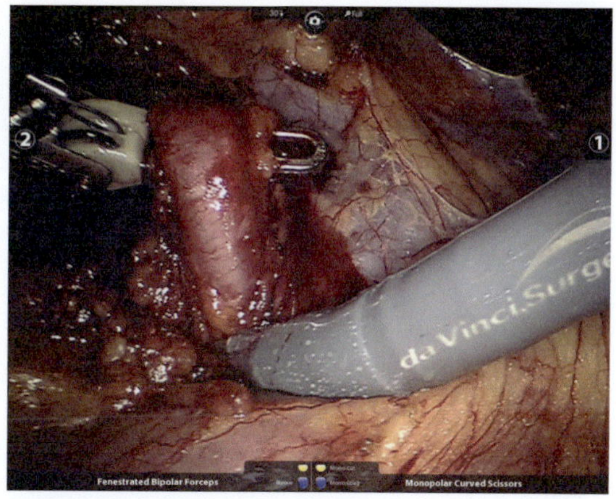

Fig. 6 Freeing the renal artery

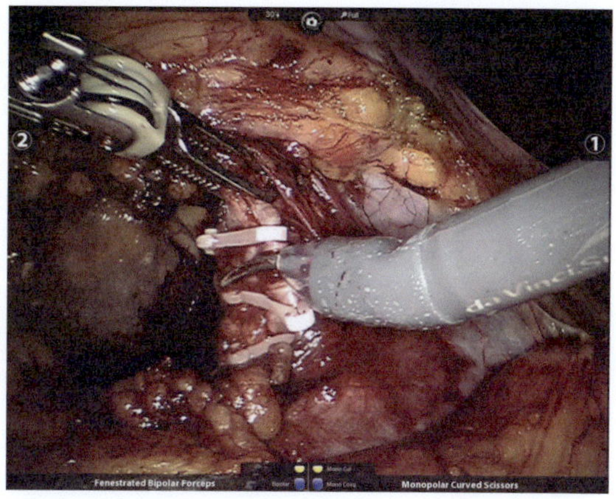

Fig. 7 Cutting off the renal artery

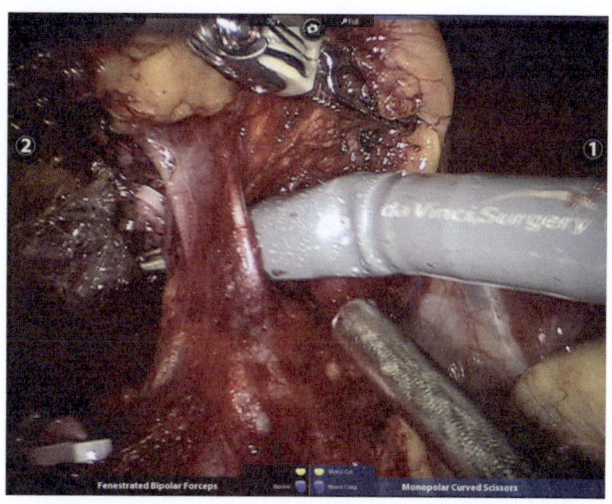

Fig. 8 Freeing the renal vein

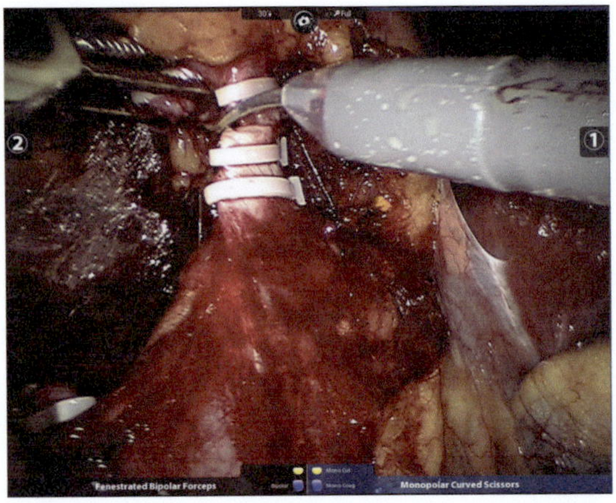

Fig. 9 Cutting off the renal vein

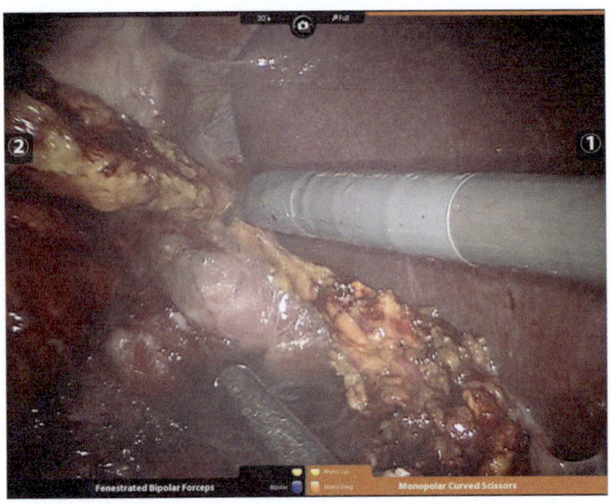

Fig. 10 Freeing the upper pole of the right kidney

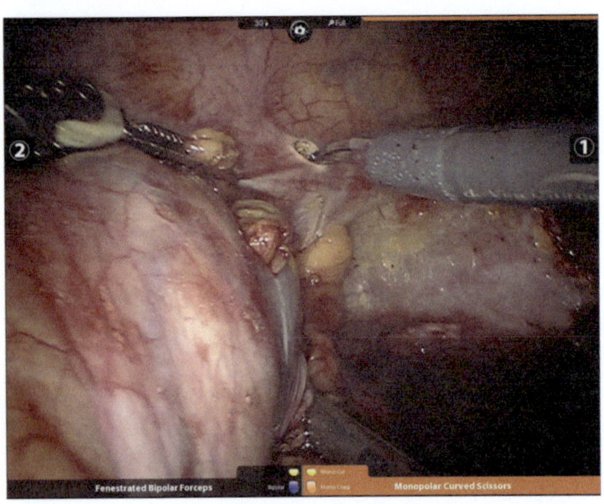

Fig. 11 Freeing the lateral and dorsal side of the right kidney

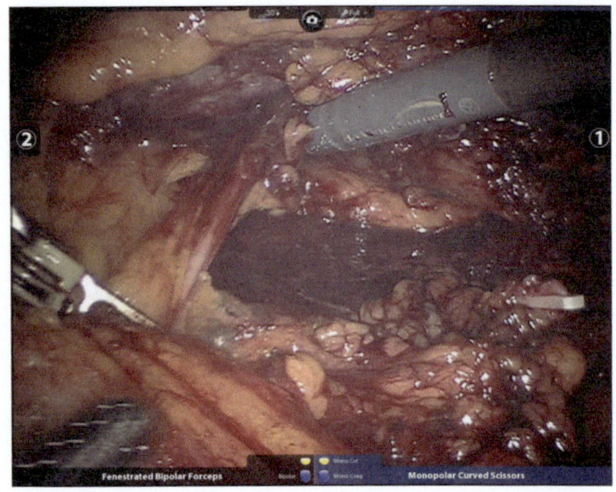

Fig. 12 Freeing the ureter

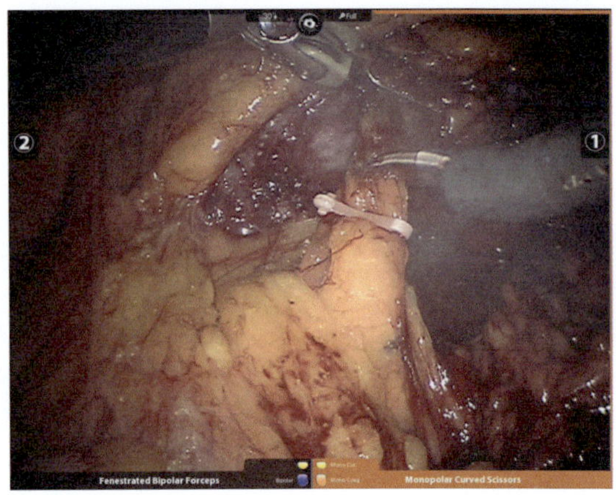

Fig. 13 Cutting off the ureter

10. After careful hemostasis, insert the specimen bag through the auxiliary hole, and place the right kidney and ureter into the bag (Fig. 14). Place the drainage tube (Fig. 15). Finally, after enlarging the auxiliary hole incision, the specimen is completely removed.

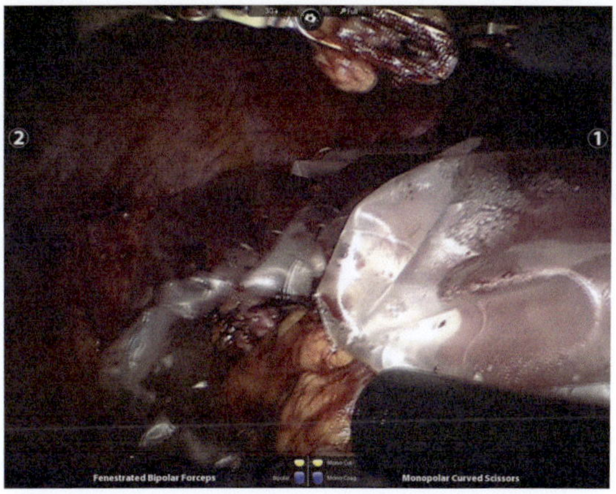

Fig. 14 Placing the kidney into the specimen bag

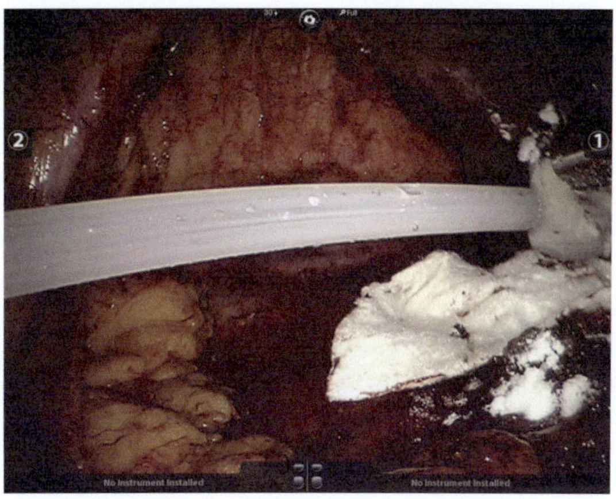

Fig. 15 Placing the drainage tube

Expert Comments

1. Choice of robot: Robotic surgery has the advantages of stable and flexible operation and more precise suturing. However, in radical nephrectomy, its advantages are not obvious compared to traditional laparoscopic surgery, and there are shortcomings such as high cost and long preparation time for surgery. But compared to other types of robotic surgery, robotic radical nephrectomy is simpler, with lower risk. For doctors who have just started robotic surgery and have not yet passed the learning curve, they can gradually become familiar with and adapt to robotic operations through such surgeries.
2. Choice of surgical approach: Consistent with traditional laparoscopic surgery, robot-assisted laparoscopic radical nephrectomy can also be performed via the abdominal or retroperitoneal approach. However, because the abdominal approach can provide a more spacious operating space and more anatomical markers, it is more convenient and safer for beginners. But for those who are proficient in robot operation, or doctors with less experience in the abdominal approach, the retroperitoneal approach to radical nephrectomy is also feasible.
3. Handling of renal hilum vessels: In radical nephrectomy, the handling of renal hilum vessels is a relatively high-risk surgical step. During the process of freeing and denuding the vessels, it is necessary to maintain a certain degree of tension in the renal hilum vessels, and the robot system lacks force feedback, so care must be taken to be gentle during operation to avoid vascular tear caused by instrument collision. In addition, sometimes the patient may have multiple renal arteries at the same time. After freeing and disconnecting a single renal artery, clamping the renal vein may cause renal bleeding, affecting the surgical field. Therefore, it is necessary to carefully read the film before surgery and predict the number and course of renal arteries through imaging examinations, and during surgery, before ligating the renal vein, make sure to carefully check the renal hilum to ensure that all renal arteries have been disconnected.

Kidney Surgery: Case 24 Robot-Assisted Laparoscopic Retroperitoneal Partial Nephrectomy of the Left Kidney

Jie Dong

Chief Complaint

A left kidney mass was found during a physical examination 20 days ago. Male, 70 years old. The patient underwent a urinary system ultrasound during a physical examination 20 days ago, which showed a moderate echo in the middle of the left kidney, measuring approximately 4.5 cm × 2.6 cm × 3.2 cm, with a regular shape, clear boundary, slightly protruding outward, and uneven internal echo. CDFI: peripheral and internal dot and strip blood flow signals. A left kidney mass was considered, and further examination was suggested. Subsequently, an enhanced abdominal CT was performed, which showed a slightly high-density round mass in the middle of the left kidney, with a strip of low-density shadow inside, a plain CT value of about 37 HU, unclear boundary, and a size of about 3.1 cm × 2.8 cm. The arterial phase was significantly enhanced during the enhanced scan, and the venous phase and delayed phase exited (Fig. 1). Malignant lesions were considered, with a high possibility of clear cell carcinoma. PET-CT examination suggested a slightly high-density nodule on the posterior lip of the left kidney, with a diameter of 2.9 cm, slightly increased radioactive uptake, SUVmx5.3, suggesting further examination to rule out malignant lesions. The patient denied symptoms such as fever, frequent urination, urgency, dysuria, back pain, afternoon fever, night sweats, gross hematuria, etc. He was admitted to our hospital for further surgical treatment.

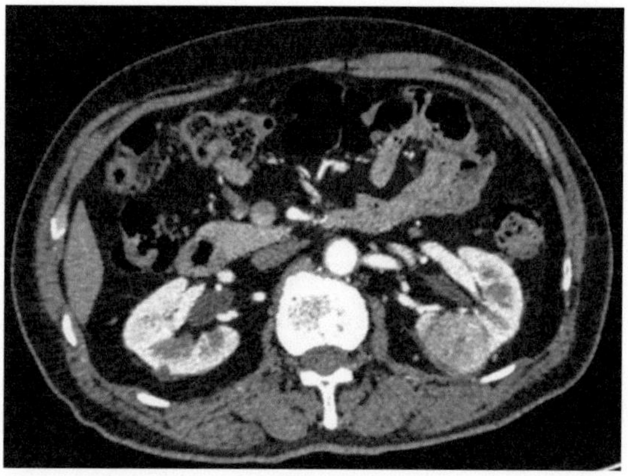

Fig. 1 Enhanced abdominal CT

Supplementary Information The online version contains supplementary material available at https://doi.org/10.1007/978-981-96-8598-1_26.

J. Dong (✉)
Beijing Union Medical College Hospital,
Beijing, China

Y. Zhang, X. Zhao (eds.), *Laparoscopic Surgery in Urology*,
https://doi.org/10.1007/978-981-96-8598-1_26

Past History

Diagnosed with bradycardia for more than 10 years, with an average heart rate of 55 beats/minute, no special treatment.

Physical Examination

No special findings in the heart, lungs, and abdomen and no percussion pain in both renal areas.

Imaging Data (Fig. 1)

Preoperative Assessment

The patient's radiological examination suggests a left kidney tumor, with a diameter of approximately 3.5 cm, and a high likelihood of malignancy. Considering the patient's clinical data, the diagnosis of left kidney tumor is basically clear, with the possibility of renal cancer and a clinical stage of cTlaN0M0. The indications for surgery are clear. Further outpatient assessment of cardiopulmonary function showed no obvious abnormalities. No evidence of distant metastasis was found on lung CT. Renal blood flow imaging suggests normal perfusion and function of both kidneys, with a GFR of 89.25 ml/(min·1.73 m^2), of which the left kidney GFR is 42.21 ml/(min·1.73 m^2) and the right kidney GFR is 47.04 ml/(min·1.73 m^2). The surgical method is robot-assisted laparoscopic partial nephrectomy of the left kidney.

Surgical Procedure

1. The retroperitoneal upper urinary tract surgical position is adopted. The surgical side is marked in the ward before surgery. Intubation general anesthesia is used. A urinary catheter is placed. Routine disinfection and draping are performed.
2. Establish the retroperitoneal cavity and place the upper urinary tract surgical channel. This surgery uses four ports.
3. Clean the extraperitoneal fat (Fig. 2), identify the peritoneal reflection, and longitudinally open the renal fascia on the dorsal side of the peritoneal reflection, revealing the psoas major muscle and the perirenal fat capsule (Fig. 3).
4. Fully free the perirenal fat capsule along the surface of the psoas major muscle and push it toward the abdominal side (Fig. 4). Locate the medial arcuate ligament on the surface of the psoas major muscle, and find and free the left renal artery at the symmetrical position of the ligament and the medial edge of the psoas major muscle (Fig. 5).

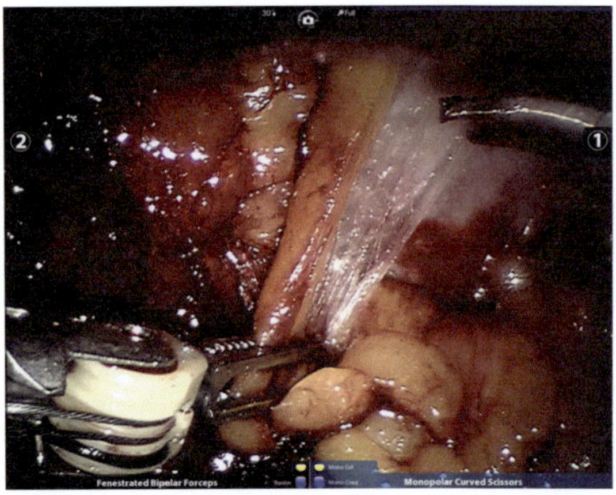

Fig. 2 Freeing the extraperitoneal fat

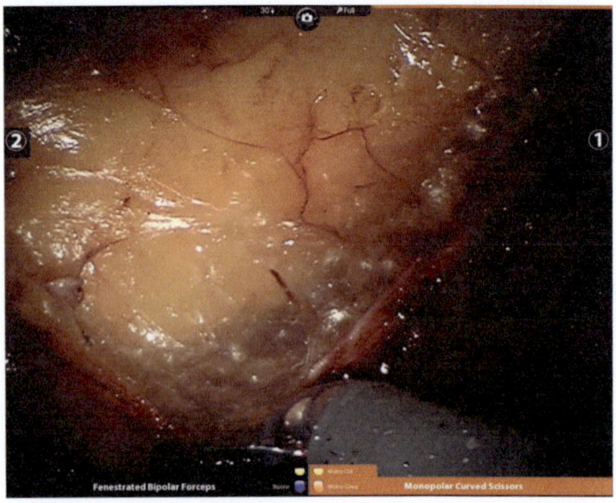

Fig. 3 Opening the renal fascia

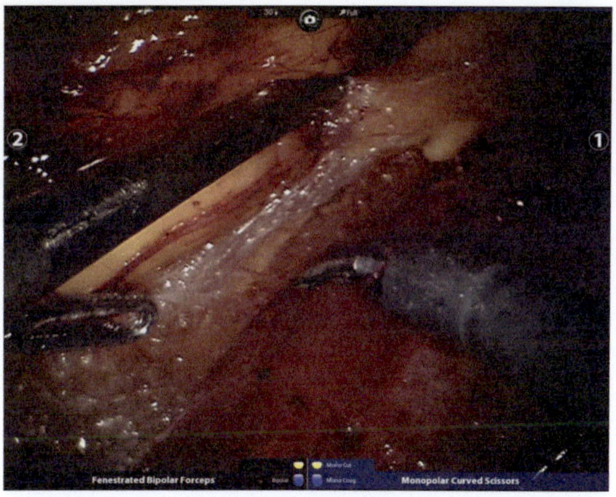

Fig. 4 Pushing the kidney toward the abdominal side

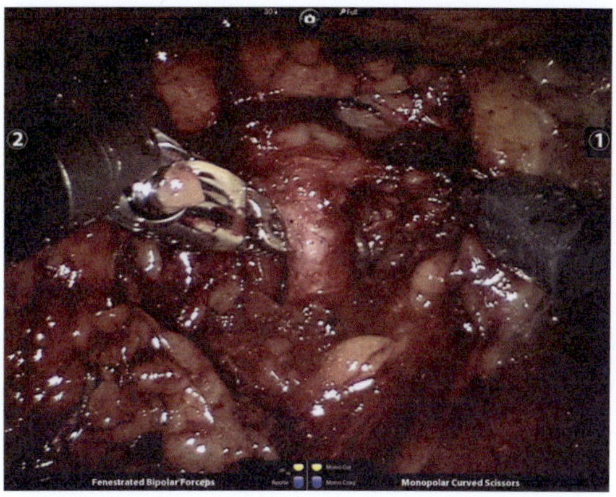

Fig. 5 Freeing the renal artery

5. At a position close to the peritoneum, longitudinally split the renal fat capsule, free the left kidney, and expose the tumor (Figs. 6 and 7).
6. Use a vascular occlusion clamp to block the renal artery (Fig. 8). Cut the renal parenchyma 0.5 cm from the edge of the tumor, and use a combination of blunt and sharp methods to free the base of the tumor while avoiding damage to the vessels and collecting system as much as possible (Fig. 9).
7. Replace the right arm with a needle driver. Use a layered suturing method, 3–0 V-Loc thread for continuous suturing of the tumor base (Fig. 10), tighten it, and then use 1–0 V-Loc thread for continuous suturing of the wound.

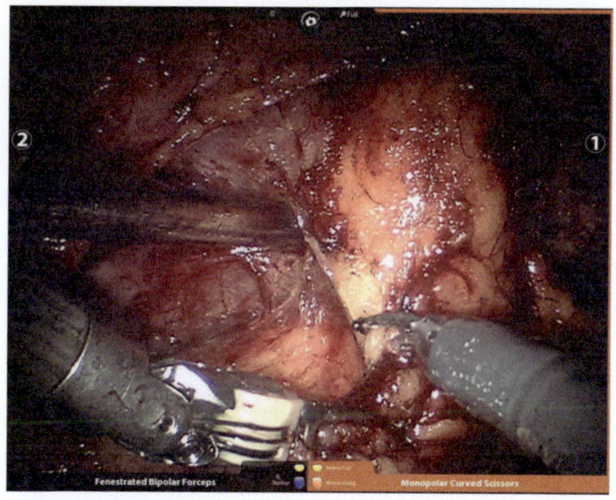

Fig. 6 Freeing the kidney

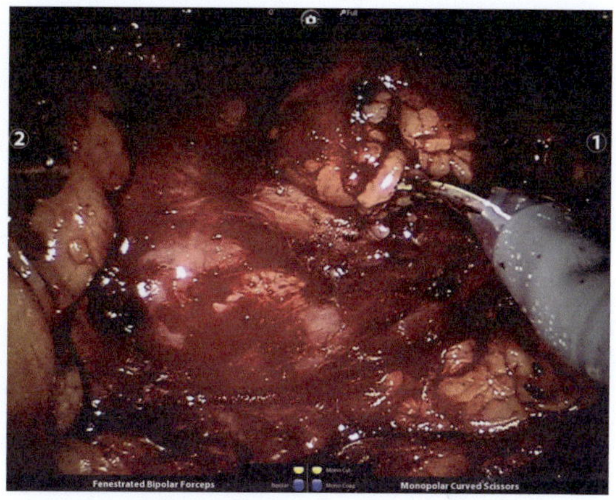

Fig. 7 Exposing the tumor

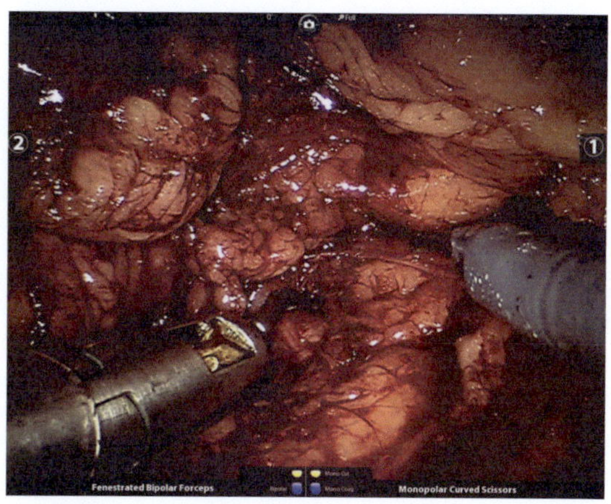

Fig. 8 Blocking the renal artery

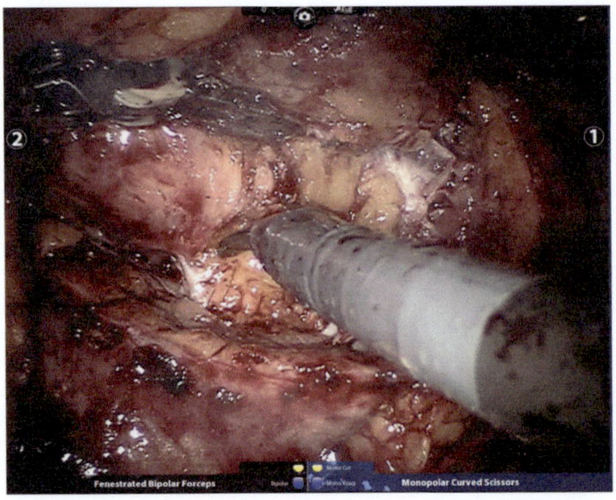

Fig. 9 Removing the tumor

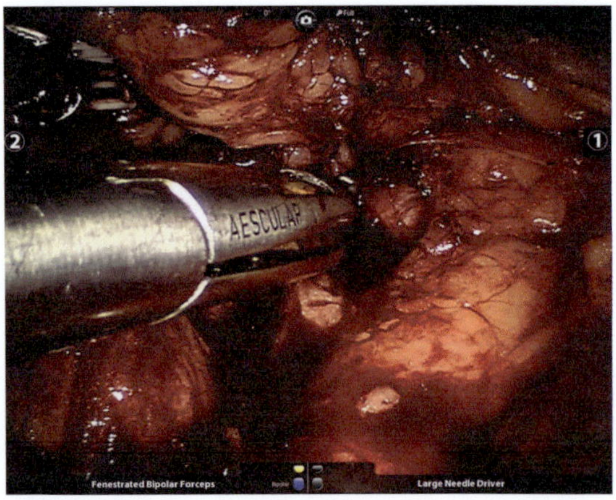

Fig. 12 Removal of arterial occlusion

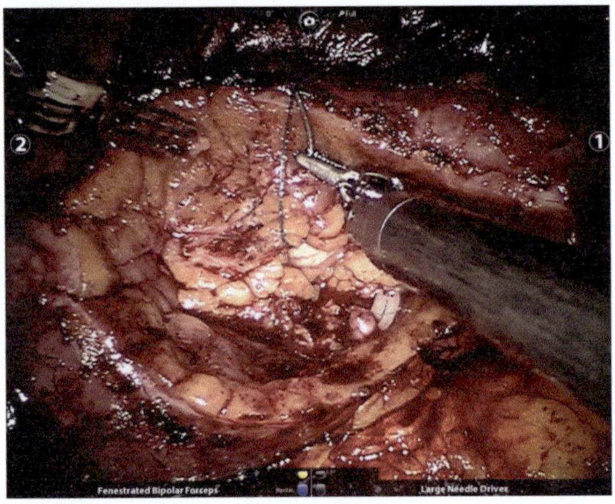

Fig. 10 3–0 V-Loc suture at the base

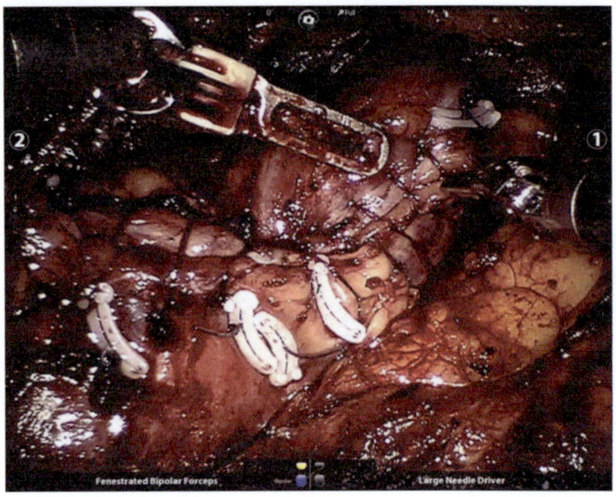

Fig. 13 Checking the wound

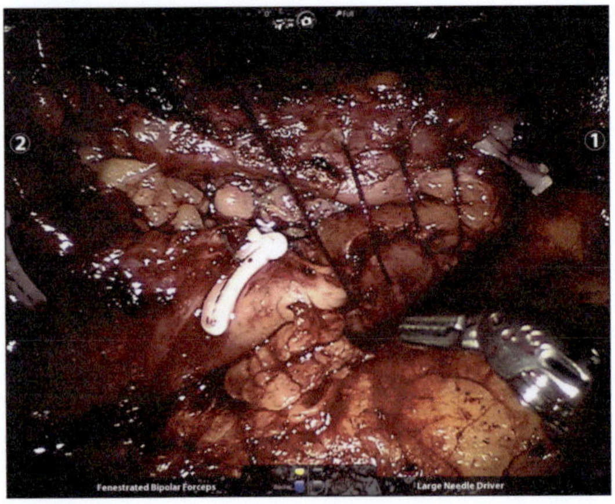

Fig. 11 1–0 V-Loc suture of the wound

The thread end is fixed with Hem-o-lok (Fig. 11).

8. Remove the arterial occlusion clamp, and check for active bleeding in the renal hilum and renal wound (Figs. 12 and 13).
9. Insert a specimen bag through the auxiliary hole, and place the left kidney tumor in the bag (Fig. 14). Place a drainage tube (Fig. 15). Finally, after enlarging the auxiliary hole incision, the specimen is completely removed.

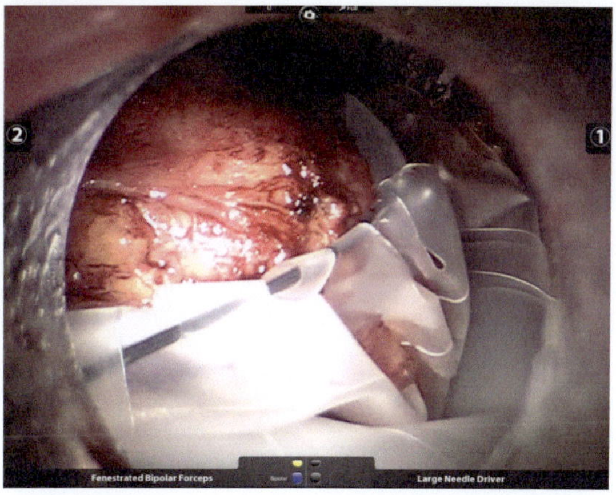

Fig. 14 Tumor loaded into specimen bag

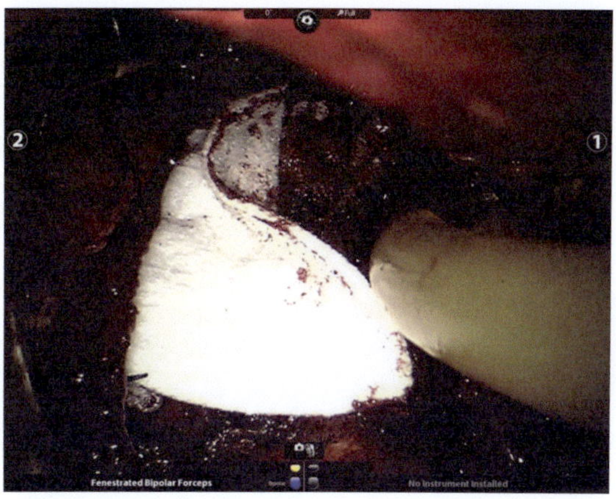

Fig. 15 Placement of drainage tube

Expert Commentary

1. Placement of the robotic trocar: Because the space in the retroperitoneal cavity is small, the expansion of the space is very important before placing the robotic trocar. An airbag can be used to push the peritoneum as far as possible toward the abdominal side, and the robotic trocar can be placed at the edge of the peritoneal fold under direct vision, maximizing the use of the operating space in the retroperitoneal cavity. At the same time, if the trocar is placed too deep, it may cause difficulty in operating near the trocar, so when placing the trocar, the first marking line on the sheath can be seen.
2. Choice of surgical approach: Consistent with traditional laparoscopic surgery, robot-assisted laparoscopic partial nephrectomy can also be performed via the abdominal or retroperitoneal approach. Presently, the robot's flexible manipulator makes tumor removal and wound suturing more flexible, greatly reducing the restriction of tumor location on the approach. Because the retroperitoneal approach is more direct and has less impact on the intestinal tract in the abdomen, faster postoperative recovery, etc., our department prefers to use the retroperitoneal approach for robot-assisted partial nephrectomy. However, for tumors in the upper pole and anterior lip, there are certain visual and operational blind spots in the retroperitoneal approach, and we tend to use the abdominal approach. Of course, the choice of surgical approach also needs to be combined with the patient's own conditions and the doctor's experience for comprehensive judgment.
3. Handling of renal pedicle vessels: During partial nephrectomy, the degree of renal artery occlusion determines the clarity of the interface. Some patients have premature or multiple renal arteries, which may cause the surgeon to mistake the freed branch or one of the renal arteries for the main renal artery, resulting in unsatisfactory occlusion. In addition, it may also be due to the incomplete occlusion of the artery occlusion clamp. Therefore, when the occlusion is unsatisfactory, if it is confirmed that there are no other branch arteries, you can try to use two occlusion clamps side by side on the renal artery to achieve complete occlusion.
4. Wound suturing: For the suturing of the wound after partial nephrectomy, especially when the wound is relatively deep, it is recommended to use a layered suturing method. The inner layer mainly closes the small openings of the blood vessels and collecting system formed during tumor removal. It also reduces the tension of the wound by suturing the inner layer of renal medulla and then achieves complete hemostasis and reconstruction through suturing of the outer layer of the

wound. In robotic surgery, doctors should fully utilize the advantage of the robot's flexible manipulator arm to make the suturing process more precise, which also helps to shorten the ischemic time of the kidney. However, due to the lack of force feedback in robotic operations, there may be problems with sutures being too loose or too tight or cutting renal parenchyma during suturing. It is necessary to summarize experience in actual operations and compensate for the lack of touch through vision.

Kidney Surgery: Case 25 Laparoscopic Retroperitoneal Radical Surgery for Left Renal Pelvic Carcinoma

Wenda Wang

Chief Complaint

Dark urine for 2 months and hematuria for 3 weeks.

Medical History

Female, 59 years old. Two months ago, the patient developed unexplained dark urine. She sought treatment at another hospital and received traditional Chinese medicine treatment, but the effect was unsatisfactory. She developed painless hematuria 3 weeks ago, accompanied by tubular casts, without fever, urinary urgency, urinary frequency or pain during urination. She then presented to the emergency department of our hospital. Ultrasound examination showed separation of the left renal collecting system with hypoechoic foci inside (please combine with other imaging examinations) and hypoechoic lesions in the bladder, which were considered blood clots. The emergency department administered oral Yunnan Baiyao capsules for hemostasis and performed continuous bladder irrigation. After the color of the irrigation fluid gradually cleared, bladder irrigation was stopped. For further diagnosis and treatment, she visited our outpatient department. Enhanced CT of the chest, abdomen, and pelvis showed a lesion in the left renal pelvis, about 2.0 cm × 1.0 cm in size, with low enhancement on the enhanced scan; malignancy cannot be excluded (Figs. 1 and 2). For further diagnosis and treatment, the outpatient department admitted her to the hospital with a preliminary diagnosis of renal pelvis tumor.

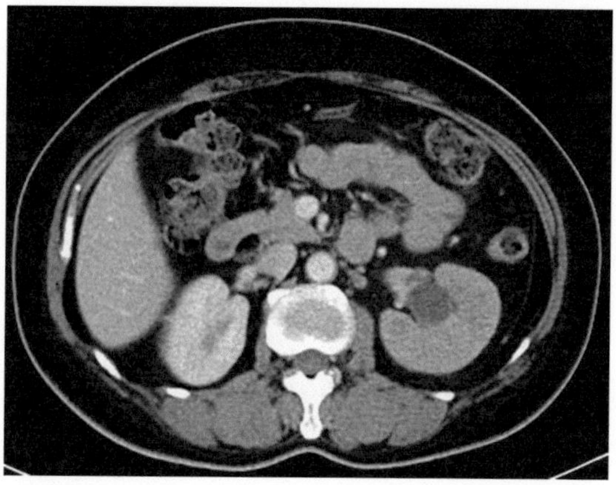

Fig. 1 Abdominal enhanced CT (arterial phase)

Supplementary Information The online version contains supplementary material available at https://doi.org/10.1007/978-981-96-8598-1_27.

W. Wang (✉)
Beijing Union Medical College Hospital,
Beijing, China

Y. Zhang, X. Zhao (eds.), *Laparoscopic Surgery in Urology*,
https://doi.org/10.1007/978-981-96-8598-1_27

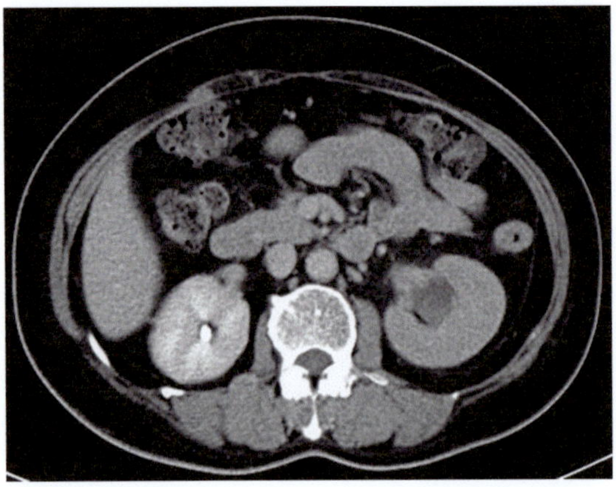

Fig. 2 Abdominal enhanced CT (excretory phase)

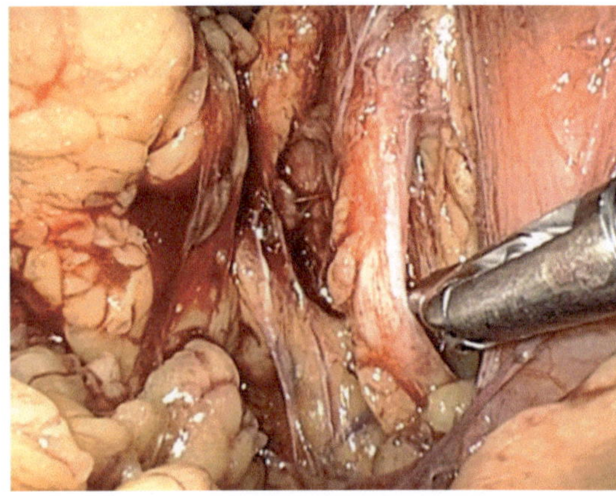

Fig. 3 Surface of the psoas major muscle revealing the ureter

Past History

History of cervical squamous cell carcinoma for more than a year, with previous treatment involving radiotherapy and chemotherapy.

Physical Examination

No special findings in the heart and lungs; no bulging in both renal regions; no percussion tenderness; no tenderness along the course of both ureters; and no bladder distension.

Imaging Data (Figs. 1 and 2)

Preoperative Assessment

The patient's imaging examination suggested a lesion in the left renal pelvis, about 2.0 cm × 1.0 cm in size, with low enhancement on the enhanced scan; malignancy cannot be ruled out. Combined with the patient's clinical data, the diagnosis of left renal pelvis tumor is basically confirmed, and renal pelvic carcinoma is suspected. The indications for surgery are clear.

The outpatient department further assessed the cardiac and pulmonary function, and no obvious abnormalities were found. Chest CT showed no evidence of distant metastasis. Renal blood flow imaging suggested that the GFR of both kidneys was 72.05 ml/(min·1.73 m^2), with the GFR of the right kidney being 52.30 ml/(min·1.73 m^2), and the GFR of the left kidney being 19.75 ml/(min·1.73 m^2). The patient had severe pelvic adhesions due to previous radiotherapy and chemotherapy for cervical cancer. After fully communicating with the patient and her family about the condition, it was planned to perform laparoscopic left nephrectomy combined with partial left ureterectomy.

Surgical Procedure

1. The retroperitoneal upper urinary tract surgical position was adopted. The surgical side was marked in the ward before surgery. Endotracheal intubation general anesthesia was administered. A urinary catheter was placed. Routine disinfection and draping were performed.
2. After establishing pneumoperitoneum, the upper urinary tract surgical access was placed. Four ports were used in this operation.
3. After cleaning the extraperitoneal fat and identifying the peritoneal reflection, a longitudinal incision was made in the renal fascia on the dorsal side of the peritoneal reflection to expose the psoas major muscle and the renal fat capsule. The ureter was located on the sur-

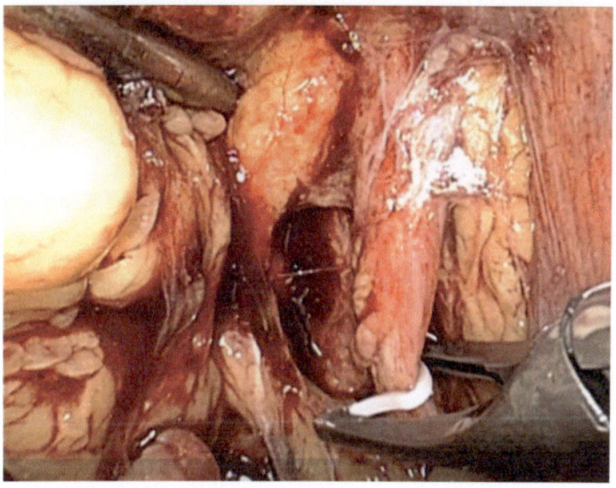

Fig. 4 Obstruction of the ureter

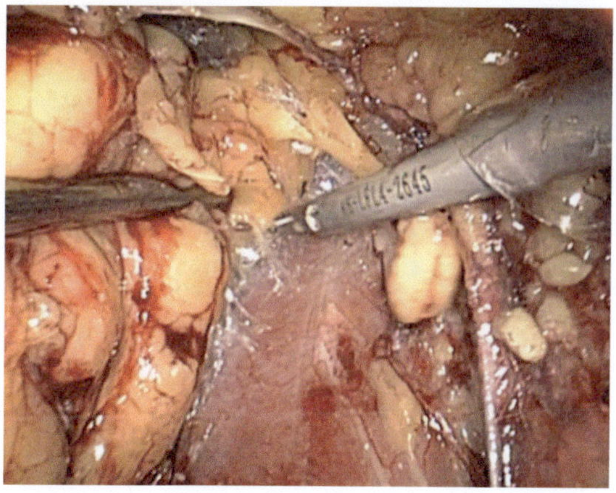

Fig. 5 Freeing the perirenal fat along the surface of the psoas major muscle

face of the psoas major muscle (Fig. 3), and the ureter was clamped with a Hem-o-lok (Fig. 4).

4. Along the surface of the psoas major muscle, the perirenal fat capsule is fully freed and pushed toward the abdominal side (Fig. 5).
5. Locate the medial arcuate ligament on the surface of the psoas major muscle, then find and free the left renal artery and vein at the symmetrical position of this ligament and the inner edge of the psoas major muscle (Fig. 6).
6. Sever the left renal artery and renal vein separately (Figs. 7 and 8).
7. Free the kidney from the peritoneum on the outside of the perirenal fat capsule (Fig. 9).
8. Free the left ureter, expose the accompanying gonadal vein, and protect it (Fig. 10). Use a Hem-o-lok clip to obstruct the upper end of the ureter again (Fig. 11).
9. Considering the patient's advanced age, anemia, etc., try to free the left ureter downward as much as possible via the retroperitoneal approach, use a Hem-o-lok clip to clamp the ureter near the site where the left ureter crosses the external iliac artery, and transect the ureter (Figs. 12 and 13).
10. Continue to free the perirenal fat capsule on all sides (Fig. 14); no tumor invasion of the renal pelvis or adrenal gland was observed during the operation. Therefore, considering

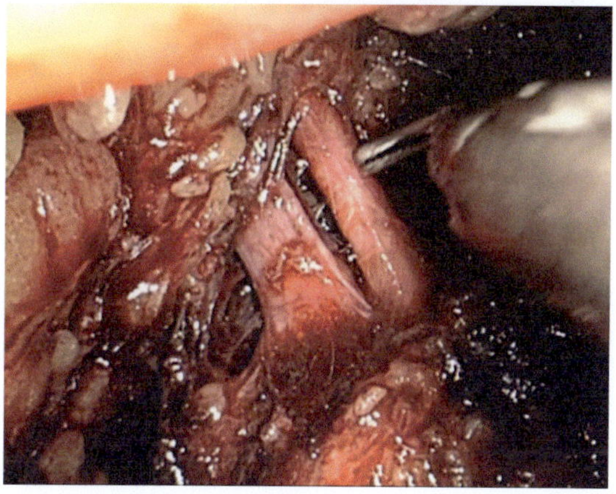

Fig. 6 Freeing the renal artery and renal vein

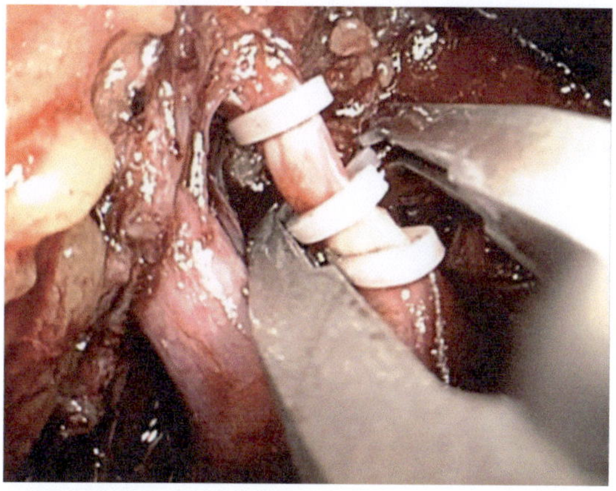

Fig. 7 Severing the renal artery

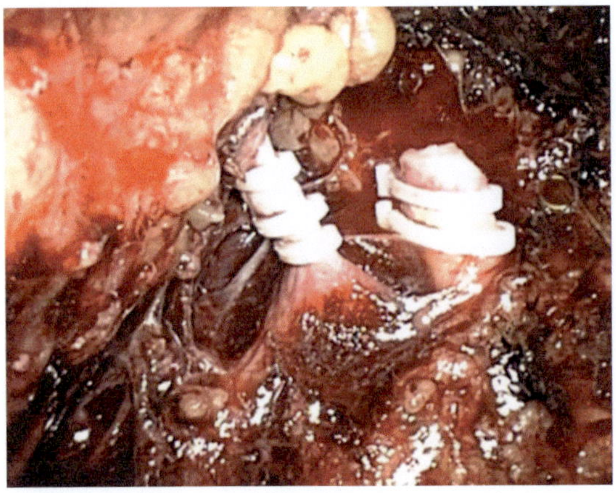

Fig. 8 Severing the renal vein

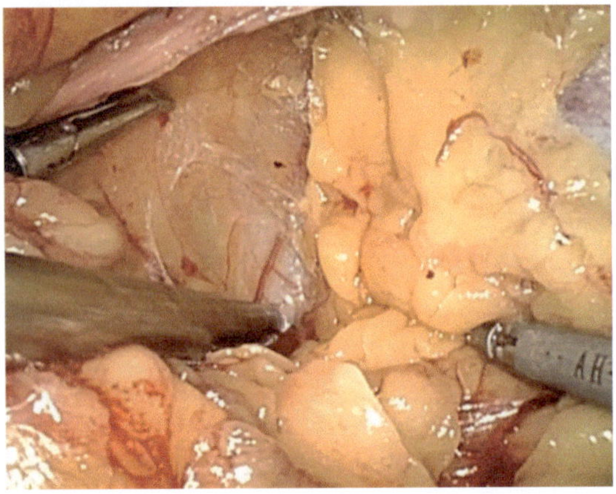

Fig. 9 Freeing the perirenal fat and peritoneum

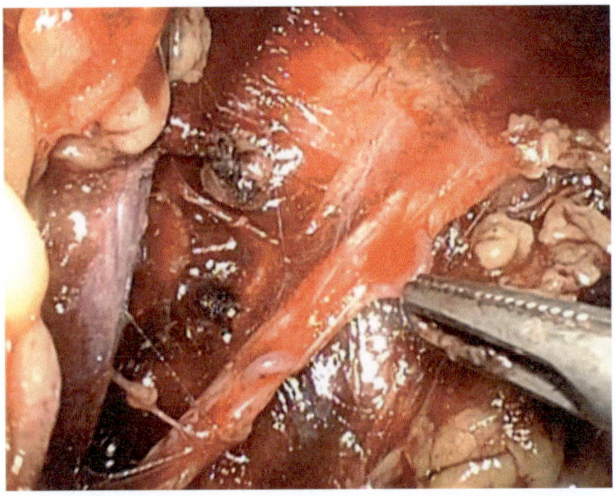

Fig. 10 Freeing the ureter and protecting the gonadal vein

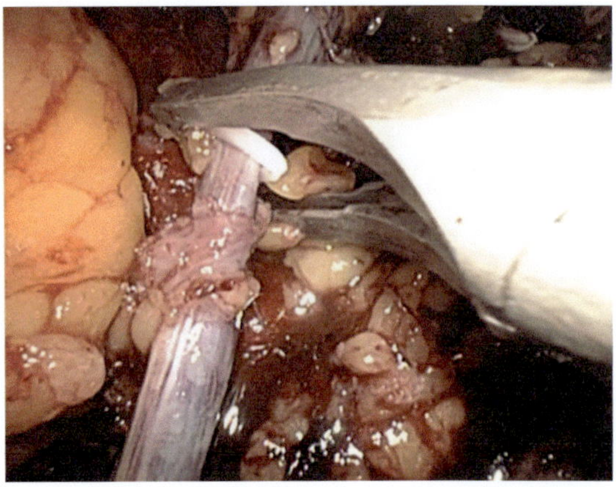

Fig. 11 Obstructing the upper end of the ureter

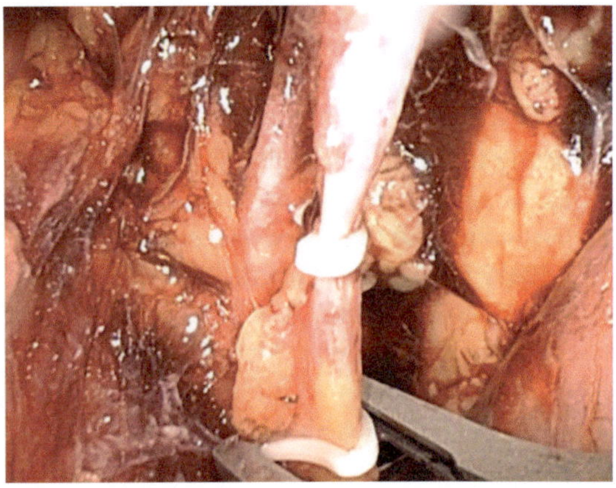

Fig. 12 Freeing the ureter downward as much as possible and obstructing it again

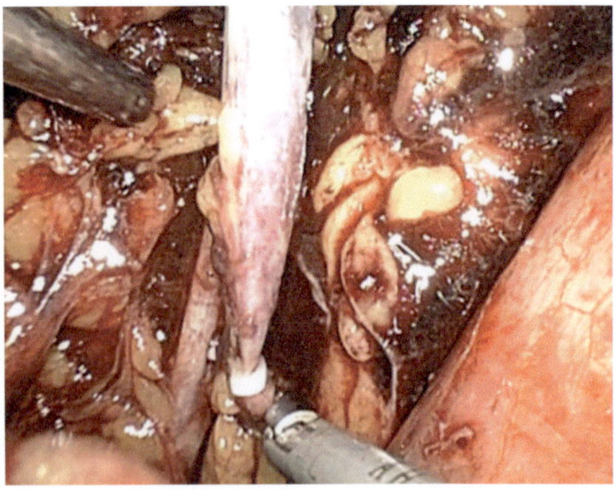

Fig. 13 Cutting off the ureter

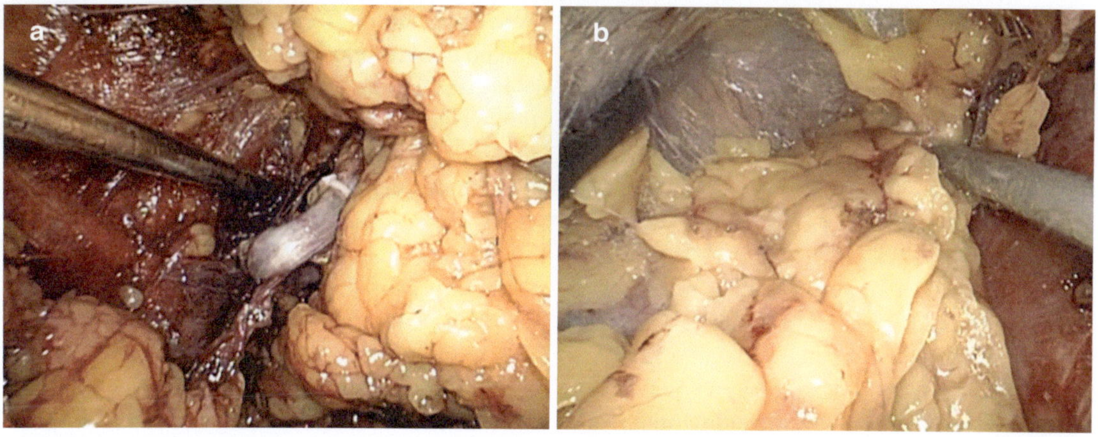

Fig. 14 (**a**) Freeing the perirenal fat capsule (I) (**b**) Freeing the perirenal fat capsule (II)

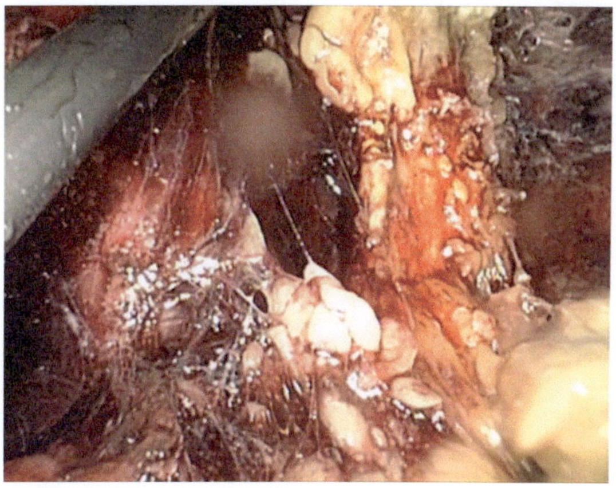

Fig. 15 Preserving the adrenal gland

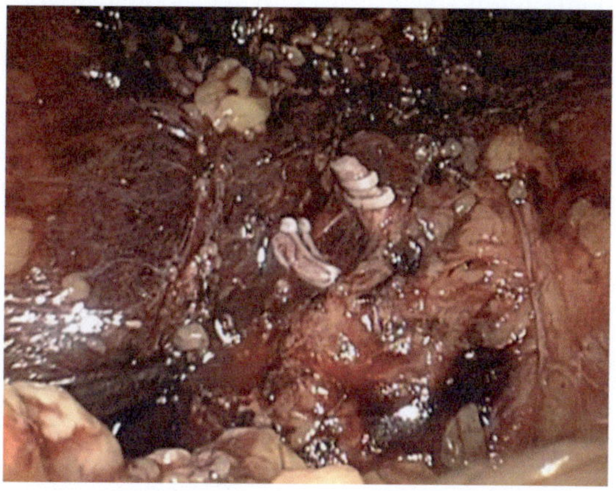

Fig. 16 Checking the ends of the renal hilum vessels

the patient's condition, the ipsilateral adrenal gland was preserved (Fig. 15).

11. After the kidney is completely freed, inspect the stumps of the renal hilar vessels, adrenal gland, etc., and achieve thorough hemostasis (Figs. 16 and 17).
12. After careful hemostasis, insert the specimen bag through the auxiliary port, and put the

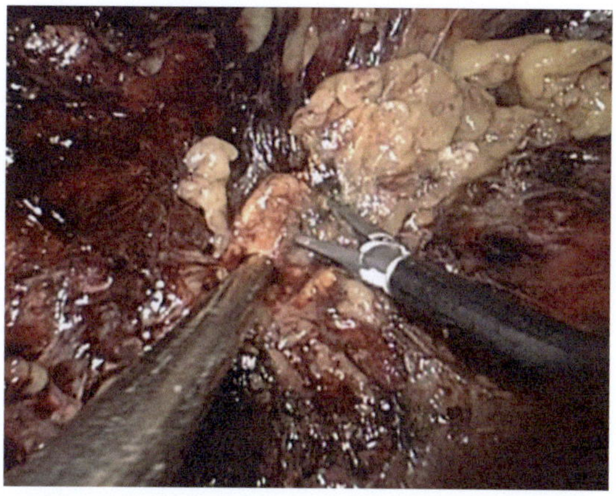

Fig. 17 Checking the adrenal gland area

left kidney and ureter into the bag. Place a drainage tube. Finally, after enlarging the auxiliary port incision, the specimen is completely removed.

Expert Commentary

The patient was diagnosed with a renal pelvis mass due to hematuria, and renal pelvis carcinoma was suspected based on imaging findings. The surgical resection range for renal pelvic carcinoma includes the kidney, the entire ureter, and the portion of the bladder surrounding the ureteral orifice. Upper urinary tract epithelial carcinoma rarely metastasizes to the adrenal gland. When the tumor is confined to the renal pelvis and no adrenal abnormalities are found preoperatively and intraoperatively, routine adrenal resection is not necessary. Because the patient had previously undergone radiotherapy and chemotherapy for cervical cancer, severe pelvic adhesions were present. Therefore, left nephrectomy combined with partial left ureterectomy was performed. During the operation, the ureter was dissected at a lower level and occluded to prevent the intraoperative downward spread of tumor cells. The traditional retroperitoneal approach was adopted with the patient in the lateral position. Intraoperatively, the ureter was dissected as far distally as possible, and transected at the site where it crosses the iliac vessels.

Bladder Surgery: Case 26 Laparoscopic Total Cystectomy

Zixing Ye

Chief Complaint

Diagnosed with bladder cancer for over a year, TURBT 1 year and 5 months post-operation, 1 month after neoadjuvant therapy.

Medical History

Male, 46 years old. The patient sought treatment at an hospital in June 2021 due to gross hematuria. Ultrasonography of the urinary system suggested a bladder tumor (details unknown), so he came to our hospital. CTU suggested a tumor about 1.1 cm in diameter on the left wall of the bladder, with no other obvious abnormalities. Cystoscopy showed a wide-based tumor on the left wall of the bladder, 1.5 cm in diameter. In August 2021, he underwent transurethral resection of bladder tumor under general anesthesia. Pathology: High-grade stromal invasive urothelial carcinoma of the bladder, no muscle invasion. After the operation, he underwent 15 times of BCG instillation therapy, with no discomfort. Regular follow-ups showed no abnormalities. In April 2022, the cystoscopy showed a wide-based lump on the left wall of the bladder and around the ureteral orifice, about 1.5 cm in diameter; CTU: A patchy high-intensity shadow was seen around the left wall of the bladder and around the left ureteral orifice; the larger one was about 0.9 cm in diameter, with a filling defect in the excretory phase, suggesting a recurrence of bladder cancer. Therefore, he underwent transurethral resection of bladder tumor in May 2022. Pathology: High-grade stromal invasive urothelial carcinoma, no muscle invasion, suggesting a recurrence of bladder cancer. After ruling out contraindications to chemotherapy, he began gemcitabine + cisplatin neoadjuvant intravenous chemotherapy in July 2022 and has completed two courses so far, with good tolerance. Recently, the patient's follow-up chest and abdominal enhanced CT suggested scattered micronodules in the lower lobes of both lungs as before, and the left wall of the bladder and the left ureteral orifice were slightly thickened with abnormal enhancement, which was more obvious than before (Fig. 1). The patient was admitted to our hospital for radical cystectomy.

Supplementary Information The online version contains supplementary material available at https://doi.org/10.1007/978-981-96-8598-1_28.

Z. Ye (✉)
Beijing Union Medical College Hospital, Beijing, China
e-mail: yezixing@pumch.cn

Y. Zhang, X. Zhao (eds.), *Laparoscopic Surgery in Urology*,
https://doi.org/10.1007/978-981-96-8598-1_28

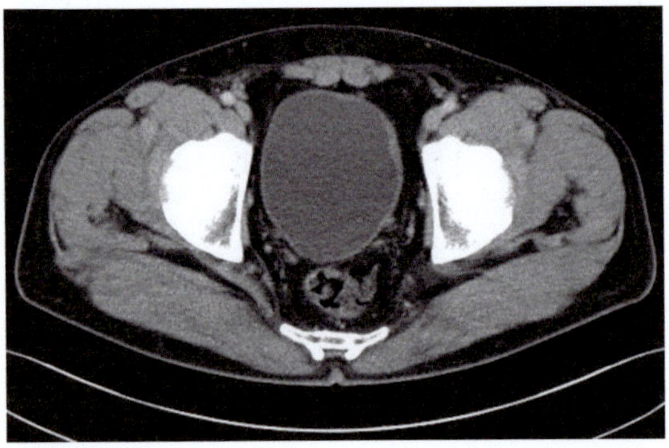

Fig. 1 Bladder enhanced CT: Thickening of the left wall of the bladder with abnormal enhancement

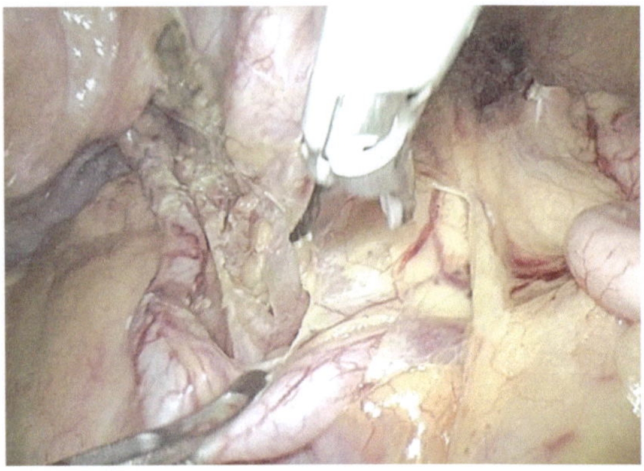

Fig. 2 Free the right ureter

Past History

Hypertension for 13 years, up to 160/100 mmHg, oral telmisartan 80 mg qd. Blood pressure was controlled well. Hyperlipidemia for 13 years, presently taking rosuvastatin 5 mg qn.

Physical examination: Vital signs stable, no special findings on heart, lung, and abdominal examination, and no filling or tenderness in the bladder area.

Image Data (Fig. 1)

Preoperative Assessment

The patient presently was diagnosed as high-grade urothelial carcinoma of the bladder, T1N0M0. The bladder cancer recurred after BCG instillation. No metastasis was observed and the radical cystectomy was considered. The surgical method is laparoscopic radical cystectomy + ileal conduit.

Surgical Process

1. After successful anesthesia, the patient is placed in the supine position, followed by routine disinfection and draping.
2. After establishing pneumoperitoneum, 10 mm trocars are placed 2 cm below the umbilicus on the left and right sides of the rectus abdominis, and 5 mm trocar is placed at the McBurney's point.
3. Explore the abdominal organs, incise the posterior peritoneum at the right ureter crossing the iliac vessels, incise to find, and free the right ureter as far down as near the bladder; the proximal ureter is freed about 10 cm for future use. Pay attention to protect the blood supply of the ureter (Fig. 2). Dissect the right external iliac artery, internal iliac artery, and obturator lymph nodes (Figs. 3 and 4). The left ureter and lymph nodes are treated in the same way.
4. Lift the bladder upward, display and open the bladder rectal fossa (Fig. 5), free the posterior wall of the bladder to the junction with the prostate transect the vas deferens, and free the seminal vesicle.
5. Lift the vas deferens and seminal vesicle upward to keep the Denonvilliers' fascia under tension, incise the Denonvilliers' fascia to expose the pre-rectal fat tissue, and free it toward the front of the rectum to the tip of the prostate, separating the prostate from the rectum (Fig. 6).
6. Free the anterior wall of the bladder (Fig. 7), and expose the posterior pubic space, suture the DVC with 3–0 V-Loc (Fig. 8); free both

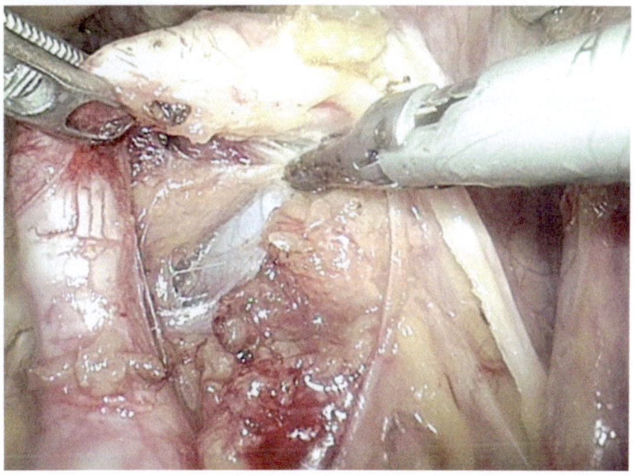

Fig. 3 Dissect the lymph nodes beside the iliac vessels

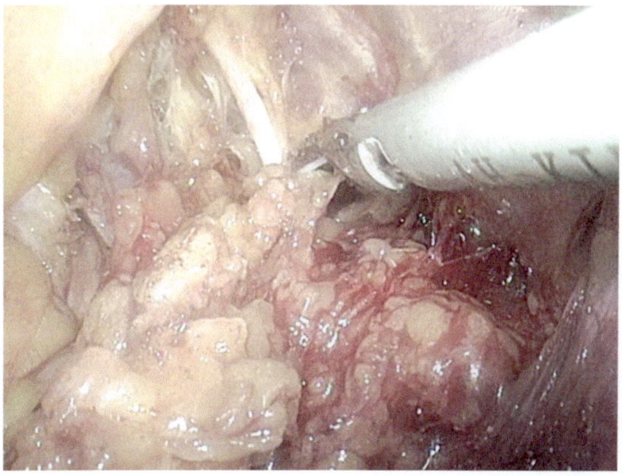

Fig. 4 Dissect the lymph nodes beside the obturator nerve

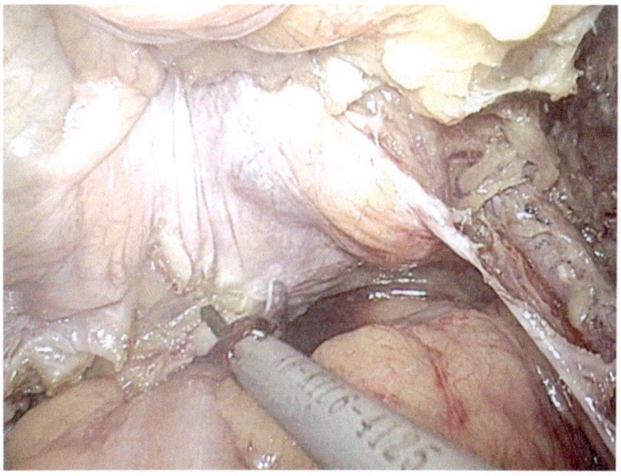

Fig. 5 Open the bladder rectal fossa

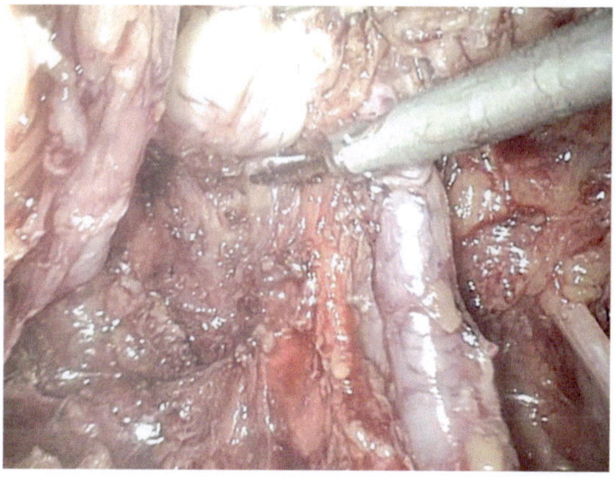

Fig. 6 Free the seminal vesicle gland, and free toward the tip of the prostate in front of the rectum

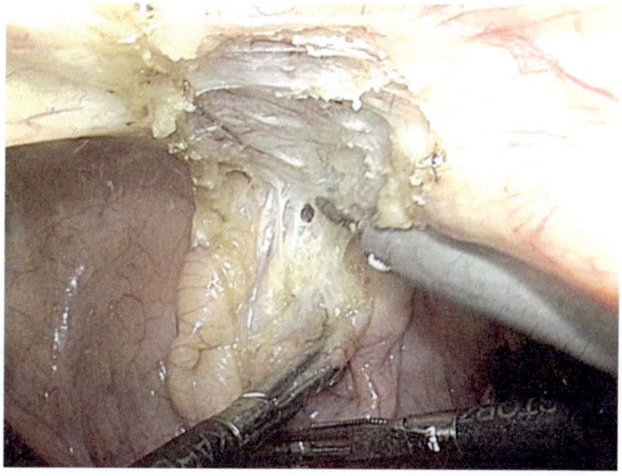

Fig. 7 Free the anterior wall of the bladder

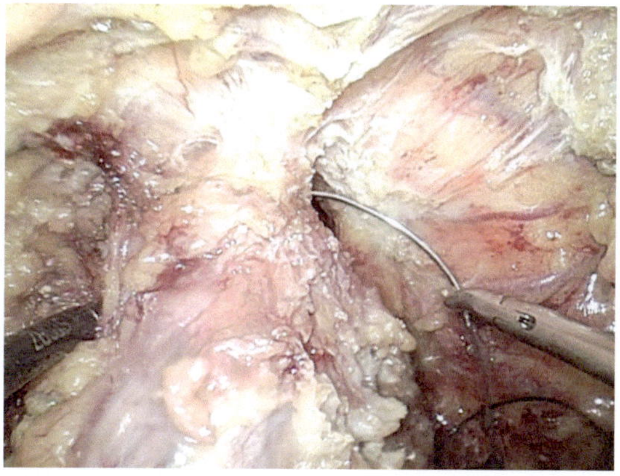

Fig. 8 3–0 V-Loc suture DVC

sides of the prostate, and incise the deep dorsal vein of the penis.

7. Transect the bilateral bladder ligaments and prostate ligaments to the tip of the prostate.
8. Transect the bilateral ureters near the bladder; remove the bladder, seminal vesicle, and prostate together; extend the incision below the umbilicus for about 6 cm; and remove the specimen.
9. Prepare a section of the ileum about 15 cm long, about 15 cm proximal to the ileocecal valve, preserving the mesenteric blood supply. The ileum is reconstructed to restore its continuity with an end-to-end anastomosis, the mesentery is sutured to prevent internal hernia. A single J-tube is placed in each of the bilateral ureters, and the distal ends of the two ureters are each anastomosed end to side with the proximal end of the ileum section.
10. The ileal conduit ostomy opened in the right lower abdomen. The incision was closed.

Expert Commentary

Radical cystectomy is a complex surgery, and has a high risk of complications.

1. Freeing the ureter: The ileal conduit ostomy opens at the lower right abdomen, it is necessary to free the left ureter completely. It should also be noted that freeing the ureter too long may affect the blood supply to the ureter and cause the ureter torsion.
2. Freeing the bladder pedicle and the prostate pedicle: During the procedure, the assistant maintains the tension of the Denonvilliers' fascia by pulling the seminal vesicle in the opposite direction and transects the pedicle blood vessels close to the prostate capsule. For patients with high requirements for urinary control and sexual function, the NVB can be divided bluntly.

Bladder Surgery: Case 27 Cystoscopy Combined with Laparoscopic Cystic Paraganglioma Resection

Guoyang Zheng

Chief Complaint

Increased blood pressure and headache after urination for over a year, bladder tumor discovered 4 months ago.

Medical History

Female, 31 years old. The patient started to have episodic headaches in March 2021, accompanied by high blood pressure, no palpitations or heavy sweating, mostly occurring after urination or activity. The highest blood pressure during an episode reached 200/110 mmHg, and the symptoms could relieve themselves within 10 minutes. She went to a local hospital for a complete brain MRI, echocardiography, and other examinations, but no obvious abnormalities were found. The patient was given oral antihypertensive drugs for symptomatic treatment, but the blood pressure control was not good. In August 2021, she further underwent an adrenal enhanced CT examination at another hospital and found a left adrenal tumor, about 1.4 cm × 0.9 cm in size. On August 5, 2021, she underwent laparoscopic total resection of the left adrenal gland at another hospital. The pathology of the other hospital: left adrenal ganglioneuroma. The consultation result of our hospital pathology department: (left adrenal gland) adrenal tissue can be seen around the ganglion tissue. After the operation, the patient's high blood pressure slightly relieved, but there were still episodic high blood pressure and headaches, mostly occurring 5–10 minutes after urination. In December 2021, she visited our urology outpatient clinic; completed a chest, abdomen, and pelvis enhanced CT examination; and found a nodular soft tissue density shadow on the left rear of the bladder, with a smooth, clear edge, uniform density, CT value of about 42 HU, and the largest cross section of about 21 mm × 15 mm. The posterior wall of the bladder showed compression changes, the enhanced scan was uniformly enhanced, and the venous phase CT value was about 68 HU, considering the possibility of benign lesions (Figs. 1 and 2). Complete adrenal medulla whole body imaging examination: Soft tissue nodule in the left posterior wall of the bladder, with increased radiotracer uptake, considered to be a paraganglioma. The completion of 18F-MFBG PET/CT examination suggests increased radiotracer uptake in the left posterior wall of the bladder. Endocrine tests suggest a blood NM level of 2.28 nmol/L (1), considered to be diagnosed as bladder paraganglioma. Starting from January 26, 2022, the patient began oral

Supplementary Information The online version contains supplementary material available at https://doi.org/10.1007/978-981-96-8598-1_29.

G. Zheng (✉)
Beijing Union Medical College Hospital,
Beijing, China

Y. Zhang, X. Zhao (eds.), *Laparoscopic Surgery in Urology*,
https://doi.org/10.1007/978-981-96-8598-1_29

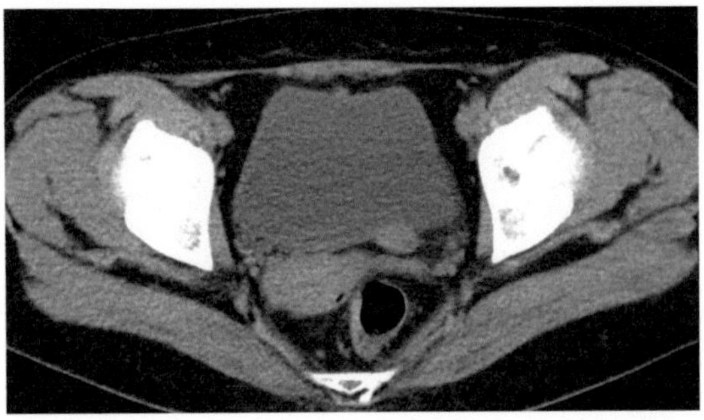

Fig. 1 Abdominal and pelvic enhanced CT (plain scan phase)

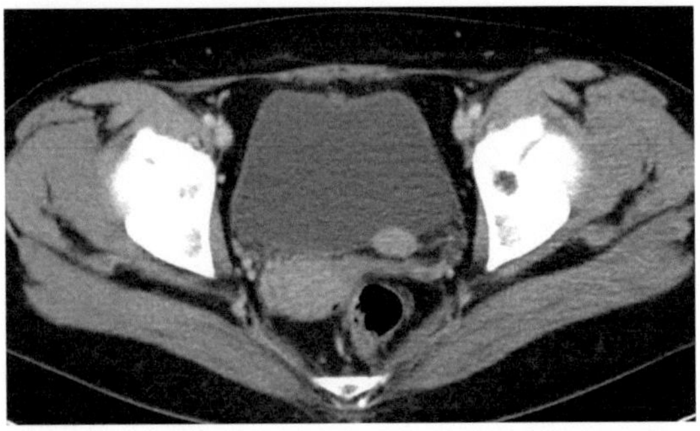

Fig. 2 Abdominal and pelvic enhanced CT (arterial phase)

administration of phenoxybenzamine, with a starting dose of 5 mg bid, presently gradually increased to 10 mg bid. The patient's paroxysmal headache symptoms have improved, with no palpitations, heavy sweating, no cold limbs, no cold extremities, mild nasal congestion, warm limbs, and stable blood pressure and heart rate monitoring. The patient was admitted to the hospital for further surgical treatment.

The patient's recent mental state, sleep, and appetite are good, bowel movements are normal, and the patient has gained about 2 kg since starting medication.

Past History

Generally healthy.

Physical Examination

Clear consciousness, good spirit, blood pressure 108/86 mmHg, heart rate 92 beats/min, no special findings in heart, lung, and abdominal examination; no mass or tenderness in both renal areas, no tenderness in the course of both ureters, no tenderness in the suprapubic area, and no palpable full bladder.

Imaging Data (Figs. 1 and 2)

Preoperative Assessment

The patient's abdominal and pelvic enhanced CT examination suggests a soft tissue nodule with enhancement in the posterior wall of the bladder, about 2.1 cm × 1.5 cm in size. MIBG examination shows radiotracer uptake, suggesting the possibility of paraganglioma. Endocrine tests suggest elevated blood NMN levels, combined with the patient's clinical manifestations of paroxysmal hypertension and headache after urination, considered to be diagnosed as bladder paraganglioma; the diagnosis is basically clear, and the indications for surgery are clear.

Further supplementary assessment of cardiopulmonary function: no obvious abnormalities were found. Preoperative oral administration of phenoxybenzamine was fully prepared, blood pressure and heart rate were stable, and there were no episodes of orthostatic hypotension or hypertension. The surgical method is laparoscopic combined with cystoscopic removal of bladder paraganglioma.

Surgical Procedure

1. The patient is positioned in the supine/lithotomy position, with general anesthesia. Routine disinfection and draping (Figs. 3 and 4).

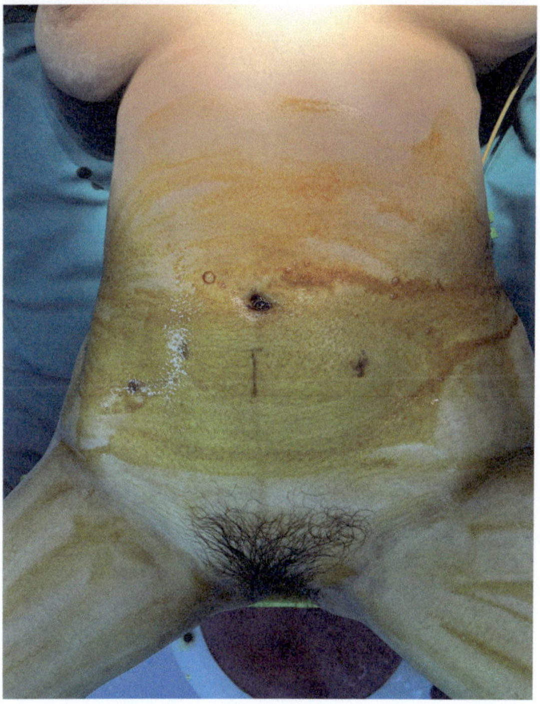

Fig. 3 Abdominal puncture position

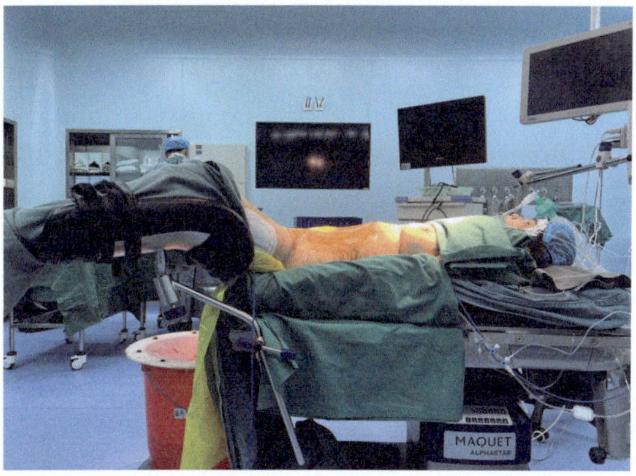

Fig. 4 Patient position

2. Establish pneumoperitoneum through the abdominal approach, and insert the laparoscopic surgical sheath; this operation uses four ports (5 mm and 10 mm each two).
3. Identify the peritoneal reflection, recognize the bladder position (Fig. 5), insert the cystoscope sheath and 30-degree cystoscope into the urethra in turn, retrogradely insert the Fr 6 ureteral stent tube along the guidewire to the left ureteral orifice, find the tumor position under the cystoscope, and identify the cystoscope light source position under the laparoscope (Fig. 6).

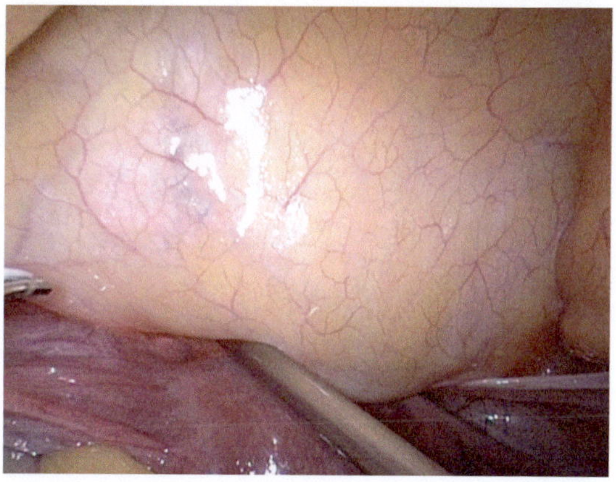

Fig. 5 Identify the bladder under laparoscopy

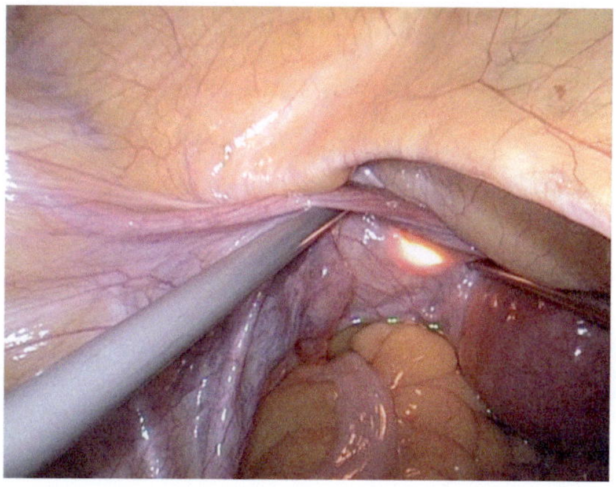

Fig. 6 Find the tumor under the cystoscope, and identify the cystoscope light source under laparoscopy

4. Under the guidance of a cystoscope, an ultrasonic knife is used to mark the tumor range at the peritoneal reflection on the bladder surface along the tumor edge. The instrument touches the tumor for feedback assistance, and the marked range is confirmed jointly under laparoscopy and cystoscopy (Fig. 7).
5. Under the guidance of a cystoscope, the peritoneum and bladder wall are cut layer by layer along the marked area, and the tumor is completely removed, taking care to avoid damaging the ureter (Figs. 8 and 9).

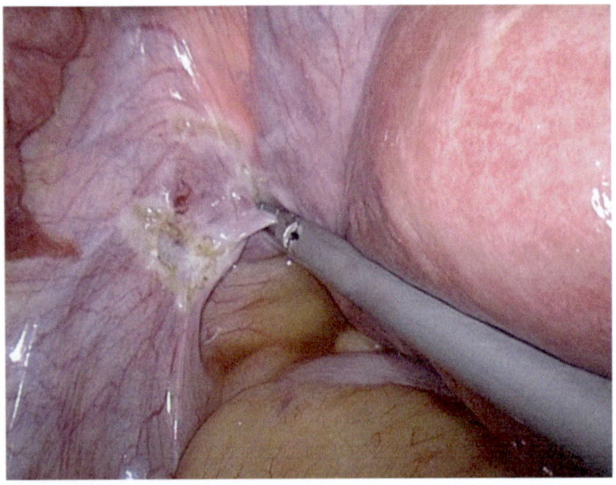

Fig. 7 Bilateral joint positioning mark

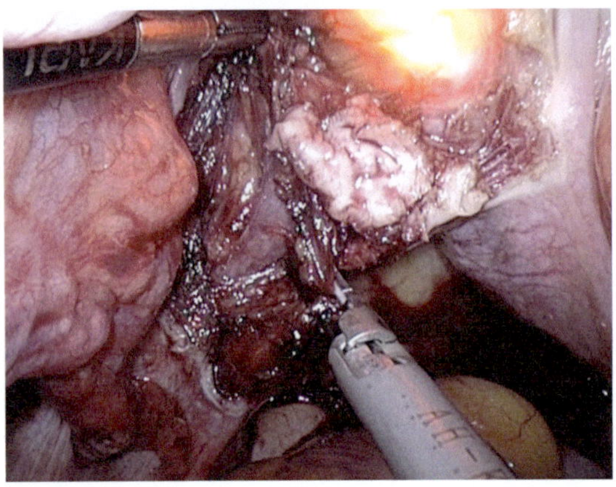

Fig. 8 Layer-by-layer cutting of the peritoneum and bladder wall

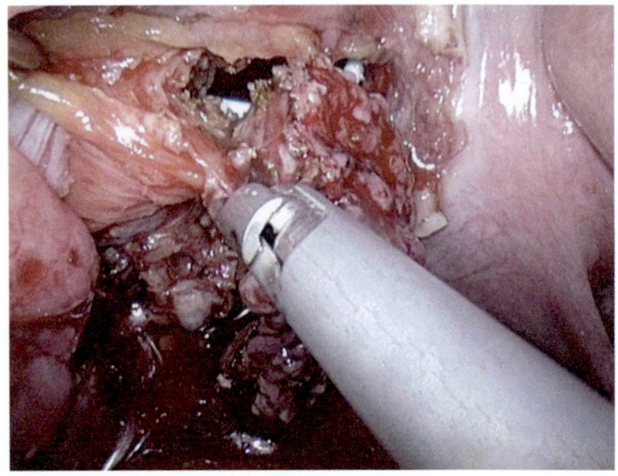

Fig. 9 Tumor removal

6. The tumor is placed in a specimen bag. Use 3-0 V-Loc thread to continuously suture the entire layer of the bladder wall. It is recommended to start the suture from the lowest point of the wound, continuously suture toward the top of the bladder, and ensure the alignment of the bladder mucosa during suturing, avoiding suturing to the ureteral orifice or ureteral stent (Fig. 10).
7. Perform a bladder water injection test to check for urine leakage from the wound, then use 3-0 V-Loc thread to continuously suture and close the peritoneum (Fig. 11), check the wound for active bleeding, place a drainage tube, and remove the specimen (Fig. 12).

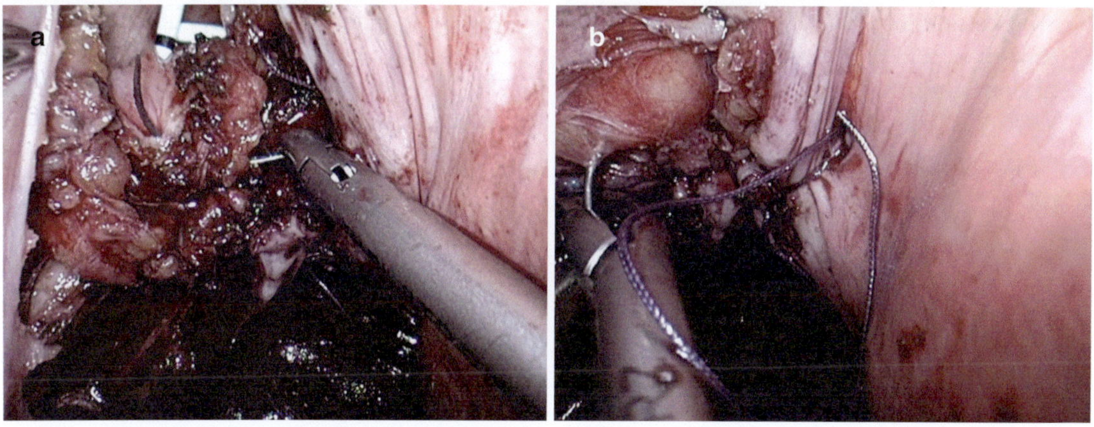

Fig. 10 (**a**, **b**) Continuous suturing of the bladder incision

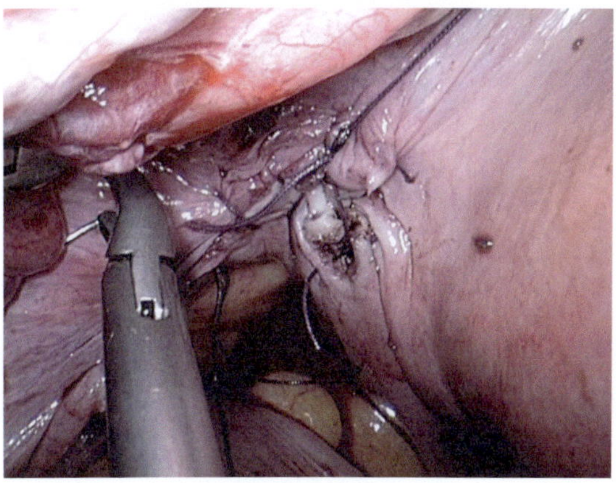

Fig. 11 Closing the peritoneum

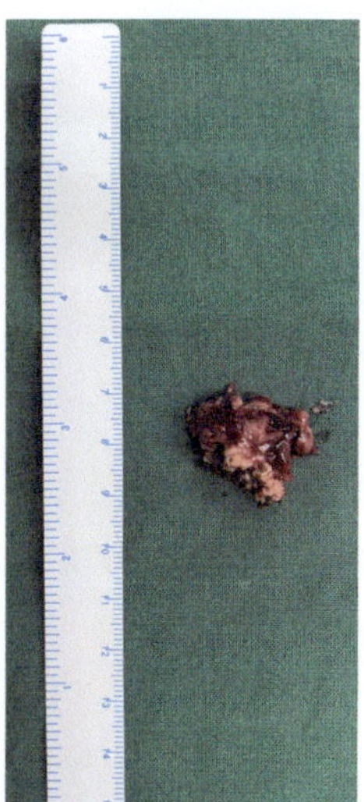

Fig. 12 Tissue specimen

Expert Comments

1. The importance of preoperative diagnosis and drug preparation: The diagnosis of pheochromocytoma/paraganglioma should improve the enhanced CT imaging examination of the abdomen and pelvis to avoid missing the discovery of bladder paraganglioma. Endocrine tests and nuclear medicine examinations such as MIBG should be improved to assist in the diagnosis of paraganglioma. Preoperative α-receptor blockers should be used for sufficient drug preparation to avoid excessive fluctuations in hemodynamic indicators during surgery. Close cooperation with the anesthesiologist is required during the operation to maintain the patient's hemodynamic stability.
2. Tumor positioning and removal: Since bladder paragangliomas are usually small in size, the difficulty of the operation lies in the accurate positioning of the tumor. It is difficult to accurately locate the tumor position by simply observing through laparoscopy. It is recommended to combine cystoscopy for tumor positioning and mark the tumor range with the feedback effect of instrument touch. It is recommended to leave a ureteral stent during the operation to avoid damaging the ureter during the process of tumor removal or wound suturing. The tumor should be thoroughly removed to avoid leaving tumor tissue.

3. Wound suturing: During suturing, attention should be paid to the tight alignment of the bladder mucosa. It is recommended to start suturing from the lowest point of the wound toward the more mobile bladder top in order. After the suturing is completed, a bladder water injection test should be performed to avoid urine leakage due to loose suturing.

Bladder Surgery: Case 28 Cystoscopy Combined with Laparoscopy for Removal of Bladder Foreign Body

Jiaquan Zhou

Chief Complaint

Intrauterine contraceptive device inserted 26 years ago, bladder foreign body discovered 4 months ago.

Present Illness

Female, 52 years old. The patient had an intrauterine contraceptive device inserted 26 years ago for contraception and did not pay attention to the device afterward. Nine months ago, she experienced discomfort and pain during urination without any obvious cause, no hematuria, no lumbar soreness or pain, and no fever or chills, and did not take it seriously. Four months ago, due to aggravated pain during urination, a color Doppler ultrasound at an outside hospital suggested an abnormal echo within the bladder wall. Further CT scan suggested an abnormal dense focus next to the bladder, about 3.5 cm, considering the possibility of ectopic intrauterine contraceptive device in the bladder. She came to our hospital for treatment, and a re-examination with color Doppler ultrasound suggested a strong echo mass on the right side of the bladder wall, not excluding the possibility of ectopic contraceptive device, and a plain film of the lower abdomen suggested a "T"-shaped dense shadow on the left side of the pelvis. Outpatient treatment with levofloxacin oral anti-infection treatment was given, and the symptoms of painful urination have improved.

Supplementary Information The online version contains supplementary material available at https://doi.org/10.1007/978-981-96-8598-1_30.

J. Zhou (✉)
Beijing Union Medical College Hospital,
Beijing, China

Past History

None special.

Marital and Childbearing History

Married and gave birth at an appropriate age, G3P1.

Menstrual History

Menarche at 15 years old, menstrual period of 7 days, menstrual cycle of 28 days, last menstruation at 50 years old.

Y. Zhang, X. Zhao (eds.), *Laparoscopic Surgery in Urology*,
https://doi.org/10.1007/978-981-96-8598-1_30

Physical Examination

Vital signs stable, no special findings on auscultation of the heart and lungs, no bulging in both renal areas, no percussion pain, no tenderness along the course of both ureters, no bladder filling, and no tenderness.

Auxiliary Examination

1. Vaginal gynecological color Doppler ultrasound: Strong echo seen on the right wall of the bladder, about 1.2 cm long, accompanied by acoustic shadow, and no obvious abnormalities in the uterus and both adnexal areas (Fig. 1).
2. Abdominal and pelvic CT scan: "T"-shaped high-density shadow can be seen on the upper right wall of the bladder; the boundary with the bladder wall is unclear (Fig. 2).
3. Lower abdominal plain film (prone position): "T"-shaped dense shadow seen on the right side of the pelvis (Fig. 3).
4. Cystoscopy: A cord-like structure was visualized beneath the bladder mucosa on the right top side wall of the bladder, about 2 cm long, with stone formation on the surface, and embedded in the bladder wall (Fig. 4).

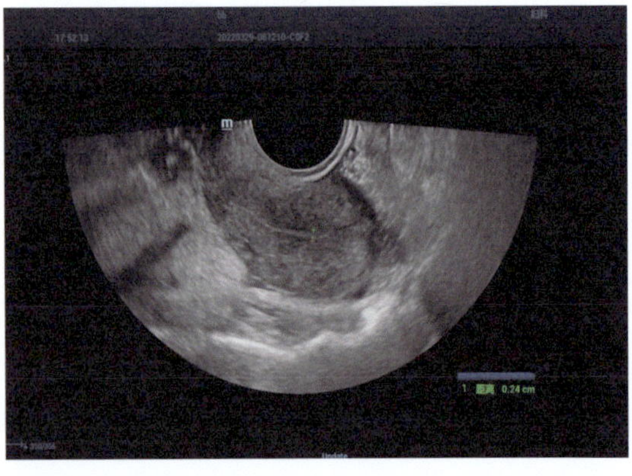

Fig. 1 Bladder wall hyperechoic mass (color Doppler ultrasound examination)

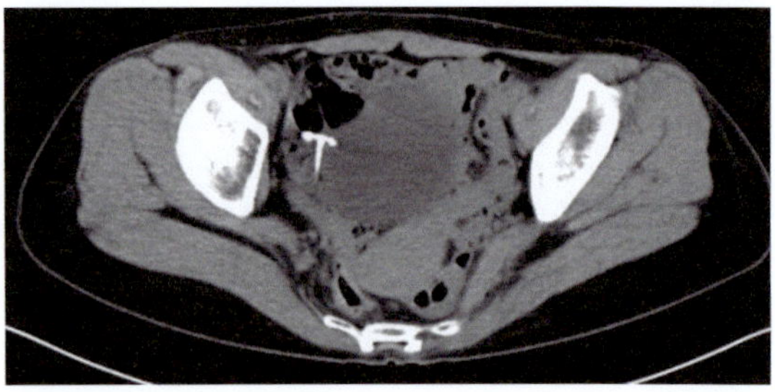

Fig. 2 Abdominal and pelvic CT

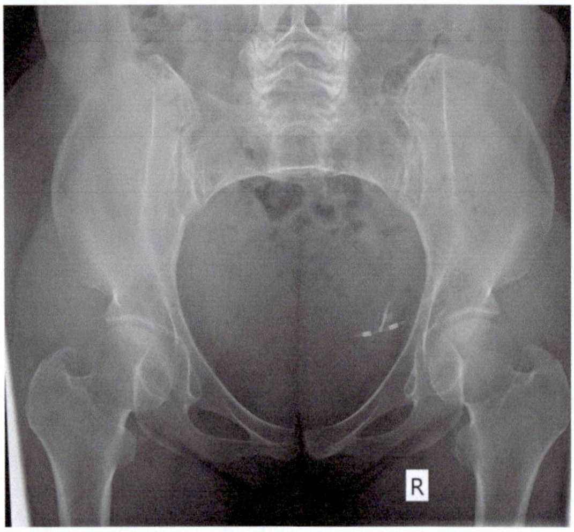

Fig. 3 Lower abdominal plain film

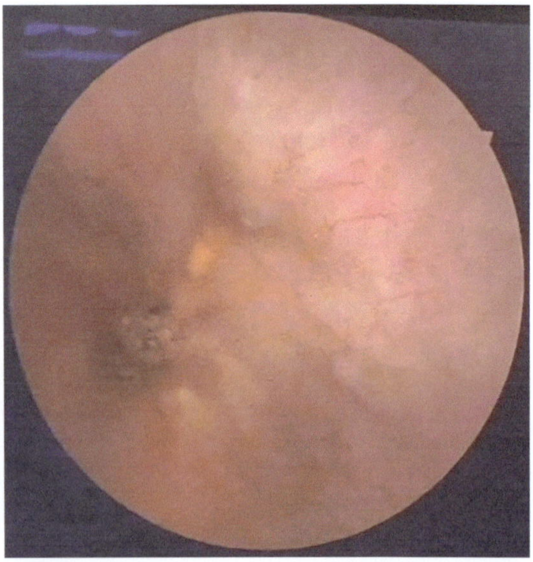

Fig. 4 Cystoscopy

Preoperative Assessment

The patient had symptoms of painful urination during the course of the disease, suggesting the presence of urinary tract infection. After outpatient treatment with levofloxacin tablets, the symptoms of painful urination improved, and no increase in urinary white blood cells was found in the routine urine test. Preoperative assessment of heart and lung function showed no obvious abnormalities.

Considering the patient's medical history, past history, and results of imaging examinations, it is considered to be an ectopic intrauterine contraceptive device (IUD) in the bladder. It is planned to perform laparoscopic removal of the bladder foreign body through the abdomen. Intestinal preparation was given 1 day before the operation.

Surgical Procedure

1. The patient was placed in the supine position and intubated under general anesthesia; a urinary catheter was inserted, and routine disinfection and draping were performed.
2. An incision was made at the upper edge of the navel, a 10 mm trocar is inserted as an observation hole, pneumoperitoneum is established, and under direct vision, a 5 mm and 10 mm trocar are respectively inserted at the outer edge of the rectus abdominis on both sides, 2 cm below the navel, as operation holes.
3. Under laparoscopy, the relationship between the ectopic IUD and the bladder wall is observed. The IUD is seen to be located on the right side of the top wall of the bladder, with the surface covered by peritoneum showing scar-like changes. The uterus is normal and far from the foreign body (Fig. 5).
4. The peritoneum on the right side of the bladder is cut along the outer edge of the ectopic IUD, revealing the right wall of the bladder (Fig. 6).

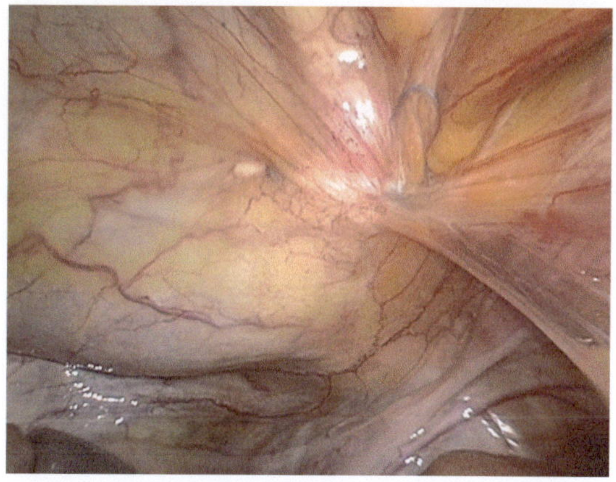

Fig. 5 Position of the ectopic IUD under laparoscopy

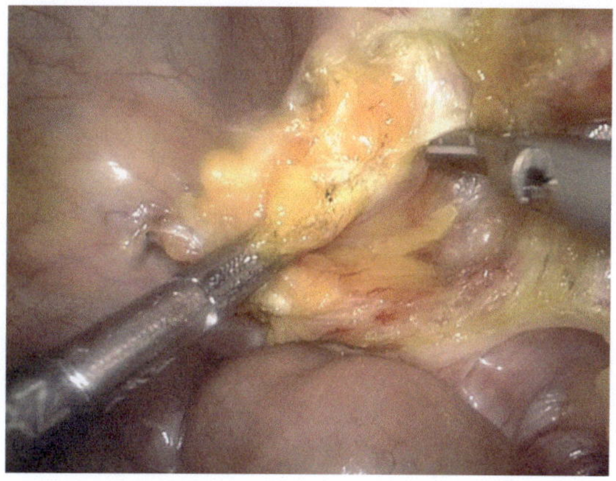

Fig. 6 Opening the peritoneum

5. The peritoneum is cut along the other edges of the ectopic IUD, revealing the surrounding bladder wall (Fig. 7).
6. The bladder wall is cut open, revealing the bladder cavity (Fig. 8). A stone about 1 cm in size is seen attached to the surface of the foreign body, embedded in the bladder tissue (Fig. 9).
7. Part of the bladder wall is cut along the periphery of the ectopic IUD, and the foreign body and surrounding inflammatory tissue are completely removed. Care should be taken during the operation to avoid removing too much normal bladder wall tissue (Fig. 10).
8. The specimen is placed in a specimen bag, and the specimen bag is placed under the 10 mm trocar.

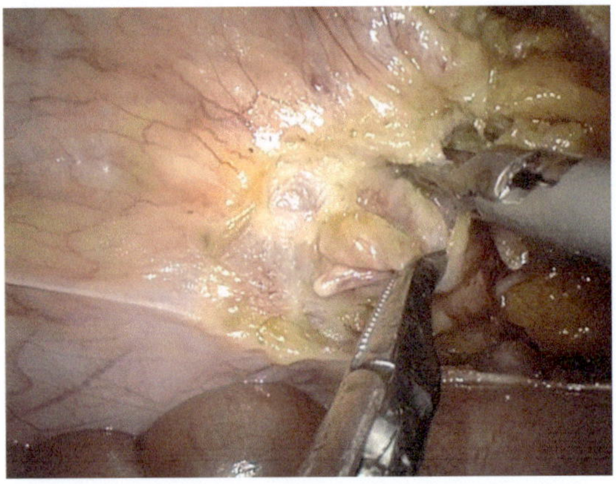

Fig. 7 Continuing to open the peritoneum

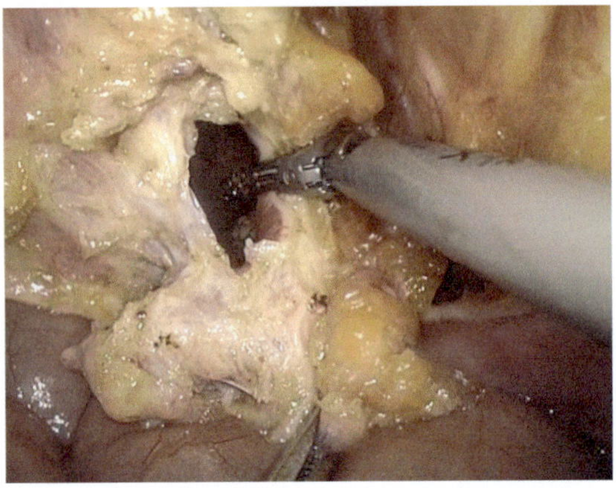

Fig. 8 Opening the bladder wall

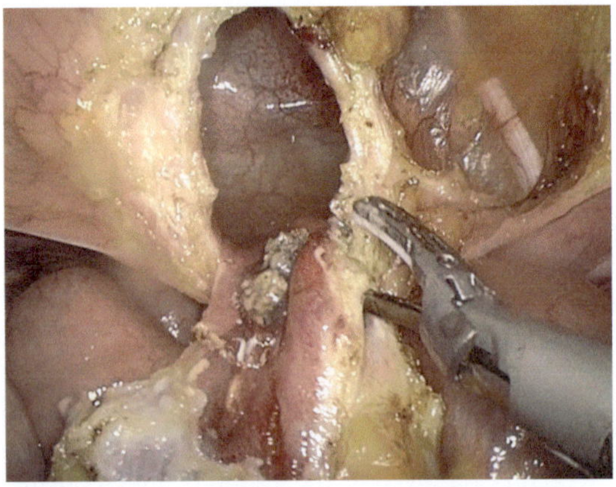

Fig. 9 Foreign body embedded in the bladder wall, with attached stone

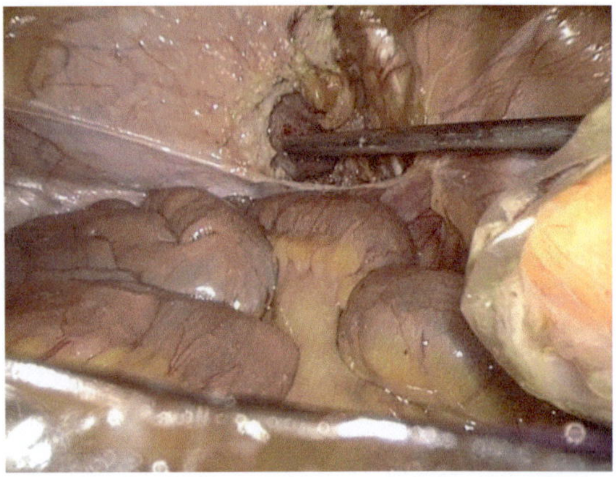

Fig. 10 Partial removal of the bladder wall

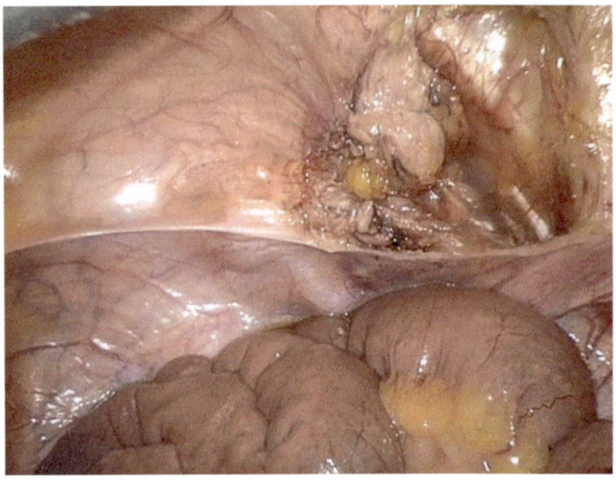

Fig. 11 Suturing the bladder wall

9. The bladder wall is continuously sutured with 3-0 V-Loc thread. If necessary, the bladder can be filled to assess whether the bladder is tightly sutured (Fig. 11).
10. The peritoneal incision is continuously sutured with 3-0 V-Loc thread (Fig. 12), and a drainage tube is placed after reserving one drainage tube hole.
11. The specimen bag is removed, the incision is sutured, and the specimen is separated outside the body. The foreign body is seen to be a "T"-shaped contraceptive device, made of plastic, relatively soft, with a tail thread attached (broken during dissection) (Fig. 13).

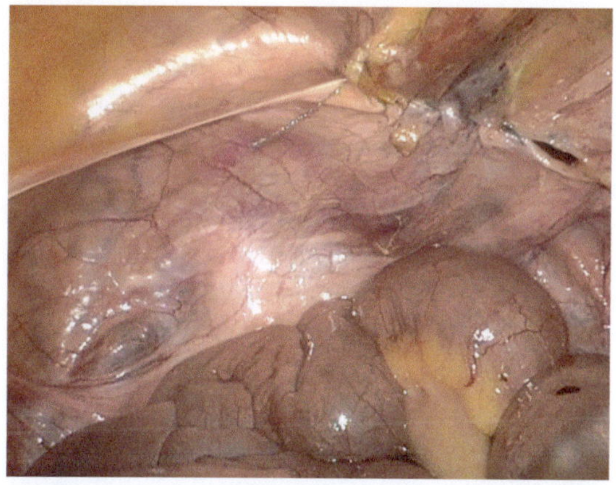

Fig. 12 Suturing the peritoneum

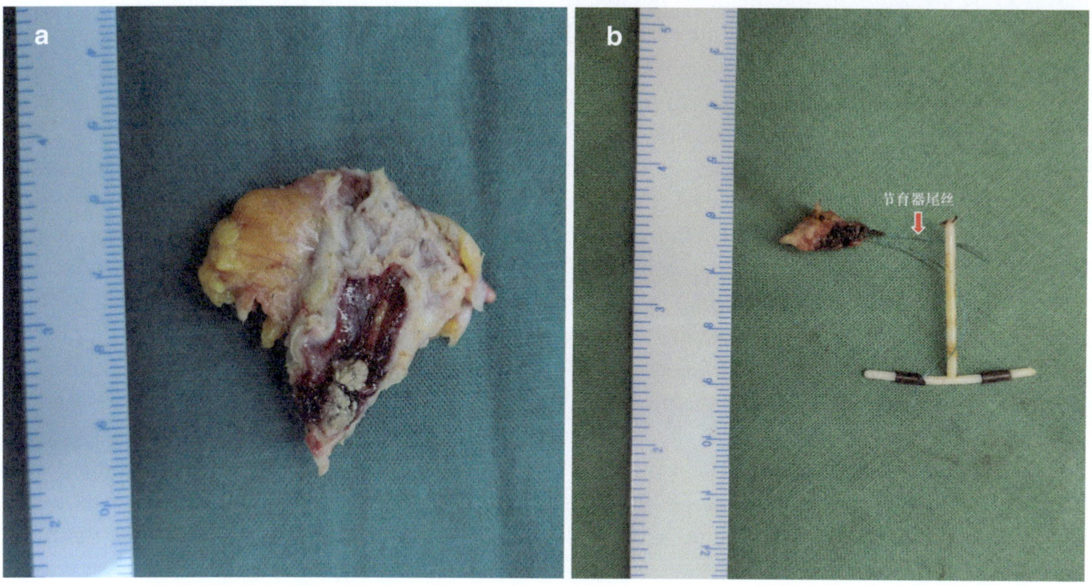

Fig. 13 IUD tail thread (removal of bladder tissue and foreign body)

Expert Comments

The mechanism of IUD displacement is presently unclear and may be related to a scarred uterus or uterine injury during IUD placement. The patient in this case had a vaginal delivery and did not have a scarred uterus. However, the patient had an IUD inserted during the lactation period 2 months postpartum, when the uterus is softer. Improper operation can easily cause endometrial injury or even direct uterine perforation, leading to IUD displacement. Normally, as the posterior wall of the bladder is adjacent to the uterus, IUD displacement in the bladder is common in the posterior wall of the bladder. However, the location of the displaced IUD in the bladder of this patient is far from the uterus, which may be related to the incomplete recovery of the uterus after vaginal delivery, the enlargement of the uterus, and its close contact with the top side wall of the bladder. In this case, the IUD is displaced out of the uterine cavity and attached to the top side wall of the bladder, and then the uterus recovers and the uterus shrinks after menopause, gradually moving away from the displaced IUD, resulting in the phenomenon of the displaced IUD being far from the uterus. However, it cannot be ruled out that the IUD may penetrate the uterus, become free in the abdominal cavity, and then be displaced to the bladder. The most common symptoms of IUD displacement in the bladder are lower abdominal pain and symptoms related to urinary tract infection, which are related to the location of the displaced IUD. The patient in this case had no obvious symptoms initially because the IUD was embedded in the bladder wall. Later, due to factors such as local chronic inflammatory response, the IUD shifted into the bladder cavity, eventually causing symptoms such as frequent urination, urgency, and pain during urination. After the IUD is exposed in the bladder cavity, it causes calcium salt deposition in the urine and local formation of wall-attached stones, further aggravating the patient's urinary irritation symptoms, and the effect of simple antibiotic treatment is not obvious. The wall-attached stone of the IUD continues to grow and forms a bladder stone. The dragging effect causes the IUD to detach from the bladder wall and eventually forms a mobile bladder stone completely free in the bladder cavity. The moving bladder stone can easily block the inner mouth of the urethra, causing the patient to have symptoms of interrupted urination, and can easily damage the bladder mucosa and cause gross hematuria. Long-term chronic inflammation stimulation of the displaced IUD can cause local urothelial squamous metaplasia and even concurrent bladder squamous cell carcinoma. The main treatment for complete bladder wall displacement of the IUD is open or laparoscopic partial cystectomy. Preoperative CT and cystoscopy are needed to assess the position of the IUD. For patients with the main body of the IUD located in the superficial muscle layer of the bladder, transurethral electrocision can also be chosen to remove the IUD. However, transurethral electrocision carries the risk of postoperative bladder perforation and urine leakage and may even require a second operation to repair the bladder. At the same time, some IUDs are not suitable for removal from the urethra due to their hard texture, large volume, or deep embedding in the bladder wall and need to be finally removed through transurethral electrocision combined with abdominal surgery. In this case, the patient was considered to have the IUD completely displaced in the right bladder wall and formed a wall-attached stone. After comprehensive consideration, laparoscopic bladder foreign body removal surgery was chosen. During the operation, it is important to completely remove the IUD and the wall-attached stone and to pay attention to the possibility of malignant lesions in the surrounding bladder wall. The bladder is sutured with full-layer continuous sutures, and reinforcement sutures can be added if necessary, and a bladder water injection test can be attempted to assess the tightness of the bladder sutures.

Prostate Surgery: Case 29 Laparoscopic Extraperitoneal Radical Prostatectomy

Zixing Ye

Chief Complaint

Elevated PSA detected for over 8 years, diagnosed with prostate cancer for over 1 month. Medical history: male, 64 years old. The patient's tPSA was found to be elevated, about 5 ng/ml, during a physical examination 8 years ago. He had nocturia three times a night, with no other significant discomfort, and did not seek treatment. He then regularly monitored his tPSA. In 2016, his tPSA was 7.63 ng/ml. He underwent a prostate biopsy at another hospital. Postoperative pathology showed small clusters of atypical glands, but he did not receive treatment. The patient continued to monitor his tPSA and was informed that it was gradually increasing (details unknown). In the past 2 years, the patient has experienced weak urination and nocturia about four times per night, without treatment. In March 2022, his tPSA was 10.57 ng/ml. The patient visited our outpatient clinic for a dynamic enhanced MRI of the prostate, which showed a mass-like lesion in the left lobe, transition zone, and peripheral zone of the prostate.

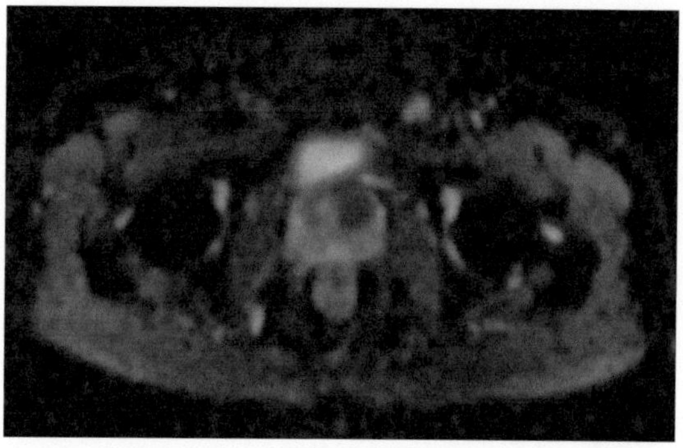

Fig. 1 Dynamic enhanced MRI of the prostate. A lesion can be seen in the left lobe of the prostate, with a reduced ADC value

The edge was blurred, T2WI showed low signal, DWI showed high signal, ADC value was reduced, and PI-RADS score was 5 points; DCE was +. It invaded the periprostatic capsule and left neurovascular bundle but did not invade the seminal vesicles, bladder neck, rectum, or pelvic floor muscles. Considering the abnormal signal in the left lobe transition zone and peripheral zone of the prostate, the possibility of prostate cancer is high (Fig. 1). The patient's tPSA was retested in May 2022 and was 13.44 ng/ml. Considering the gradual increase in tPSA, he underwent a prostate biopsy in June 2022. Pathology: Prostate adenocarcinoma (Gleason score 4 + 3, WHO grading group 3); Bone scan did not show bone metastasis. Considering

Supplementary Information The online version contains supplementary material available at https://doi.org/10.1007/978-981-96-8598-1_31.

Z. Ye (✉)
Beijing Union Medical College Hospital,
Beijing, China
e-mail: yezixing@pumch.cn

Y. Zhang, X. Zhao (eds.), *Laparoscopic Surgery in Urology*,
https://doi.org/10.1007/978-981-96-8598-1_31

locally advanced prostate cancer, he was admitted to our hospital for surgery.

Past History

Hypertension for over 10 years, highest 150/90 mmHg, presently taking oral amlodipine besylate 2.5 mg qd, blood pressure controlled at 130/70 mmHg; bilateral carotid plaques found for over 3 years, long-term oral aspirin 100 mg qd + pitavastatin 2 mg qn. Presently, aspirin has been stopped for 7 days. No other special conditions.

Physical Examination

No obvious hard nodules were palpated on digital rectal examination of the prostate, and no blood was found on withdrawal.

Imaging Data (Fig. 1)

Preoperative Assessment

The patient's prostate biopsy confirmed the diagnosis of prostate cancer, ISUP group 3, tPSA 13.44 ng/ml; dynamic enhanced MRI of the prostate suggested that prostate cancer involved the periprostatic capsule and left neurovascular bundle. Bone scan did not show bone metastasis. Presently, it is considered locally advanced prostate cancer. The indication for surgery is clear.

The surgical method is laparoscopic extraperitoneal radical prostatectomy.

Surgical Procedure

1. After successful anesthesia, the patient was placed in the supine position with the head down. Routine disinfection, draping, and urinary catheter placement were performed.
2. A vertical incision approximately 3 cm below the navel was made, and the skin, subcutaneous tissue, and anterior sheath of the rectus abdominis were incised. Blunt dissection of the posterior rectus abdominis and extraperitoneal tissue was performed with a finger, followed by trocar puncture and insertion at the points 5 cm below the navel on the left and right sides of the rectus abdominis, and above the right anterior superior iliac spine.
3. Insert a laparoscope below the navel, separate the Retzius space under the scope, and remove the fat on the surface of the prostate, bladder neck, and pelvic fascia.
4. Incise the pelvic fascia on both sides of the prostate, retract the pelvic wall muscles, and free the apex of the prostate (Fig. 2).
5. Transect the puboprostatic ligament (Fig. 3), and then use a 1-0 V-Loc suture to ligate the dorsal venous complex (DVC) (Fig. 4).
6. Identify an incise the neck of the bladder, and separate the neck of the bladder from the prostate (Fig. 5).
7. Separate the vas deferens and seminal vesicles on both sides, transect the vas deferens and pull it toward the abdominal side, expose the Denonvilliers' fascia, the fascia is tightly adhered to the rectum, and carefully separate the adhesion (Fig. 6).
8. Incise the anterior layer of Denonvilliers' fascia, and fully free the posterior wall of the

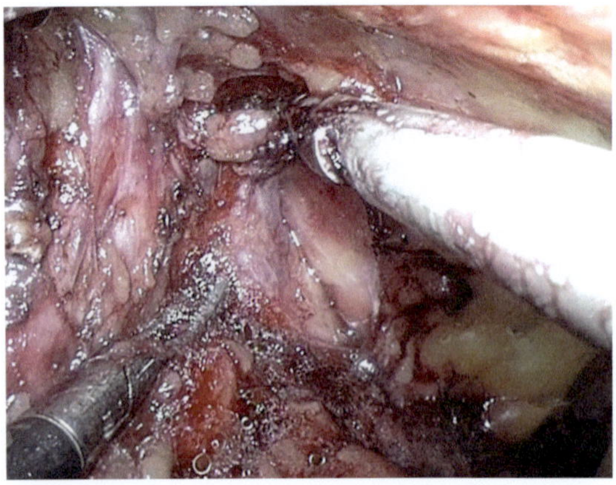

Fig. 2 Open the pelvic floor fascia and free the apex of the prostate

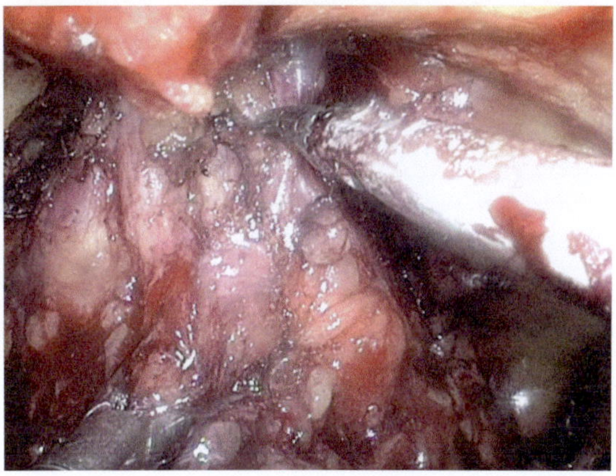

Fig. 3 Transect the puboprostatic ligament

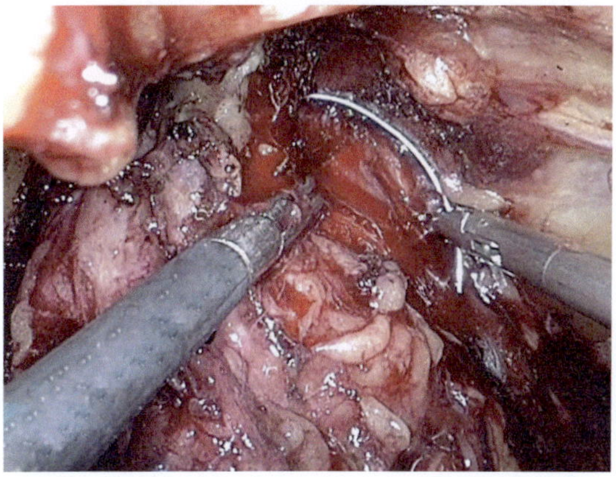

Fig. 4 1-0 V-Loc suture of DVC

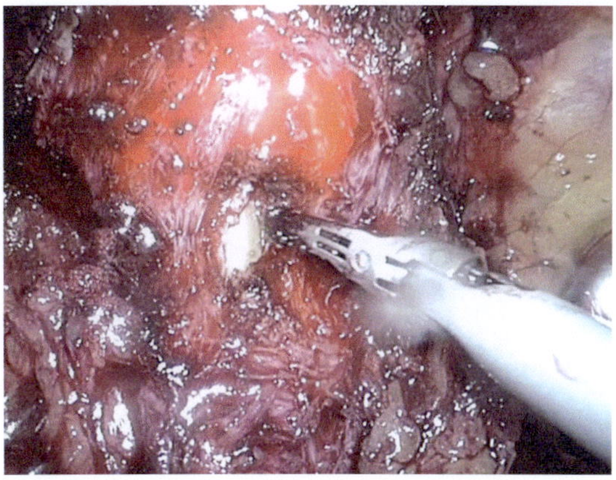

Fig. 5 Incise the anterior wall of the bladder neck to expose the urethra

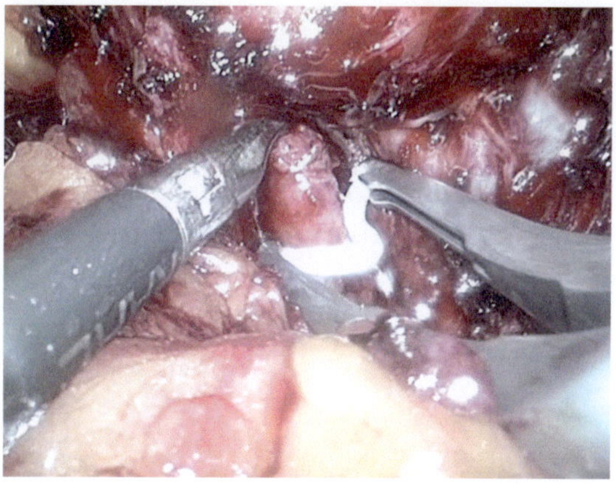

Fig. 6 Clamp and separate the right vas deferens

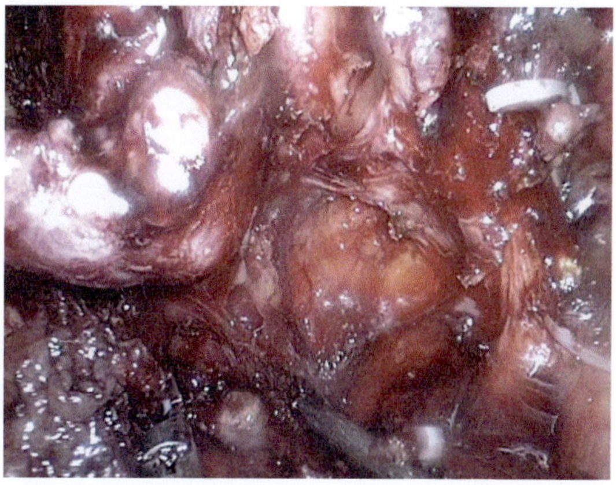

Fig. 7 After fully freeing the seminal vesicle, incise the anterior layer of Denonvilliers' fascia, and free toward the apex of the prostate

prostate towards the apex of the prostate (Fig. 7).

9. Further free along both sides of the prostate, and transect the lateral pedicle of the prostate (Fig. 8).
10. After freeing a long segment of the urethra, incise the anterior wall of the urethra close to the apex of the prostate, remove the catheter, and Transect the posterior wall of the urethra. Completely remove the prostate and seminal vesicles (Fig. 9).
11. Use a 3-0 V-Loc suture to continuously suture the urethra and neck of the bladder,

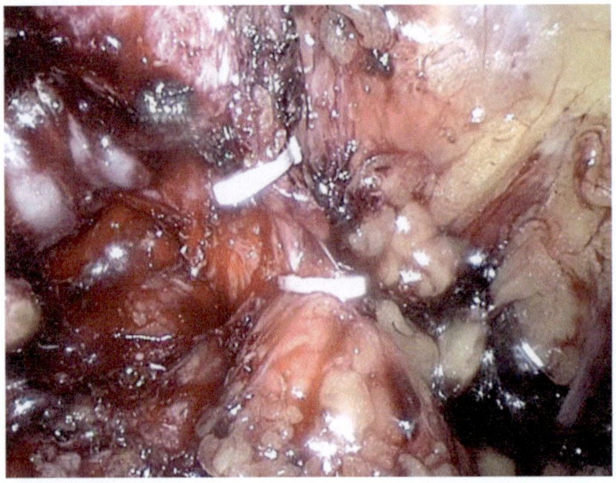

Fig. 8 Clamp and separate the lateral pedicle of the prostate

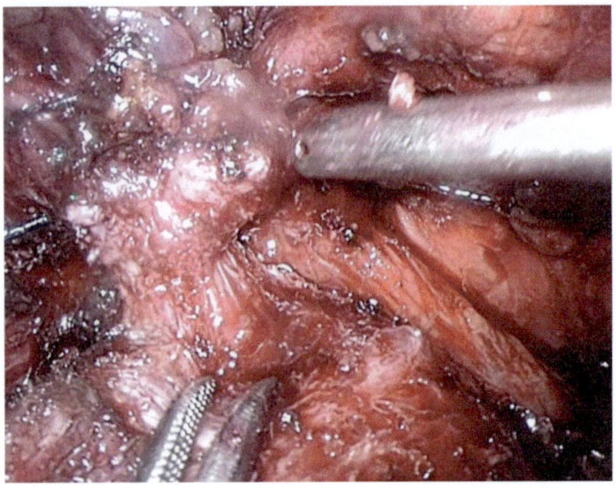

Fig. 9 Free a long segment of the urethra

completing the reconstruction of the urethra (Fig. 10). "Insert an 18-Fr double-lumen catheter into the bladder through the urethra."

12. Place a drainage tube behind the pubis close the incision, and end the surgery.

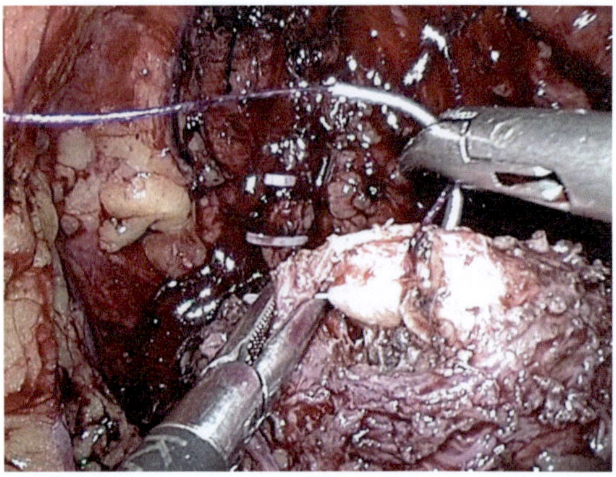

Fig. 10 Start the bladder-urethra anastomosis from the 5 o'clock direction with a 3-0 V-Loc suture

Expert Commentary

1. In terms of preserving sexual function: Interfascial and intrafascial techniques are presently the main techniques for preserving sexual function. In the intrafascial technique, the prostate is freed closely adhering to the prostate capsule, thus protecting the pelvic fascia, puboprostatic ligament, and DVC, minimizing the risk of damage to the sexual nerves. The interfascial technique, by freeing between the prostate fascia and the pelvic fascia, also well preserves the sexual nerves.
2. Protecting urinary control function: VIP techniques and veil techniques have also significantly improved the patient's urinary control function through nerve protection. In recent years, it has been found that preserving sufficient urethral length, protecting the puboprostatic complex, preserving the detrusor apron, anterior reconstruction techniques, posterior

reconstruction techniques, and bladder neck reconstruction techniques also play a very important role in protecting urinary control function. Controlling tumors, preserving urinary control function, and preserving sexual function are the goals of radical prostatectomy. In recent years, due to the gradual deepening of prostate anatomy research, some anatomical structures and surgical techniques related to function preservation have been discovered, greatly improving the functional recovery of patients after radical prostatectomy.

Prostate Surgery: Case 30 Robot-Assisted Laparoscopic Radical Prostatectomy

Yi Qiao

Chief Complaint

Elevated PSA for 3 years, diagnosed with prostate cancer for over 1 month.

History

Male, 63 years old. The patient's annual physical examination for the past 3 years has shown elevated total prostate-specific antigen (PSA-T), about 7 ng/ml (specifics unknown). On July 24, 2022, PSA-T was was 8.370 ng/ml, free/total PSA ratio (F/T) was 0.194. On July 26, 2022, prostate MRI showed abnormal signal at the 11–12 o'clock position in the transition zone of the prostate base, suggesting biopsy to rule out prostate cancer; prostate hyperplasia, inflammation; cyst in the middle of the peripheral zone of the prostate. On July 27, 2022, urinary system ultrasound suggested prostate hyperplasia with local calcification, prostate size about 3.79 cm × 4.96 cm × 2.81 cm, inner gland width about 2.38 cm, and substance echo uneven. Local strong echo mass can be seen. No obvious abnormal blood flow signal. On July 28, 2022, transrectal prostate biopsy was performed under local anesthesia, and the postoperative pathology is as follows: (left, five needles; right, five needles) prostate adenocarcinoma, Gleason score 3 + 3, WHO grouping 1. He then visited our urology outpatient clinic. Whole body bone scan: increased radiotracer uptake at the junction of the right parietal-occipital and left ninth anterior rib, benign possibility, and suggested follow-up observation; no abnormalities were seen in the rest of the whole body bone scan. The outpatient clinic admitted him for surgical treatment of prostate cancer.

Past History

Hypertension for 7–8 years, taking amlodipine besylate 5 mg qd; chronic obstructive pulmonary disease for 7 years, presently inhaling budesonide/formoterol 320 μg qd; diabetes for over 1 month, taking metformin 0.5 g bid; cervical spondylosis for 3 years, intermittently taking ibuprofen. In 1989, he underwent bilateral nasal polyp removal surgery, and in 1990 he underwent left epididymal cyst removal surgery.

Supplementary Information The online version contains supplementary material available at https://doi.org/10.1007/978-981-96-8598-1_32.

Y. Qiao (✉)
Beijing Union Medical College Hospital, Beijing, China

Y. Zhang, X. Zhao (eds.), *Laparoscopic Surgery in Urology*,
https://doi.org/10.1007/978-981-96-8598-1_32

Physical Examination

Rectal examination revealed an enlarged prostate, tough in texture, no obvious nodules being felt, no obvious tenderness, and no blood on withdrawal. No other obvious abnormalities were observed.

Imaging Data

None.

Preoperative Assessment

After admission, preoperative assessment was completed, including coagulation, infection screening (eight items), full liver + full kidney + full lipid, full blood cell analysis, and electrocardiogram that showed no obvious abnormalities. Consult the anesthesiology department for evaluation. Consult the endocrinologist to help stabilize the patient's blood sugar during the perioperative period. After excluding surgical contraindications, according to the patient's condition, it is planned to perform robot-assisted laparoscopic radical prostatectomy.

Surgical Process

1. The supine position with the head down and feet up is adopted. The surgical side is marked in the ward before surgery. General anesthesia with endotracheal intubation is used. Routine disinfection and draping.
2. At the lateral edge of the rectus abdominis at the umbilical level on both sides, above the anterior superior iliac spine on the right side, an 8 mm robot trocar is placed, connected to the robot's first, third, and fourth arms, and robot instruments are placed, respectively. An auxiliary hole is punctured above the left anterior superior iliac spine.
3. Under the microscope, the anterior abdominal wall peritoneum is separated and cut to enter the space behind the pubic bone, the extraperitoneal fat tissue is freed, the pelvic wall muscles are pushed open, and the prostate apex is freed.
4. Cut off the puboprostatic ligament, and suture the dorsal vein complex of the penis with 1-0 V-Loc thread.
5. Identify and cut open the neck of the bladder, and separate the neck of the bladder from the prostate (Figs. 1 and 2).
6. Cut off the vas deferens on both sides and separate the seminal vesicle gland. During this process, pay attention to identify the seminal vesicle artery and fully coagulate to stop bleeding (Figs. 3 and 4).
7. Cut open the Denonvilliers' fascia, and separate the posterior wall of the prostate to the apex of the prostate (Fig. 5). During the process, pay attention to protect the anterior wall of the rectum to avoid injury.
8. Further free along both sides of the prostate, ligate with Hem-o-Lok cut off the prostate pedicle, and free the gland on both sides to the apex of the prostate (Fig. 6). The prostate pedicle needs to be fully freed. During the opera-

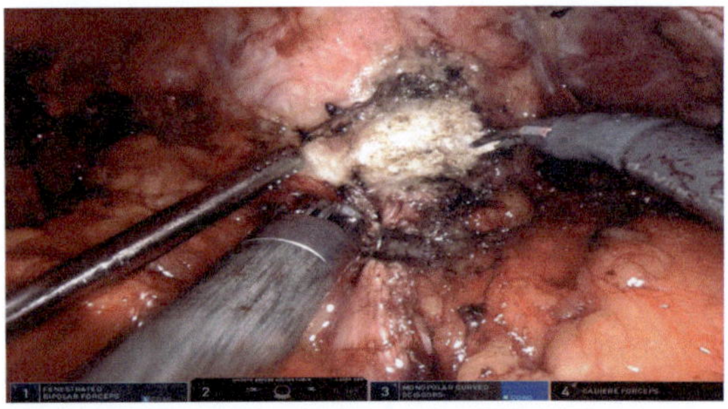

Fig. 1 Identify and cut open the neck of the bladder

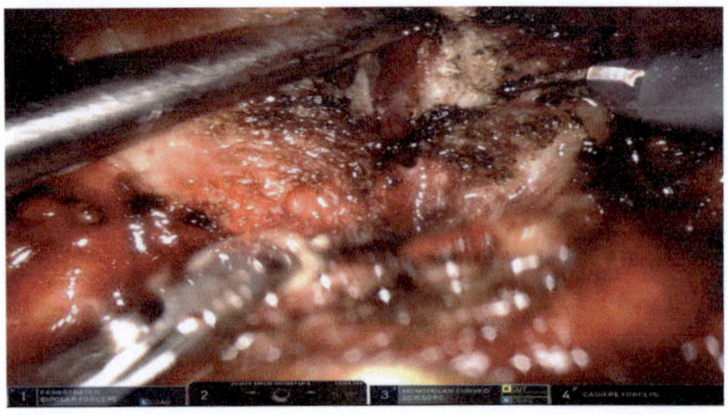

Fig. 2 Separate the neck of the bladder and the prostate

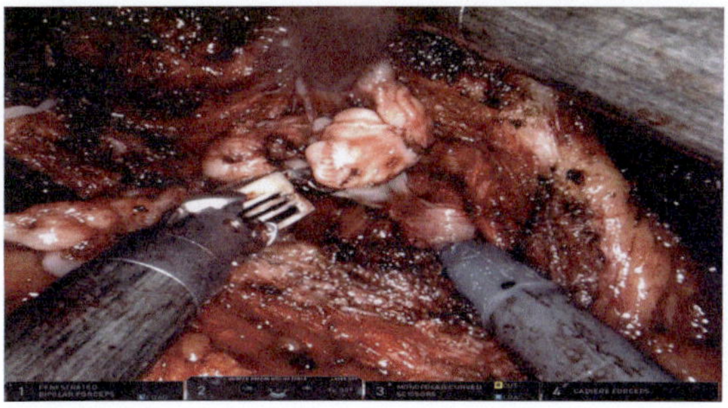

Fig. 3 Separate the seminal vesicle gland

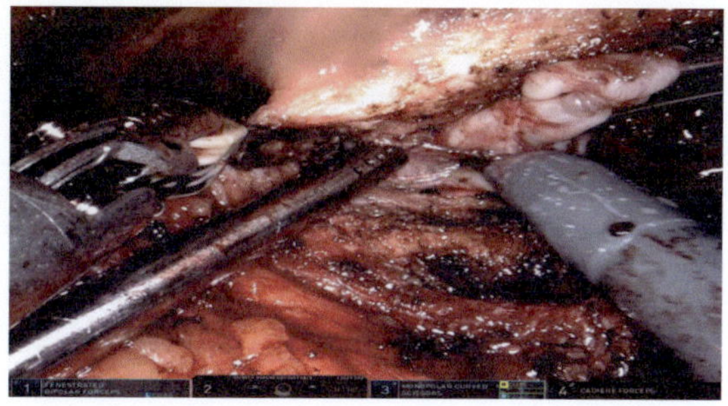

Fig. 4 Cut off the vas deferens

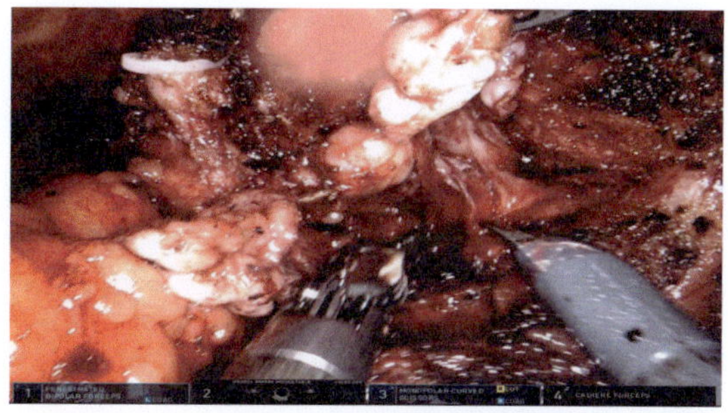

Fig. 5 Separate the posterior wall of the prostate

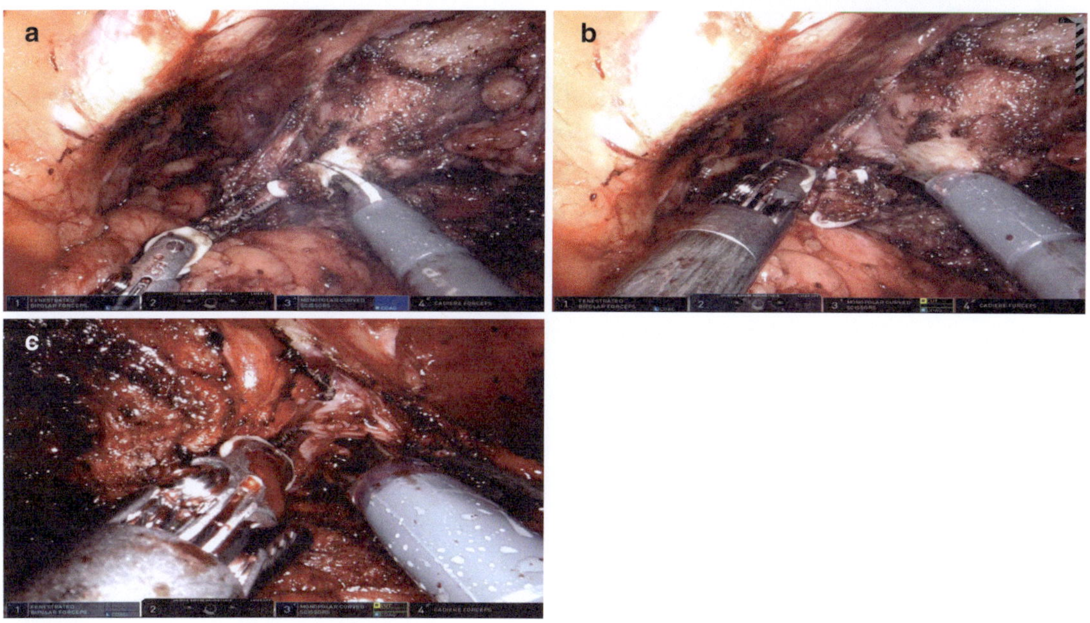

Fig. 6 (**a**, **b**, **c**) Cut off the prostate pedicle

tion, the tissue is often too thick due to insufficient freeing of the pedicle, which cannot be closed with Hem-o-lok, and there is obvious bleeding after separation. This operation uses the VIP technique of intracapsular radical prostatectomy, effectively preserving the integrity of the sexual nerves and the patient's ability to control urination.

9. Below the dorsal vein of the penis and at the apex of the prostate, the urethra is exposed

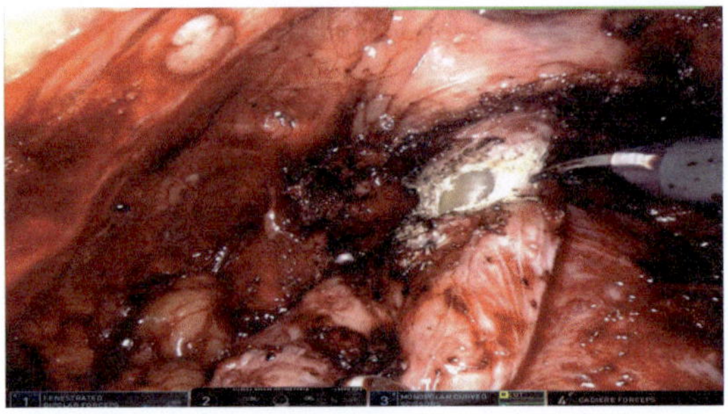

Fig. 7 Cutting off the prostate and urethra

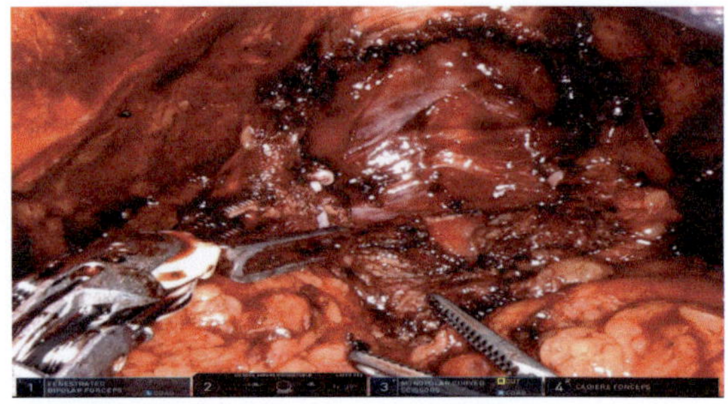

Fig. 8 Complete removal of the prostate

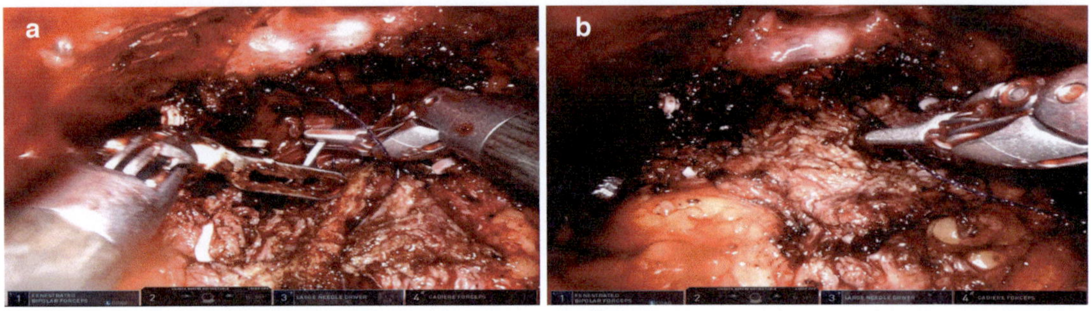

Fig. 9 (**a**, **b**) Suturing the bladder neck and urethra

and cut off, retaining about 1 cm of urethral tissue, and the prostate is removed (Figs. 7 and 8). Then use 3-0 V-Loc thread to continuously anastomose the neck of the bladder with the end of the urethra (Fig. 9). The anastomosis is satisfactory, and an 18Fr double-lumen catheter is placed into the bladder through the urethra. After careful hemostasis and ensuring no active bleeding, the specimen is removed. A pelvic drainage tube is placed, the layers are sutured, the incision is closed, and the operation is completed.

Expert Comments

1. Choice of surgical procedure: The patient in this case has a PSA-T of 8.370 ng/ml, F/T 0.194. MRI suggests the possibility of prostate cancer. The biopsy diagnosis is prostate adenocarcinoma (five needles on the left, five needles on the right), Gleason score 3 + 3, WHO Grade Group 1. Overall, the patient has low-risk prostate cancer. Considering the patient's age of 63 is not advanced, the choice of surgical procedure should ensure complete tumor removal while preserving sexual function and urinary control as much as possible. Therefore, the VIP technique is chosen to maximize the preservation of sexual nerves and urinary control.
2. Treatment of the prostate pedicle: The prostate pedicle should be fully mobilized before being clamped with Hem-o-lok. Clinically, it is common to see severe bleeding after disconnection due to insufficient treatment of the pedicle, thick tissue, and inability of Hem-o-lok to clamp. Therefore, the following two points should be noted in the treatment of the pedicle: (1) The pedicle should be fully mobilized before clamping to achieve a satisfactory thickness. (2) An appropriate size of Hem-o-lok can be chosen; at this time, a large (gold) Hem-o-lok is suitable.

MIX
Papier aus verantwortungsvollen Quellen
Paper from responsible sources
FSC® C105338

If you have any concerns about our products,
you can contact us on
ProductSafety@springernature.com

In case Publisher is established outside the EU,
the EU authorized representative is:
Springer Nature Customer Service Center GmbH
Europaplatz 3, 69115 Heidelberg, Germany

Printed by Libri Plureos GmbH
in Hamburg, Germany